W9-CCL-832

The Natural Remedy Book for Women

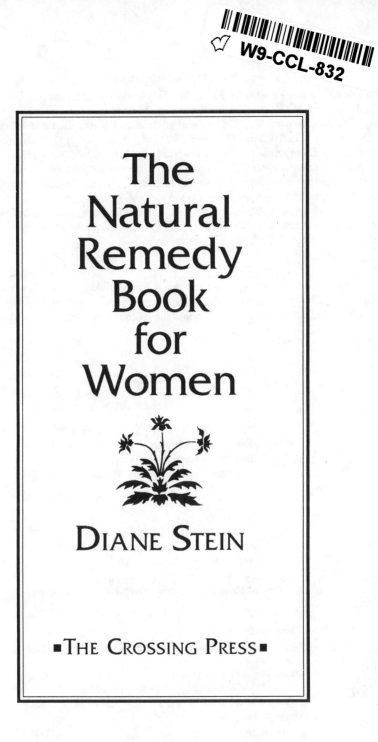

DIANE STEIN

■THE CROSSING PRESS■

Acknowledgments

I would like to thank the following for their help in reviewing this book for accuracy. Dr. Cindy Brown, M.D., checked medical facts, homeopathy, and added some valuable suggestions of her own. Miah LeCroy, herbalist and aromatherapist, reviewed the herb and aromatherapy material. Tony Crescenzi, N.D., of Vita-Ganics in St. Petersburg, Florida, made sure I did my naturopathy homework. Diana Grove, L.M.T., provided articles on healing women's dis-eases, on dong quai and on osteoporosis, and Sylla Sheppard-Hangar provided charts and information on aromatherapy. Eileen Sullivan offered valuable suggestions on heart dis-ease and obesity.

Special thanks to Elaine and John Gill of The Crossing Press for believing in my work and pushing me to "make it definitive," and to the many others at the press for making this book possible. I thank you and appreciate you all.

Note: Healing and medicine are two different fields, and the law requires this disclaimer. The information in this book is not medicine but healing, and does not constitute medical advice. In case of serious illness consult the practitioner of your choice.

For Sue

Copyright © 1992 by Diane Stein
Cover illustration and design by AnneMarie Arnold
Interior illustrations by Amy Sibiga
Interior design by Amy Sibiga
Printed in the U.S.A.

Library of Congress Cataloging-in-Publication Data

Stein, Diane 1948-
    The natural remedy book for women / by Diane Stein.
        p.   cm.
    Includes bibliographical references.
    ISBN 0-89594-526-6 (cloth) -- ISBN 0-89594-525-8 (pbk.)
    1. Women--Health and Hygiene. 2. Holistic medicine. I. Title.
RA778.S7968 1992
613'.04244--dc20
                                              91-43567
                                                CIP

Contents

Introduction
Women and Natural Healing

Almost everyone has her horror story of the medical system — illnesses and complications that natural healing could have prevented. Many women have shared with me their stories. One was prescribed antibiotics for a sore throat; she broke out in hives from the medication and developed a vaginal infection that recurred monthly for over a year. Monostat given for the vaginal infection stopped it temporarily but it continued to recur. Then she began to have skin rashes from the monostat. A week on the herb echinacea would have stopped the sore throat without other consequences; odorless garlic (Kyolic) stops vaginitis and rashes.

Another woman, experiencing her second normal pregnancy, trained to have natural childbirth. At delivery, her doctor performed a caesarean, refusing to honor her pre-agreed upon wishes though there were no complications. With the attitude of birth as a natural process and a midwife in attendance, this woman's experience would have been healthier, both emotionally and physically, for herself and her baby.

A woman having an uncomfortable menopause induced by a hysterectomy was given estriadol injections and developed breast cancer a few months later. Estriadol is a drug used for estrogen replacement therapy when the ovaries have been removed. Her gynecologist admitted that the hormone was a likely cause of cancer. With natural healing—the herbs dong quai or black cohosh, vitamins E and B-6—the hysterectomy may not have been required. One in six women over the age of forty-five experiences this surgery in the United States. Three quarters of these hysterectomies, along with eighty percent of the caesarean section births, are unnecessary. Too much estrogen is a known cause of breast cancer. Herbs, vitamins, aromatherapy or homeopathy will relieve most women's menopause symptoms, cancer free, and keep their bodies intact.

Another woman was placed on psychoactive drugs for a "mental disorder" that was later discovered to be early diabetes. Twice the number of women as men are prescribed mood altering medications, often without proper diagnosis of the problem. If a woman admits to being stressed, as virtually everyone in modern society is, she is more likely to be placed on tranquillizers than checked further. In holistic healing, enough questions would be asked to rule out simple depression in this woman. If her depression were treated, it would be with non-addictive or even non-ingested methods; the question would be, "What changes does she need to make in her life, attitude or habits?" With depression treated or ruled out, the early diabetes could be helped with eucalyptus, geranium and juniper fragrances, kelp tablets, yarrow or dandelion tea, chromium, and a whole foods, sugar free diet. Diabetes caught early can often be managed without drugs.

In every workshop on healing I hear similar stories from women. The medical system's insistence on invasive techniques and unnecessary, overly potent synthetic drugs with dangerous consequences is a pattern constantly repeated. A woman comes to western medicine reasonably whole and leaves it with organs removed or more dis-ease than she came with. Some of the doctor-caused illnesses are fatal. Others bring needless discomfort, pain, fear, expense and surgeries that would otherwise have been unnecessary. If a remedy is simple and harmless it is considered too unsophisticated to use by today's technological standards. The patient as a person, particularly as a woman, with a right to comfort and health in the easiest way possible, is not considered. Her wishes for her own well-being, as in the case of the woman with the unneeded caesarean, are all too often ignored.

Natural or holistic healing has a very different attitude, that treats the woman as a person, as a whole Be-ing. Small dis-eases are treated before they escalate to more serious ones, and the remedies are natural and without devastating side effects. Holistic remedies do not create more dis-ease. They are simple products usually found in nature (or the healthfood store) with simple effects. They are vitamins or foods, herbs or homeo-pathic tablets, aromas to place in the environment or to use in massage; they are pressure points or the energies of gemstones or flowers. Health is seen in terms of overall well-being—physical, emotional, mental and spiritual. Usually holistic remedies are not prescribed by doctors, but are chosen by the woman herself based on her own self-knowledge and informed decisions. They are an antidote to technology out of balance, a return to the ways of the earth and the Goddess, and they are effective.

I have my own horror stories. On Christmas night, 1973, I discovered blood in my urine. There was a lot of it, bright red, though there was no pain or discomfort beyond some abdominal bloating. When the bleeding continued with increasing frequency, I became frightened and went to a hospital emergency room, no other help being available on a holiday night. My clothes were taken away and I was given a hospital gown with no warmth or privacy. I sat in a freezing cubicle for several hours, terrified and totally ignored, watching a screaming man being treated for a gunshot wound and another for a drug overdose. Other cubicles were filled. At just about dawn a non-English speaking intern came and kept addressing me by someone else's name. I was unable to make him understand. Finally I found a nurse who sent the intern out and catheterized me, and told me that most likely the bleeding was nothing to worry about. She brought me a blanket.

The hospital admitted me but would give no further information. The bleeding had long since stopped. I was injected with iodine for x-rays. A surgical procedure was done to flush out the infection and dilate the urethra, and I was sent home on antibiotics the second day. "It's just cystitis," someone told me. "Women get it on their honeymoons." No one told me that cystitis means a bladder infection or that forty percent of women experience it recurrently at some time in their lives. I was not sexually active at the time, and it was not explained that intercourse can be a factor but only one of many factors. When cramps and frequency of urination without bleeding occurred again within a month I went back to the urologist and was given more antibiotics. I was incontinent from the surgical procedure, the infections recurred every month with my menstrual periods, and I began to have vaginal infections. I caught every cold and flu that went around that year. I was on antibiotics most of the time, lost thirty pounds from the nausea they induced, and was totally miserable. The expense of all the doctor visits and prescriptions was more than I could pay.

After many months of this, a woman came into the office where I worked and overheard me complaining. She said, "Why don't you just drink cranberry juice?" I asked her what she was talking about and she said that a sixteen ounce glass of cranberry juice taken hourly at the first sign of a bladder infection would stop it. She said that drinking buttermilk would also help. It would prevent the antibiotics from causing vaginal infections. It was the first connection between antibiotics and vaginitis that I had heard about. Since it was the vaginal infection I had at the time, I began with the buttermilk and it worked. The next time I felt the bladder infection starting I tried the cranberry juice and it also worked. I stopped the antibiotics and had no need to return to the urologist.

Sometime later I ran into him on the street. I told him about the cranberry juice and buttermilk, and asked him if he'd known about these things. "Of course," he said.

"Well, why don't you tell people about them and save them some misery?" I asked him.

"That stuff's just an old wives' tale," he said. "We can't tell people that."

But the old wives' tale worked. I discovered for myself what I later knew as Kegel exercises and they repaired the incontinence. I regained my weight and health. It was my first encounter with holistic healing and my awakening about medicine. I had no idea at the time that there are similar remedies for every dis-ease.

The information being reclaimed by women on holistic healing methods is only now becoming readily available. The Inquisition and the American Medical Association politics did their jobs well, from the thirteenth century to the present, to submerge this women's heritage information and keep it from popular use. Women's self-empowerment is not on the patriarchy's agenda, and we are only at the beginning of natural healing's re-emergence today.

I had one more personal run-in with the medical system, ten years after the cystitis. When my office first computerized I began to get sick, and it took over two years of trips to doctors to diagnose the problem as migraines. It took longer than that to diagnose the cause of the increasing migraines, nausea, dizziness, vision aberrations and eventual passing-out spells. I was prescribed a series of migraine relief and prevention medications, all of which only made me sicker. I experienced an almost nonstop migraine cycle, slightly lessening on weekends and holidays for close to three years. My male boss sent me for psychiatric testing, on threat of losing the job, and it was the woman psychologist there who informed me of the dangers of computers for some dyslexics—just this type of sickness from the blinking screens. I am dyslexic.

When I finally left the job, the migraines and blackouts lessened but did not stop, and I was physically and emotionally run down and exhausted. I attended my first Michigan Women's Music Festival a few weeks later (August, 1983) and was introduced to a new world. For the first time I was informed about the factors of nutrition, spinal misalignment, stress, constipation and hypoglycemia in causing migraines. I learned about other problems of women's health with computers, and about dyslexia. In several workshops I learned about herbs, vitamins, meditation and crystals, and about the growing network of women healers. Without a job, I no longer had insurance to pay for the medical system, and medicine was no longer available to me.

I went home and learned to meditate, to work with crystals and gemstones, to fix herb teas of scullcap, hops and catnip, to use lavendar fragrance, and take calcium-magnesium tablets. I became a vegetarian and threw out the sugar and junkfoods. Within months the migraines and blackouts ceased. I was fully sold on natural healing by this time and sought to learn as much about its methods as I could. Learning and using the information to help myself and others has been the focus of my life since that time. I never went back to office work; the Goddess holds me in her hand.

In this time of transition and change for the planet, I believe holistic healing to be a major part of the future of medicine. With the increase in and dependence upon costly high technology, medical care has priced itself beyond many people's means. In the United States, where over-technology has become the trend, only people with health insurance have access to most medical care. Unlike Britain's nationalized medicine, health insurance here is available to limited parts of the population—those employed by large companies or with the ability to afford more than $200 per month per person to pay for it. Without such insurance, being in the hospital costs thousands of dollars a day.

Poor people, who are mostly women and children (both white and nonwhite), may have access to Medical Assistance, but fewer and fewer are deemed eligible for the service and the coverage is minimal. Medicare was designed to provide hospital insurance for the elderly and disabled, but accessory costs are putting it out of reach for many and the coverage is also increasingly limited. Over thirty-seven million Americans fall between the cracks, being neither rich enough nor poor enough to have any coverage at all. In times of need, the hospitals may turn them away.

Even those with medical insurance find that their coverage is increasingly challenged and limited by the corporations that provide it, not as a service but to make big money. It is the insurance companies that decide who will have health care in America in the 1990s. They are also the force that lobbies against a National Health Insurance. Women have always been deprived in any patriarchal politics, and the politics of health care is definitely a women's issue. As the cost of medical technology goes up, fewer and fewer women will have access to it. There will be an increasing need for inexpensive and effective self-help alternatives.

Technology is also a human issue, reaching far beyond the price of the gadgetry. Women are patients in the medical system twice as frequently as men, visiting doctors twice as often and being hospitalized twice as much. Women are also half as tolerant as men to being treated like robots. The modern medical model sees the human body as a machine comprised of moving parts; if a part fails, remove it or replace it, or jump-start it with drugs. The overall effect on the person that "part" belongs to is not relevant. A doctor who specializes in hearts knows nothing about arthritis. A doctor that specializes in bones doesn't know how to treat a skin rash. Women expect to be treated as whole people, as human, and the increasing tendency toward drugs, surgeries and diagnostic gadgets turns them off. Such medicine does not serve women's needs. Rather than submit to machines with no answers, that treat one body part at a time, they look for other methods of healing.

Women are also increasingly aware of the damage done them by patriarchal culture—the medical system being a typical example—and they are taking back their power as a human right. In today's medicine, the patient has no say about her body or what's done to it. She is handed a pill, scheduled for surgery, and is given no information upon which to base an informed consent. The doctor (who is still usually male) knows best and will not stand for questioning. His methods are the only ones legally available, and they often leave women sicker than when they walked through his office door. The older generation's judgment (or training by doctors) that a doctor is second only to god, is slipping as women's horror stories grow in number. Women today are looking for more control and empowerment over their bodies and wellness. They want methods that do not intimidate them, that treat them with respect, that offer more than a covering up of symptoms, and that make them feel better. Only outside the traditional medical system are these methods to be found.

With technology becoming financially out of reach for so many, and so highly dehumanizing and condescending even to those who can afford it, new ways to approach wellness are needed. Add to these factors the increased need for healing on a depleted and polluted planet, the level of physical, mental and emotional stress every inhabitant of the earth lives under, and the lack of enough health practitioners to provide for all who need them, the situation becomes apparent. Unless alternatives to the standard medical system are found and used, many people will be without any health care at all. As costs mount and the economy declines, as both population and dis-ease increase and health insurance coverage becomes more restrictive, the situation approaches crisis. It is a crisis that will only escalate in coming years, and a crisis facing women and children first.

Natural healing is the bridge to fill the gap, a way for women to have effective health care inexpensively while taking their own initiative and empowerment. The self-help focus teaches women how to do it themselves, and when personal knowledge fails there are women of greater expertise to help. The attitude in women's healing is one of mutual giving and responsibility. Healing is not something done "to" but is done "with" another person, and the woman experiencing the healing has as much say (or more so) as does the healer or expert. With self-help information in many methods becoming available, women now have a choice of which methods to use.

The methods of holistic/alternative healing are not the synthetic drugs that cause side effects, but are natural substances that are powerful, proven and safe. There are no surgeries or organ transplants—the natural methods include naturopathy (foods like cranberry juice and buttermilk); plant matter (herbs, fragrances and flower essences); gemstones; vitamins and minerals, cell salts and amino acids that are intrinsic components of human body chemistry; homeopathic remedies that employ minute amounts of organic or inorganic substances; acupressure, a form of touch healing; and emotional awareness of the inner factors that cause dis-ease. These are the methods discussed in this book but are only a sampling of what is available.

Natural healing methods are used at the very beginning of dis-ease to take care of small matters before they become large ones. Their aim is to prevent the need for standard medical care, not to refuse it when necessary. An herb or vitamin will not set a broken bone or remove a hot appendix, but they add to the speed of healing once such surgeries are done. With holistic methods to turn to early, many things that would otherwise become medical emergencies are healed before they become serious. With less use of synthetic drugs and unnecessary interventions, the medical system takes over only where actually needed and where technology becomes appropriate. Women start with simple healings and gain in expertise, taking control of their wellness with increasing knowledge and empowerment.

Cost is also much less an obstacle in natural healing. The most expensive of vitamins or supplements will generally run under fifteen dollars, and most dried herbs cost about a dollar an ounce. Herb capsules and tinctures are usually under ten dollars for a month's supply. The most complex of self-help healing therapies, using several vitamins along with herbs or other methods, will probably cost less than thirty dollars a month. Cell salts and homeopathic remedies are even less expensive, under five dollars for a large amount. Flower and gemstone essences can be made at home, and pressure point therapy requires only one's hands. Aromatherapy fragrances usually cost under five dollars. Most cities have health food stores where the remedies are easily available, and a list of resources is given at the end of this book. Professionals offering natural healing methods as a service charge a variety of fees, but most still cost less than conventional doctors.

Natural healing is not new to planet earth, but was the original system of medicine in every country. In Europe, before the Inquisition burned nine million women between the thirteenth and seventeenth centuries, holistic healing was the state of the art in western medicine. With the churches' help, the beginning male medical system removed their competition—the witches, midwives and healers—and had nothing to replace them with in the way of physical knowledge. (They continued to do this in cultures worldwide as missionaries.) Since the end of the witch burnings, women's remaining information on herbal and alternative methods has been degraded as "old wives' tales by dirty midwives," and much that was vital and valuable has been lost. Along with the knowledge, what has been sacrificed is women's ability to take care of themselves.

Promising newer methods have been struck down along with proven old ones. Homeopathy operates on a par with standard medicine throughout the world, but the American Medical Association (AMA) was formed a hundred years ago to drive it from the United States. At one time, more than half of all medical doctors in America were homeopaths. Health food stores that sell vitamins, supplements, herbs and other natural remedies are harrassed and restricted today by the government's Food and Drug Administration (FDA) that is working in the interest of drug corporation profits. Most holistic healers run the risk of prosecution for "practicing medicine without a license." The patriarchal system of technological medicine, synthetic drug manufacturers and health insurance companies wants a full monopoly on women's bodies. They have made their methods the only ones by law.

But more and more women are refusing the cost, danger and invasive practices of standard medicine and are turning to natural healing. They are reclaiming old knowledge and adding to it, learning the parameters of methods beyond the legislated medical system. As their work continues and they learn, their healing becomes highly effective. Alternatives are proving their value and ability for healing beyond any doubts. In many cases, natural methods succeed where medicine fails, and in every case holistic healing returns women's bodies to their real owners, creating empowered, healthy women.

The women's movement that started in the 1960s is coming of age, and the politics of health and healing remain central to it. Freedom of choice for women's bodies has always been a major issue and quality health care is a part of that freedom. Creating wellness, caring for each other, building community and living together in peace are necessary if both women and the planet are to survive. Quality humane health care is essential to all and is not available under the current patriarchal world order. It is up to women to create it for ourselves and our children by taking it into our own hands. Along with fighting laws and systems that oppress women, the reclaiming of self-help knowledge and its use is vital and essential. In a high-tech world of stress and misogyny, of pollution and corporate greed, human survival is at stake.

The information in this book lists fifty dis-eases of interest to women and a variety of natural remedies for healing them. With many choices given, the individual chooses the methods and remedies that seem the most appropriate to her. While every method at once is not useful, there is an eclectic approach here that says a woman may use herbs and vitamins, acupressure and gemstones, fragrance and foods together if she wishes.

She may try one of the choices or several, but the emphasis is on simplicity. Information on using each of the healing methods follows, and specific remedies and directions are given for each illness under that illness' listing. The most effective or easiest remedies are indicated.

A list of ten healing methods is represented by the remedies. These have been mentioned before but include:

1. Vitamins and Minerals
2. Herbs
3. Naturopathy
4. Homeopathy and Cell Salts
5. Amino Acids
6. Acupressure
7. Aromatherapy
8. Flower Essences
9. Gemstones and Gem Essences
10. Emotional Healing

Other methods not included in this book but that are recommended include Reiki, chiropractic or osteopathic adjustments, neuromuscular massage, bodywork, touch healing, aura work, colors, acupuncture, and gestalt therapy. There are many methods of natural healing, and many individual choices. In every case, the remedies used here were chosen for safety, effectiveness and availability. I have used most of them personally, and have experience with all of the methods discussed.

No attempt has been made to offer solutions to every human dis-ease. This would not be possible in a single book. While no book or self-help method will replace the need for standard medicine, this one seeks to give women other methods and choices so that technology, surgery and synthetic drugs are needed less often. The remedies are proven by time and experience, and when used early enough in the dis-ease process they usually work. When they fail after fair trial, for whatever reason, other help should be sought. Take notice too, of the emotional sources of dis-ease; valuable keys to healing are presented in them. Natural healing works with the whole human—body, emotions, mind and spirit—and coming to terms with the emotions surrounding an illness is often all that is needed to heal it.

New Moon in Gemini
May 14, 1991

Methods

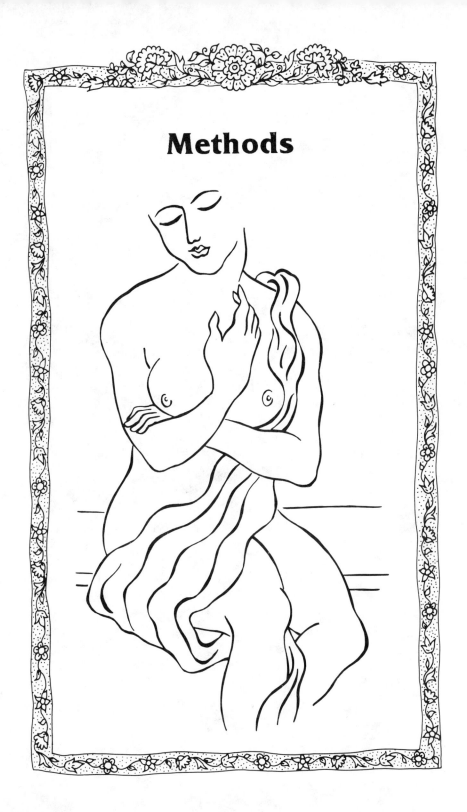

Vitamins and Minerals

Vitamins and minerals are intrinsic components of the body's chemistry, and they are necessary for life. They are essential nutrients, called micronutrients because of the minute amounts required. Vitamins regulate metabolism and release the energy produced by food digestion. They are coenzyme precursors, regulating and working with enzymes to catalyze all of the processes of the body. Minerals also participate in enzymatic processes. They are needed for blood and bone formation, the formation and chemistry of body fluids, and the maintenance of nerve function and the entire nervous system.

Both vitamins and minerals are primarily obtained from foods. Vitamins are either not made in the body or are made in inadequate amounts. Since water soluble vitamins are excreted through the urine, they must be taken in daily. These vitamins include vitamin C and the full B-complex. Oil soluble vitamins are stored for a period of time in the liver and fatty tissues. Vitamins A, D, E and K are oil soluble. Because water soluble vitamins are excreted and not stored, actual overdoses are not possible though there may be some discomfort from major excesses. Oil soluble vitamins can be overdosed (except for vitamin E), but the extent of toxicity has been highly over-emphasized by those who disparage vitamins.

Minerals come from the soil that is the body of the planet, entering plant matter first on the food chain. Herbivorous animals and human vegetarians obtain their minerals from eating plants. Meat eaters obtain their minerals from the bodies of herbivores. Thus women obtain minerals from eating plants, meat, poultry or fish. There are two types of minerals: trace minerals and macro (bulk) minerals. Trace minerals are needed in very minute quantities but those quantities are essential. They include zinc, iron, copper, boron, manganese, chromium, germanium, selenium and iodine. Macro minerals, needed in larger amounts, include calcium, magnesium, sodium, potassium, and phosphorus. The most frequent nutritional deficiencies for women are the minerals calcium and iron and the B-vitamins folic acid and B-6. Minerals are stored in bone and muscle tissue, but only massive amounts taken over long periods of time will cause toxicities.

Ninety-eight percent of women (and slightly less of men) are deficient in the B-complex vitamin folic acid, and ninety percent of women are deficient in vitamin B-6. Calcium deficiency affects seventy-three percent of women, zinc deficiency fifty-seven percent of women, and iron deficiency is experienced by sixty percent of women.[1] Folic acid is essential for the formation of blood, as is B-6, and B-6 is vital for metabolism of amino acids and protein. Many women's pre-menstrual stress is caused by these vitamin deficiencies, and women on the contraceptive pill are particularly at risk. Calcium is needed for bone, muscle and nerve formation and function, as well as for milk production in lactating mothers. Calcium deficiency is also implicated in pre-menstrual nervous tension, water retention, muscle spasms of the legs and osteoporosis. Zinc regulates the immune system, the healing of organs and wounds, and the development of healthy skin and hair. Iron produces hemoglobin, the oxygen-carrying component of red blood cells. Women with heavy menstrual flows often have iron deficiency anemia.

Vitamin and mineral deficiencies are a major factor in women's health. Yet, if vitamins and minerals come from food, why is this so even in women who eat healthy diets? Why is vitamin and mineral deficiency increasing as a factor in women's dis-ease? Vitamins and minerals are nutrients essential to human life. The food chain begins with plants' absorption of minerals from the soil. The soil is the earth, the planet, that is now depleted and polluted to the crisis point. Women's vitamin and mineral deficiencies begin with the depleted earth, the nutrients that are no longer available for plants to assimilate from the soil. Depleted plant nutrition means depleted nutrition all along the food chain.

Earth's soil is mineral deficient from farming practices like over-cropping and single-crop farming. Soil erosion is a worldwide crisis that continues to remove needed minerals from the soil and from food plants. Chemical replacement fertilizers are often not nutrients that can be assimilated by humans or animals eating plants grown with them. Chemicals are used by today's agribusiness farmers to stimulate plant growth, create attractive appearance, and extend shipping and shelf-life at the expense of the nutritional value (and taste) of the crops. Pesticides are highly over-

[1]Michael Van Straten, ND, DO, *The Complete Natural Health Consultant* (New York, Prentice Hall Press, 1987), p. 12. I am attempting to keep footnotes to a minimum in this book. See the bibliography for a full list of source references.

used on today's farms, the residues of which are present in all food and contaminate the water tables. Extended shipping time from picking to eating further depletes the vitamin content of foods, as does preservation by chemicals, dyes and additives. Irradiation reduces the vitamin content by twenty to eighty percent.

Food that was grown and eaten a hundred years ago, or even fifty years ago, contained the essential vitamins and minerals for good health. Today's chemicalized and refined food does not. Because of this, most women are vitamin and/or mineral deficient in some way, and I consider a *good* (not cheap but *good*) daily multiple vitamin and mineral supplement a *must* for everyone. This simple step alone goes a long way toward prevention of dis-ease, and often the addition of it to the diet is enough to heal many women's health problems. Choose a quality healthfood store supplement, not one from the supermarket, and take it with meals. My own choice is Schiff's Single Day, but there are many others of good quality. A balanced calcium-magnesium supplement is needed by most women, also.

Vitamins and minerals suggested for healing in this book start with the assumption that you are taking a daily multiple vitamin and mineral tablet. Many vitamins require others taken with them to work and the multiple provides these in proper balance and quantity. Calcium, for example, requires small amounts of vitamins A, C, and D, as well as iron, phosphorus and an amount of magnesium that is half the amount of the calcium. Each of the B-complex vitamins requires the rest of the B-complex to activate it. Vitamin E requires selenium, manganese and inositol in small amounts. Supplement amounts of a vitamin or mineral used alone can cause an imbalance that functions like the deficiency it is meant to heal. The vitamins and minerals present in a multiple prevent this. The amounts of each suggested supplement require a balance of others.

The Food and Drug Administration (FDA) has set up a list of vitamin and mineral amounts called the RDA, Recommended Dietary Allowances, and bases its watchdogging of supplements on these amounts. The figures, however, were founded on very little nutritional research and at best are only what is required to prevent a nutritional deficiency dis-ease such as scurvy or pellagra. Vitamins and minerals are needed in much greater quantities than the RDA limits for optimal health, and greater amounts yet may be needed to correct an illness or deficiency. It is also important to remember that each individual has her own body requirements that may be different from other women's or the norm. A chart is provided comparing the RDAs for the most common vitamins and minerals with the amounts recommended for women's good health. For specific dis-eases, the amounts

Vitamins and Minerals [2]

Vitamin/ Mineral	RDA Adult Amount	Recommended for Women of Average Weight		
		Age 22–25	Age 36–60	Over 60
A	5000 IU	20,000 IU	20,000 IU	20,000–30,000 IU
D	400 IU	800 IU	800 IU	800–1200 IU
E	30 IU	200–400 IU	400–1200 IU	800–1200 IU
C	60 Mg	1000–5000 Mg	1000-5000 Mg	1000–5000 Mg
B-1 (Thiamine)	1.5 Mg	100–200 Mg	150–300 Mg	200–300 Mg
B-2 (Riboflavin)	1.7 Mg	50–100 Mg	100–300 Mg	150–300 Mg
B-3 (Niacin)	20 Mg	200–1000 Mg	200–1000 Mg	400–2000 Mg
B-5 (Pantothenic Acid)	10 Mg	100–200 Mg	100–200 Mg	100–200 Mg
B-6 (Pyridoxine)	2 Mg	200–600 Mg	300–800 Mg	100–600 Mg
B-12 (Cyano-cobalamine)	6 Mcg	25–75 Mcg	25–75 Mcg	25–75 Mcg
Biotin	0.3 Mg	0.3–0.6 Mg	0.3–0.6 Mg	0.3–0.6 Mg
Choline		250–1000 Mg	250–1000 Mg	250–1000 Mg
Folic Acid (B-9)	0.4 Mg	2–5 Mg	2–5 Mg	2–5 Mg
Inositol		500 Mg	500–1000 Mg	1000 Mg
PABA		100 Mg	100 Mg	200 Mg
F (EFA-Essential Fatty Acids)		10–20 Gm	10–20 Gm	10–20 Gm
Calcium	0.6 Gm	1–2 Gm		
Phosphorus	0.5 Gm	1–2 Gm		
Iodine	45 Mcg	150–300 Mcg		
Iron	15 Mg	20–60 Mg		
Magnesium	70 Mg	400–800 Mg		
Copper	0.6 Mg	2–4 Mg		
Zinc	5 Mg	15–30 Mg		

[2]Diane Stein, *All Women Are Healers*, (Freedom, Ca, The Crossing Press, 1990), p. 163.

suggested may vary from those given. The chart is from my book *All Women Are Healers* (The Crossing Press, 1990).

Here is a very quick run-down of vitamins and minerals and their uses in women's healing. For more complete information, see *All Women Are Healers*, as well as James Balch, MD, and Phyllis Balch, CNC, *Prescription for Nutritional Healing* (Avery Publishing Group, 1990) and Velma Keith and Montene Gordon, *The How-To Herb Book* (Mayfield Publishing, 1984).

Vitamin A is an antioxidant. It protects the body from pollutants, aging and cancer, and boosts the immune system. It is effective in nightblindness and eyestrain, in rough or dry skin and hair, acne, eczema, angina, recurrent colds, flus or infections, and impaired sense of smell. Vitamin A may help or heal gastric ulcers, boils, allergies, hay fever, respiratory infections, hyperthyroidism, emphysema and any dis-eases of the skin, hair, eyes, teeth and gums. It may delay heart attacks in high risk women, and is important for weight gain, children's growth and bone formation.

Beta-carotene is converted to vitamin A in the liver and the vitamin may be taken in this form. Hypothyroid or diabetic women, however, may be unable to convert beta-carotene adequately. Vitamin A should not be taken in large amounts by women with liver dis-ease, and women on the pill may need less vitamin A than others. If you are pregnant, take no more than 25,000 IU per day. Adults have taken as much as 100,000 IU a day of vitamin A, and infants up to 18,000 IU a day for many months without toxicity. Beta-carotene is water soluble and cannot be overdosed, and vitamin A also comes in a water soluble dry form.

The B-Complex is a group of vitamins that need to be taken together, rather than as individual vitamins used alone. In a deficiency situation, take the full B-complex or a multiple vitamin that contains it, then add the individual B supplement needed. Unlike vitamin A, these are water soluble vitamins with no toxicity, but too much can result in diarrhea, constipation or nightmares (B-6) for some women. Reducing the dosage stops these side effects immediately. B-vitamins are helpful for mental and nervous disorders, depression, insomnia, stress and anxiety. They are useful in pre-menstrual tension, migraines, epilepsy, candida albicans, asthma, anemia and allergies. Vegetarians, women on antibiotics and women on diuretics especially need B-complex. AZT, the primary drug used in AIDS, drains B-vitamins from the body. B-vitamins are energy balancing calmatives, useful for the skin, eyes, hair, liver and nerves.

Vitamin B-1 (Thiamine) enhances circulation, digestion, blood formation, mental attitude, heart function, the muscles and the central nervous system. It is helpful in motion sickness, dental postoperative pain, shingles, brain damage, fatigue, mental confusion, heart dis-ease, and numb hands or feet. Taken every three or four hours on camping trips, it repels mosquitos, particularly when started (in less amounts) a few weeks before. Women who are pregnant, nursing or on the pill, women with multiple sclerosis, and women who smoke or have digestive problems need more B-1. Antibiotics, sulfa drugs, caffeine, alcohol, sugar, estrogen, a high carbohydrate diet, and heat all decrease thiamine levels in the body. B-1 is essential for anyone with central nervous system dis-ease or damage.

Vitamin B-2 (Riboflavin) is a major antistress vitamin. It is needed for red blood cell formation, the production of immune system antibodies, cell metabolism, growth, iron absorption, and the metabolism of proteins, fats and carbohydrates. Riboflavin helps prevent birth defects and is important in pregnancy, vision and eye fatigue, cataracts, anemia, digestive problems, eczema, sores on mouth, lips or tongue, oily skin, exhaustion and depression. It prevents hair loss, dandruff, and vaginal itching, is an anti-cancer agent and helps carpal tunnel syndrome (with B-6). Vegetarians, diabetics and women on anti-ulcer diets, as well as women on the pill or who take strenuous exercise need more B-2. The vitamin is destroyed by light, cooking, antibiotics and alcohol. It may decrease the effect of some cancer drugs. Cracks and sores at the corners of the mouth are an indication of riboflavin deficiency.

Vitamin B-3 (Niacin) is necessary for circulation and the function of the nervous system; it aids metabolism of carbohydrates, fats and proteins, and aids digestion by producing hydrochloric acid in the stomach. Niacin reduces cholesterol in the blood and lowers high blood pressure. Vertigo, headaches, constipation or diarrhea, backaches, bad breath, stress and insomnia are helped by B-3. Schizophrenia may be a niacin deficiency dis-ease, as well as autism in children, hostility, paranoia and personality changes.

The niacin flush—B-3's tendency to cause a temporary heating, tingling, flushing and reddening of the skin—starts about fifteen minutes after taking it and has an important use for women who have migraines. I describe the sensation as the "the hotflash of your life," but it is harmless and short term (about 15–20 minutes). With daily use of niacin, the effect lessens in a few days and finally disappears. At the earliest start of a migraine, a dose of 50 mg niacin (nicotinic acid form) induces this flush, which dilates the blood vessels, increasing blood circulation to the brain and head, and stops the cycle. If the first 50 mg does not cause the flush, take a second one in about fifteen minutes. One or two usually are enough.

To take B-3 without the flush use niacin*amide*; it is not useful for migraines but can replace niacin/nicotinic acid for other dis-eases. Women with gout, peptic ulcers, glaucoma, liver dis-ease, diabetes or who are pregnant should use vitamin B-3 conservatively. The amino acid l-tryptophan is converted to niacin in the body.

Vitamin B-5 (Pantothenic Acid) is the major anti-stress vitamin for women, and important help for those who are hypoglycemic or suffer from adrenal fatigue. The vitamin is needed for the production of adrenal hormones (including natural cortisone) and in the formation of immune system antibodies. It aids in the metabolism of vitamins and foods for energy and the functioning of the gastrointestinal tract. Pantothenic acid is a safe and drugless stimulant—use 500 mg twice a day with meals, increasing to up to 2000 mg a day if needed. There are no known toxicities and no side effects, but avoid at bedtime.

B-5 is concentrated in the body organs and is needed by every body cell. Indications for this vitamin include peptic or gastric ulcers, head-aches, hair loss, eczema, skin disorders, respiratory disorders, impaired motor coordination, anemia, cataracts, thyroid dis-ease, depression, anxiety, fatigue and postoperative shock. A furrowed tongue is an indication of B-5 deficiency, and arthritis, sinusitis, hay fever and allergies may be deficiency dis-eases of pantothenic acid. For allergies take 1000 mg each of B-5 and vitamin C twice a day with meals.

Vitamin B-6 (Pyridoxine) is essential for both physical and mental health and is intrinsic to more body functions than any other vitamin, mineral or nutrient. Brain function, red blood cell formation, the central nervous system, absorption of fats and proteins, immune system function and the synthesis of DNA and RNA all require this vitamin. Pyridoxine is an anti-cancer agent and protects the heart; it reduces arteriosclerosis and kidney stones, arthritis, allergies, asthma and pre-menstrual syndrome. B-6 is also useful for women who have hypoglycemia, epilepsy, ulcers, anemia, AIDS, diabetes (check blood levels frequently; it may reduce insulin need), insomnia, anxiety, irritability and general or muscular weakness.

Women on the contraceptive pill need increased amounts of pyridoxine to prevent phlebitis. The vitamin is also essential in pregnancy to aid morning sickness and prevent toxemia and leg cramps. Many women's pre-menstrual anxiety and water retention can be reduced or eliminated with B-6, and ninety percent of both men and women in the United States are deficient in it. Carpal tunnel syndrome may be a B-6 deficiency dis-ease, and antidepressants or estrogen increase women's need for this vitamin. (For carpal tunnel syndrome, try B-2 with B-6.) If pregnant use no more than 50 mg a day. The vitamin is water soluble and nontoxic but overuse can cause nightmares.

Vitamin B-9 (Folic Acid) is another serious deficiency for women, involving about ninety-eight percent. Uterine cervical dysplasia (suspicious Pap smear) often responds to a supplement of folic acid. If you are a vegetarian, pregnant, anemic, insomniac or depressed, you probably need more of this vitamin. B-9 is needed for energy production and brain function, cell division, protein metabolism, embryonic and fetal development, and normal growth. Neural tube defects and spina bifida in infants can be reduced by sixty to seventy percent by the mother's use of folic acid in very early pregnancy or at the time of becoming pregnant. The vitamin is a coenzyme in DNA synthesis. It helps in heavy menstrual bleeding and hemorrhaging in childbirth, aids nursing, helps in tissue repair, regeneration and debilitation. It increases intelligence and with vitamin B-5, can return color to greying hair. Folic acid is generally used with vitamin B-12 and often with B-6. Oral contraceptives, estrogen, dilantin, sulfa drugs, alcohol or high use of vitamin C increases women's need for this vitamin. If you are a smoker, folic acid may decrease your risk of lung cancer; use it along with vitamin A/beta-carotene. Avoid high doses longterm if you have hormone-related cancer or convulsive disorder.

Vitamin B-12 (Cyanocobalamin) prevents nerve damage and anemia, and aids in cell and blood formation, proper digestion, fertility and growth. Women who are longterm vegans are susceptible to B-12 deficiency. Persons with AIDS on AZT, elders, and those with digestive disorders are also often deficient. B-12 is useful for women with menstrual difficulties, nervousness, insomnia, memory loss, depression, fatigue, some skin problems, asthma, schizophrenia, heart palpitations, abdominal difficulties, and difficulties of pregnancy or lactation. Hormone use, gout medications, anticoagulant drugs and potassium supplements may block the absorption or increase the need for this vitamin. B-12 is taken by doctor's injections or sublingually (under the tongue) as it is not easily assimilated through the digestive tract. The symptoms of B-12 deficiency anemia, presenting all at once, are: reduced sensory perception, jerky limb motion, arm and leg weakness, trouble walking and speaking, memory loss, hallucinations, eye disorders and digestive disorders.

Vitamin B-13 (Orotic Acid) metabolizes B-9 and B-12, but is not readily used or available in the United States. Some better multiple vitamin-mineral combinations contain it. It may help multiple sclerosis.

Vitamin B-15 (Pangamic Acid) is an antioxidant; it increases cell life and immunity, and is useful in angina, asthma, high cholesterol and fatigue. Also known as DMG (dimethyl-glycine), it is used by athletes to reduce oxygen debt. The vitamin prevents some glandular and nerve disorders and is helpful for women in sobriety—it reduces alcohol cravings and protects against cirrhosis of the liver.

Vitamin B-17 (Laetrile) is banned by the FDA, but used in Mexico and other countries. A controversial substance, it is reputed to be a cancer cure, while opponents say it is worthless. The high cyanide content of apricot pit kernels, apple seeds and other fruit seeds is the vitamin's source. Suggested use is five to thirty apricot kernels taken through the day. One in three women in the United States will die of cancer, and one in nine women will develop breast cancer in her lifetime. Cancer is big business for the medical system and drug industry, and natural cures are suppressed as not profitable. Much more research is needed on B-17 but does not seem to be happening, and women who want laetrile treatment cannot get it here.

It should also be noted that vitamins B-13, B-15, and B-17 are not accepted as vitamins by the establishment (which calls them "pseudovitamins"). They have been largely ignored for research, and compared to other vitamins are almost unknowns. Likewise, choline, inositol and PABA, usually listed as B-complex vitamins, are not strictly vitamins, but called vitamin-like substances.

Biotin is one of the few vitamins that can be produced in the body. It is synthesized in the intestines from food, and is present in breast milk. Cell growth, fatty acid production, carbohydrate metabolism, metabolism of fats and proteins, and metabolism of all the B-complex vitamins are biotin attributes. The vitamin promotes healthy hair and skin, reduces hair loss and regulates the sweat glands, nerves and bone marrow. Seborrhea, eczema, dermatitis, dry peeling skin or cracked lips may be biotin deficiency symptoms, as well as extreme fatigue, heart dis-ease, muscle pains, depression and insomnia. Raw egg whites deplete biotin from the body, as do rancid fats, saccharine, sulfa drugs, antibiotics and estrogen. Pregnant or nursing women and women with skin problems are usually deficient.

Choline and inositol together make lecithin. Choline helps to prevent arterio- and atherosclerosis, heart failure, glaucoma, gall bladder dis-ease, circulatory problems and blood clots. It minimizes excess fat in the liver, gall bladder and heart, and aids in hormone production, brain function and memory. The vitamin is useful for nervous system dis-eases like multiple sclerosis, Parkinson's and Alzheimer's dis-ease, plus for diabetes, liver and kidney dis-ease and hepatitis. Choline is an anti-cancer agent, regulating the thymus and spleen for immune and red blood cell production.

Inositol, like choline, is also vital for preventing and aiding arterio- and atherosclerosis, and in fat and cholesterol metabolism. It helps to remove fats from the liver, reduce fibroid cysts and is necessary for brain function and assimilation of vitamins C and E. Women after menopause need more inositol and choline (lecithin), particularly Black women who have higher frequency of arterial dis-ease. Coffee drinkers and alcohol users need more inositol, as these substances deplete it from the body. Women with cerebral palsy, multiple sclerosis and other central nervous system dis-eases are helped by inositol, as well as women with vision and eye disorders, gall bladder dis-ease, diabetes, skin problems, eczema and psoriasis, hair loss and some forms of mental retardation.

PABA (Para-Amino Benzoic Acid) is the last of the B-complex and a constituent of vitamin B-5. It is an antioxidant that helps protect the skin from sunburn and skin cancer (which has increased four-fold in the last five years as a result of global ozone layer damage). PABA also aids in protein assimilation and in the formation of red blood cells. In cases of stress or nutritional deficiency, PABA can return color to greying hair. Eczema is a PABA deficiency dis-ease, and digestive disorders, fatigue, depression and irritability may be deficiency symptoms. Infertility in women, psoriasis, vitiligo and intestinal disorders are helped by PABA. Sulfa drugs may cause a PABA deficiency, and in turn the vitamin may inactivate sulfa medications. PABA should be included in your multiple vitamin-mineral supplement; most common additional amounts are 30–100 mg taken three times a day (internally). The vitamin is often found in sunscreen lotions.

Vitamin C is the important vitamin for white blood cell and immune system building, and is a major antioxidant, anti-toxin, and anti-cancer substance. C is required for tissue growth and repair, adrenal function and healthy gums. It protects the body against pollutants, infections, high blood pressure, cholesterol and atherosclerosis, bruising, bleeding and phlebitis. Vitamin C promotes wound healing and the production of interferon and anti-stress hormones. A gram (1000 mg) of vitamin C taken every hour at the start can stop a cold or bladder infection. Use a lot of water with this, and/or increase your calcium/magnesium or B-6 intake to prevent kidney stones; decrease gradually when symptoms end. C also reduces menstrual flows and heavy bleeding in menstruation (or otherwise). Mega-doses of C taken intravenously have been known to put AIDS patients into remission; HIV status has been changed from positive to negative if done early enough.[3] Schizophrenia has also been reversed with vitamin C.[4]

There are countless uses and benefits of vitamin C. Use it for bacterial and viral infections, colds, tonsillitis and ear infections, gum dis-

[3]Tom O'Connor, *Living With AIDS* (San Francisco, Corwin Publishers, 1987), Appendix C, p. 324 ff.
[4]Adele Davis, *Let's Get Well* (New York, Signet Books, 1965), p. 124.

ease and flu. Use it for hepatitis, diabetes, cataracts and eye infections, allergies and sinus, ulcers, gallstones and burn healing. Women living in inner cities or near highways need more vitamin C, and so do women who are smokers. Vitamin C may prevent Sudden Infant Death Syndrome, and women who are pregnant, nursing or on the pill, steroids or antibiotics need more of it. Alternate aspirin with vitamin C, as aspirin depletes C in the bloodstream. The vitamin can cause false results in some laboratory tests, so doctors need to be aware of it. It can also reduce the effectiveness of sulfa drugs and diabinase (for diabetes), and should be avoided by women taking radiation or chemotherapy for cancer. Pregnant women should limit C intake to 5000 mg per day or under.

At the onset of dis-ease or for serious illness or detoxification, take vitamin C to bowel tolerance for the time necessary to clear the dis-ease, then decrease the amount gradually. To determine bowel tolerance, take one or more grams of C per hour, with a lot of water, until diarrhea develops. At that point, cut back ten percent. The goal is to take as much C as possible without diarrhea, and this amount will vary with the individual and the state of her immune system. The amount of C that can be taken may vary from day to day, but surprisingly high amounts will be tolerated when they are needed. When using large amounts or in serious illness, try Ester-C—more is assimilated into the system. Take a calcium/ magnesium tablet or 50 mg of B-6 three times daily when using C in megadoses to prevent the possibility of kidney stones. Vitamin C is water soluble and nontoxic; too much results in diarrhea or nausea that stops when the amount is decreased. Many women's dis-eases can be healed with C.

Vitamin D and calcium deficiencies are major causes of osteoporosis in women. An oil soluble vitamin, natural vitamin D may be taken in very high amounts (100,000–150,000 IU daily) longterm before toxicity results, but about 800 IU per day is recommended. D is necessary for growth and for bone and tooth formation, and in the prevention of bone dis-eases. Black women in northern climates, Islamic women and nuns whose bodies are kept completely covered, women who work at night, and women living in smog laden cities are more susceptible to deficiencies. The vitamin is naturally obtained by exposure to the sun, where it forms in the skin. Supplemental D requires conversion by the kidneys and liver, and should not be taken without calcium. Women with kidney or liver dis-ease are more likely to be vitamin D deficient and to develop osteoporosis. Some cholesterol-lowering drugs interfere with absorption of vitamin D in the body, as well as antacids, mineral oil, thiazide diuretics and cortisone.

Vitamin E is essential for healing and regeneration in every part of the body, and is an antioxidant that prevents cancer and heart dis-ease. Use it for fertility, fibrocystic breasts, breast cancer, premenstrual syndrome, prevention of miscarriage, to reduce hotflashes and menopause discomfort, in pregnancy and lactation, and when on estrogen or the pill. Vitamin E is used for the healing of burns, wounds and scars and is positive before and after surgeries for internal and external regeneration. The vitamin prevents and aids cataracts, reduces blood pressure and removes cholesterol deposits from artery walls (start at 100 IU per day and increase slowly for heart and artery dis-ease). It protects women's bodies from pollution and secondary cigarette smoke and retards aging, aids migraines and visual problems, skin, hair and muscular dis-eases. Vitamin E taken in pregnancy prevents muscular dystrophy in children, and women with muscular dystrophy need high doses. Black women are especially susceptible to keloids, high blood pressure, breast cancer and arthritis, and vitamin E is a major preventive.

To maintain vitamin E levels in the blood, zinc is required with it. While a fat soluble vitamin, vitamin E is only stored in the body for a short time so that there are no toxicities in any amount. Iron and vitamin E should be taken eight hours apart, and women with diabetes, rheumatic hearts or overactive thyroids should not take high amounts.

Vitamin F (Essential Fatty Acids) is used with vitamin E as a factor in reducing cholesterol and heart dis-ease. It is an antioxidant that protects against x-ray damage and free radicals from saturated fats. Free radicals are atoms that damage cells, leading to cancer, leukemia, reduced immune function, cell fluid retention, infections, and a variety of dis-eases. Vitamin F helps the endocrine glands, especially the adrenals and thyroid. Skin dis-eases such as acne or eczema are vitamin F deficiencies, as are dry skin and hair, dandruff, diarrhea, gallstones, varicose veins, and the loss of beneficial bacteria in the intestines (which in turn cause candida over-run and dis-eases such as colitis). Essential fatty acids aid respiration, the nervous system, reproduction and blood coagulation. They can cause weight loss, but in excess cause gain. The substance is best used with vitamin E and with meals. It is composed of three items—linoleic acid, linolenic acid and arachadonic acid, and though oil soluble, has no toxicities. I listed it here as a vitamin, though the FDA does not.

Vitamin K is essential for the proper coagulation of the blood, and has a role in bone formation and preventing osteoporosis. It converts glucose to glycogen for storage in the liver, and therefore is important in sugar metabolism. The vitamin is usually available by prescription only, though it is nontoxic in natural forms; in foods it is most easily found in alfalfa and yoghurt. Vitamin K is used before surgery and childbirth to prevent hemorrhaging and for overly heavy menstrual flows, as well as to treat heart attacks. Deficiency symptoms include colitis, excessive diarrhea, nosebleeds and celiac dis-ease. X-rays, radiation, aspirin, air pollution, mineral oil, antibiotics and frozen or irradiated foods destroy it in the body. When synthetic vitamin K is used heavily in pregnancy, the infant may have a toxic reaction.

Vitamin P (Bioflavinoids) are several citrus factors that work synergistically with vitamin C and enhance its effects. They include rutin, hesperidin and citrin, and have particular benefit for the capillaries and in reducing pain, for blood circulation, cataracts, bile production, herpes, and in lowering cholesterol levels. Bioflavinoids are used by athletes to reduce bruising and bumps, as well as for back and leg pain, and they lessen the effects of prolonged bleeding. Bleeding gums, blood clots, hot flashes, ulcers, asthma, edema, varicose veins and inner ear problems (dizziness and vertigo) are helped by bioflavinoids. They are antibacterials that also help to fight infections. Bioflavinoids and C together are known as C-complex, and there should be 100 mg of bioflavinoids for every 500 mg of vitamin C. For daily use, take 1000 mg (1 gram) vitamin C with bioflavinoids in a time-release form. There are no toxicities, but high doses may cause diarrhea. Along with vitamin U below, bioflavinoids are technically not vitamins.

Vitamin U may help with ulcer healing. It is not readily available and little else is known about it. More research is needed.

Coenzyme Q10 (Ubiquinone) resembles vitamin E but is even more powerful as an antioxidant. It is not a vitamin, but is chemically similar to one. CO-Q10 retards aging and significantly boosts the immune system. It shows promise in cancer healing for reducing tumors and in leukemia for reducing the side effects of chemotherapy. Heart dis-ease and high blood pressure, high cholesterol, allergies, asthma, respiratory dis-ease, Alzheimer's, diabetes and multiple sclerosis all respond and improve with this coenzyme. Other uses include schizophrenia, obesity, candidiasis, gum dis-ease and AIDS. It is important for healing duodenal ulcers, and helps prevent cancer. There are no side effects. Keep it away from heat and light for best potency; pure coenzyme Q10 is bright yellow and has very little taste. Prices on this vary widely, but it is expensive; watch the mg amounts on the bottle. Use 30–100 mg per day.

These are the vitamins, and information on the minerals follows. Vitamins and minerals are a complex but major method of treating women's dis-eases in this book, and the length of the descriptions is justified. More dis-ease prevention is possible with knowledge of vitamins and minerals than in any other form of healing. For best results, the supplements should be taken in natural forms, rather than synthetic, wherever possible. Be careful with cheap or old vitamin E's that may be rancid. Vitamins taken in capsules or gelatin soft pills are preferred over hard-pressed tablets, as some women's bodies have difficulty in dissolving the tablets. Minerals are best in chelated form, molecularly protein bonded, as more is assimilated. Because so much is lost in digestion, much higher amounts must be taken than are actually needed. 1000 mcg equals 1 mg. 1000 mg equals 1 gram.

Minerals make up the actual structures of the body, such as bones and teeth, and deficiencies can cause serious dis-eases. Some minerals make vitamin assimilation possible, a few are toxic in excess, and most require a balance of other vitamins and minerals. Some women with extensive deficiencies or digestive problems need hydrochloric acid or digestic enzyme supplements to assimilate minerals. Mineral deficiencies affect the bones and teeth, as well as cause fatigue, menstrual problems, depression, insomnia, skin and hair problems, muscle cramps and stress intolerance.

Boron is a trace mineral often not listed in mineral information but of major importance to menopausal and postmenopausal women. In a study by the US Department of Agriculture, it was found that within eight days of adding 3 mg of boron to the diet, "postmenopausal women lost forty percent less calcium, one third less magnesium and slightly less phosphorus through their urine."[5] This has hopeful implications for women susceptible to osteoporosis and its resulting weakened and broken bones. Three milligrams is enough to take per day; avoid taking more.

Calcium is a bulk mineral and one of the most important for all women. It prevents osteoporosis, aids premenstrual stress, cramps and water retention, and halts insomnia and leg cramps. It is essential in regulating heartbeat, in blood clotting, as a preventive of colon cancer, in muscle growth and contraction, and in the transmission of nerve impulses. It is involved in DNA and RNA function and activates several enzymes.

Most women require supplemental calcium from menarche on. It is useful for any form of stress, for headaches and migraines, pleurisy, bone or tooth dis-ease, arthritis, and heart dis-ease. It decreases pain, lowers cholesterol and blood pressure, and is particularly useful in menstruation, menopause and postmenopause. Calcium deficiency symptoms include: charlie horses and muscle cramps or spasms, nervousness, heart palpitations, brittle nails, eczema, aching back or joints, rheumatoid arthritis, tooth decay, rickets, and numbness in arms or legs.[6]

To test absorption of your calcium supplement, place it in warm water and shake. If it does not dissolve within twenty-four hours, try a different brand. Most sources list calcium as nontoxic in any amount, but

---

[5]James Balch, MD and Phyllis Balch, CNC, *Prescription For Nutritional Healing* (Garden City Park, NY, Avery Publishing Group, 1990), p. 17–18.
[6]*Ibid.*, p. 18.

recommend doses under 2000 mg per day. Take a calcium supplement that includes half the amount of magnesium, traces of zinc, and vitamins A and D for the best possible absorption and activation. General Nutrition's Calcium Plus is a good one. Try calcium at bedtime as a relaxant, and take 1000–4000 mg after dental work to relieve pain. Women whose diets contain less protein need less calcium.

Chromium is a trace mineral also known as GTF (Glucose Tolerance Factor). It balances blood sugar levels, lowers high blood pressure and retards cholesterol buildup in the liver and arteries. Two thirds of Americans are either diabetic or hypoglycemic because of chromium deficiency and junkfood diets. This is an important mineral for women, and is essential for women over sixty-five. Suggested dosages are 25–250 mcg per day. There are no side effects or toxicities, but diabetics need to watch blood sugar levels as less insulin may be needed while taking this supplement.

Cobalt is a part of vitamin B-12 and longterm vegetarians (vegans) may be deficient. Obtain it through a B-complex or B-12 supplement; it helps prevent anemia.

Copper's earliest deficiency symptom is osteoporosis, a major health threat to postmenopausal women. It helps in the assimilation of iron and vitamin C, but supplements may upset the balance of zinc in women's bodies. Copper deficiencies are rare, and doses of more than 15 mg per day cause side effects. Copper aids bone, hemoglobin and red blood formation, forms elastin and is important in healing and energy, skin and hair color, the nerves and sense of taste. Get copper from a multiple vitamin-mineral supplement rather than adding it alone. Raw organic foods are high in natural copper.

Fluoride is present in fluoridated water and toothpaste, and supplements are not needed. It helps prevent tooth decay but does nothing for gum degeneration (the most frequent cause of tooth loss). Chemical fluoride may be harmful to the liver and a cause of osteoporosis. If your water is fluoridated, you are probably getting too much.

Germanium increases oxygen in the cells, tissues and organs. It is a major aid to the immune system but highly expensive. This trace mineral is important for AIDS and cancer, chronic fatigue syndrome, food sensitivities and allergic reactions, rheumatoid arthritis, high cholesterol, systemic candida, and any infectious dis-ease or low immunity situation. It is also a relaxant, anti-stress factor and mood balancer, and important for women exposed to toxic chemicals and pollutants. Women in chronic pain will benefit from germanium, as well as those with asthma or respiratory problems. There are no toxicities, and plants that contain germanium include garlic, ginseng, comfrey, aloe vera, chlorella, shiitake mushrooms, onions, barley and suma. If taking germanium capsules, expect to pay about a dollar each.

Iodine deficiency may be a factor in breast cancer, and as such it is an important trace mineral for women. Use it to regulate the thyroid and help metabolize fat. It is important in mental development and a deficiency in pregnancy may cause mental retardation in the child. Goiter, slowness and obesity are iodine deficiency symptoms. If using supplements, be sure to take natural ones. Kelp tablets are the most recommended form. Find it also in Edgar Cayce's Atomidine, 636, or Lugol's Solution. Toxicities have been cited by the FDA as a reason to restrict supplemental iodine, but 2400 mg have been given daily for as long as five years with no side effects. Too much iodine results in a metallic taste, mouth sores, swollen salivary glands, diarrhea and vomiting.

Iron is one of the major mineral deficiencies for women, with heavy menstruation as its cause. Iron produces hemoglobin, the oxygen-carrying component of red blood cells, and is required for the function of many enzymes. It is necessary for dis-ease resistance and immune system health. Iron deficiency symptoms include anemia, weakness and fatigue, debility, dizziness, irritability, brittle nails with vertical ridges, pallor, gas, nausea after meals, itching, constipation or diarrhea, hair loss, heart palpitations, poor attention span, and recurrent illnesses. When using supplements, use only organic iron called hydrolized-protein chelate, and avoid synthetic iron (ferrous sulfate). Suggested daily doses are 20–60 mg a day for women, the higher amounts in menstruation or after childbirth and for elders and growing girls. Floridix is a good supplement brand.

Do not take extra iron when having an infection, as bacteria requires iron for growth and the body will store and not utilize it. Take vitamin E and zinc eight hours apart from iron, as they interfere with iron absorption. Women with chronic candida or herpes are susceptible to iron deficiency, and those with cancer or rheumatoid arthritis will have difficulty assimilating it. Deficiencies can be caused by excessive menstrual flows, high phosphorus diet, poor digestion, ulcers, and excess use of antacids, coffee or tea. In cases of iron deficiency anemia, vitamins B-6 or B-12 deficiency may be the cause, rather than iron itself. Women with sickle cell anemia, thalessemia or hemochromatosis should not take iron. Use it carefully in pregnancy. Most women who menstruate are iron deficient.

Magnesium is necessary for the utilization of calcium, potassium and phosphorus and most women are deficient in it. It is necessary for muscle function, nerve impulse transmission and enzyme activity, prevents kidney stones and gallstones, and helps bone, tooth and tissue growth. Magnesium increases energy, helps the nerves, insomnia and depression, lowers blood pressure and helps to prevent heart attacks.

Mental confusion, fast pulse and irregular heartbeat are magnesium deficiency symptoms, as are weakness, twitching muscles and leg cramps. It protects the artery linings, is important in mineral metabolism and regulates the acid-alkaline balance of the body. Premenstrual chocolate cravings are a sign of magnesium deficiency, as is premenstrual nervous tension. Use a calcium/magnesium tablet for indigestion, but avoid any antacid right after meals.

Women who are pregnant or lactating, on the pill or taking estrogen, and who have premenstrual or menstrual discomfort need more magnesium. Alcoholics are usually magnesium deficient, and so are women who use diuretics, have frequent diarrhea, live in fluoridated or softwater areas, or take high amounts of zinc or vitamin D. Cod liver oil, too much calcium for the amount of magnesium, or a high fat or protein diet decrease the assimilation of this mineral. Magnesium requires twice the amount of calcium to work, as well as phosphorus and vitamins A and C. A good calcium/magnesium supplement will contain it all in one tablet, at about ten dollars for a three month (or more) supply. There are no toxicities.

Manganese is a trace mineral needed for protein and fat metabolism, assimilation of the B-vitamins, C and E, for balanced blood sugar, healthy nerves and immune system, and for production of breast milk. Deficiency symptoms include poor memory, poor muscle coordination and reflexes, bowed bones, dizziness, hearing problems, tinnitus (ear noises), and high blood sugar. Use it for multiple sclerosis and other muscular weakness dis-eases, epilepsy, diabetes, hypoglycemia, digestion or food assimilation disorders, fatigue, irritability, the central nervous system, and dis-eases such as Alzheimer's. Heavy milk drinkers or meat eaters may need more manganese as it is used in the production of milk and fat-digesting enzymes. Women who are pregnant or lactating will need increased amounts as well—it is essential for milk production. Use 2.5–5 mg per day; there are no toxicities. Take B-complex with manganese for a feeling of rested well-being.

Molybdenum deficiency is found in women with cancer and with gum or mouth disorders. A highly refined diet of processed foods may cause it. The mineral is used by the body in minute amounts for iron and nitrogen utilization and production of uric acid, as well as in enzyme and cell reactions. It is one of the minerals suggested for AIDS and cancer, but excessive use (over 15 mg per day) may cause gout and interfere with copper assimilation. Keep supplements away from heat or dampness.

Phosphorus works in balance with calcium and magnesium and more women are overloaded than deficient in it. The mineral is used as a chemical fertilizer and food additive, and junk foods are full of it. Too much phosphorus causes the body to over-release calcium and is a factor in osteoporosis. The mineral is necessary for utilization of vitamin D, calcium and niacin (B-3), and too much iron or calcium makes phosphorus ineffective. Tooth and gum problems, poor bone growth, arthritis, kidney dis-ease, heart contraction problems, poor appetite control, and over-weight or underweight are symptoms of deficiency. Most women do not need supplements, but if wishing to add phosphorus to your diet, use bonemeal with vitamin D, or use it in a balanced calcium-magnesium-phosphorus supplement.

Potassium may benefit women with edema, hypoglycemia, hypoadrenia, allergies, irregular heart rhythm or high blood pressure. Fasting, diuretics, diarrhea, kidney disorders or stress can cause a deficiency, as can coffee, alcohol, laxatives, cortisone and chocolate. Potassium helps prevent strokes, aids in muscle and heart muscle contraction, regulates blood pressure, balances the nervous system, and with sodium controls the body's water balance. Deficiency symptoms include continual thirst, tiredness, insomnia, poor reflexes, weak heart or muscles, constipation, hypoglycemia and poor breathing. Daily orange juice or bananas may prevent the need for supplements.

Selenium works with vitamin E as an antioxidant and has been called the anti-aging mineral. It protects against free radicals, toxins and pollutants to boost the immune system, create antibodies and strengthen the heart. It is a DNA/RNA activator, an anti-cancer agent, and relieves hot flashes. Selenium deficiency may be a factor in strokes and heart dis-ease, skin problems, infertility, early aging and muscular dystrophy. Dosage is 50–200 mcg, and though no toxicities have been discovered, avoid higher amounts.

Silicon (Silica) is a trace mineral that may protect the body from aluminum poisoning; it is important in preventing Alzheimer's dis-ease and osteoporosis. Silicon helps maintain flexible arteries and protect against cardiovascular dis-ease. It is needed for calcium absorption, bone and connective tissue formation, and for healthy nails, skin and hair. Silicon is needed more by elders, as levels decrease in the body with age. There are no reported toxicities. It is found in several herbs.

Sodium (Salt) is a major contaminant of processed foods and most women are overdosed on it continually. It is necessary with potassium to maintain the water balance and pH of the cells. Too much sodium results in high blood pressure, liver and kidney dis-ease, edema, heart failure and potassium deficiency. Deficiency symptoms include confusion, low blood sugar, weakness, lethargy and heart palpitations. Except in rare cases of heat exhaustion, few or no women need supplements.

Sulfur is part of the chemistry of amino acids, and if you are getting enough protein, you are probably getting enough of this trace mineral.

Sulfur protects the cells, stimulates bile, is an antibacterial, and aids oxidation reactions in the body. It protects against radiation and pollution to slow aging and lengthen life. Sulfur is needed for good skin and hair, and many skin creams contain it. Supplements are available, but the best source is in complete amino acids.

Vanadium is useful in lowering cholesterol and preventing heart attacks, as well as in reproductive difficulties and preventing infant mortality. Vanadium is needed for cell metabolism, and bone and tooth formation. This trace mineral is not easily absorbed and is rarely supplemented; take chromium and vanadium at different times. Smoking decreases uptake.

Zinc is necessary for proper functioning of the immune system and for all regeneration and healing. It regulates body processes, forms insulin and controls muscle contraction; it regulates the body's pH balance and the flow of enzymes in the cells, and is a factor in the synthesis of DNA. Use zinc for scaly dry skin or skin rashes, sores or boils, hair loss, acne, growth problems, too slow healing, dandruff and poor night vision. It is a factor in preventing diabetes, protecting the liver from chemicals, resisting infections and inflammations, and reducing senility and body odors. Use it for poison ivy, infertility, schizophrenia, AIDS, Alzheimer's dis-ease, hypoglycemia, arteriosclerosis, and loss of sense of smell.

Women with irregular menstrual cycles may benefit from zinc. Girls, pregnant women, women after surgery or heavy bleeding, and elder women need more zinc. Losses occur in sweating, pregnancy, nursing, diarrhea, kidney dis-ease, cirrhosis of the liver, and diabetes. A symptom of deficiency is white spots on the fingernails. Extra zinc may require extra copper, and doses over 100 mg a day depress the immune system, where doses under 100 mg enhance it. Zinc is essential for all forms of healing.

Women reading this information may find the answers to their own dis-eases right here. Vitamins and minerals are important and essential for women's well-being, and are the primary dis-ease preventive and healing method of this book. Many women's dis-eases are caused by vitamin-mineral deficiencies and are healed simply by returning the needed nutrient/s to the diet. Each of the dis-eases discussed in this book is helped by vitamins and minerals as based on the material of this section. Primary sources for vitamins in this chapter and throughout the book are: Balch and Balch, *Prescription for Nutritional Healing* (Avery Publishing Group, 1990), Dr. Ross Trattler, *Better Health Through Natural Healing* (McGraw-Hill Book Co., 1985), Adele Davis, *Let's Get Well* (Signet Books, 1965), and Diane Stein, *All Women Are Healers* (The Crossing Press, 1990).

Herbs

Where vitamins and minerals are the major form of dis-ease prevention and longterm balancing discussed in this book, herbs are the most important method for healing dis-ease situations that are acute (need attention right now). For best results, use them as early as possible in the dis-ease process (and use them along with vitamins). Unlike antibiotics and medicinal drugs, herbs work slowly and carefully. They may not cure your illness in one dose, as some doctors' pills seem to do, but they will cure it without toxic side effects and without iatrogenic (doctor- caused) threats to well-being. Because herbs contain all of the natural components of the plant, along with the specific healing factor, they work *with* the body, instead of *against* the dis-ease, boosting the immune system so the body heals itself. They treat the source instead of just masking symptoms. When used early enough and with knowledge of their properties, herbs are as effective as drugs or more so, and are pleasant to use and safe.

Herbs were the first form of healing, going back to the days when women were nomadic food gatherers, depending on the plants they found for food and medicine. Women knew the uses of every plant in their travelling area, testing them on themselves and teaching the information to others. They had herbal knowledge of painkillers, antispasmodics, tonics and cleansers, and herbs for wound and infection healing, for contraception and abortion, and for digestion and fevers. The uses of herbs have been known to every culture for millions of years, and the herb knowledge passed down to us today has the benefit of long testing and tradition. Modern drugs come on the market after a few months of limited testing and much drug company self-interest and politics. No one knows what they will really do until they are used, and sometimes not until years later, there are many unpleasant surprises. Herbs have been known for millennia, and what each plant does is well researched by time. Where in the past the only herbs available were local ones, and these are still considered the most effective, herbs from all over the world are now available. The Chinese system of healing included use of over 500 herbs as long as 5000 years ago. Today's Chinese healers use almost 6000 herbs and herbal preparations, many of them now known here.

The western synthetic drug industry, central to the attack-the-disease philosophy of the medical system, is based on early women's use of herbs. Many of the now-patented, high-priced medicinal drugs were synthesized from plant extracts women used in the past. Foxglove was used by pre-Inquisition witches to strengthen the heart, and has now been synthesized into digitalis. Native women in the American southwest used white willow bark, which in synthesized form is the active ingredient of aspirin. Nineteenth century hospital nuns used bread mold for healing infections long before penicillin was "discovered," and African women used the wild yam for fertility before it was synthesized to estrogen. Hildegard of Bingen, a nun who lived from 1098–1179, wrote an herbal that is considered the basis of western medicine, and the Egyptian healer-queens were teachers of herbs and healing before 2300 BCE.

What the medical system has done differently is to study the plant and remove from it the active ingredient which is believed to cause the healing. They then design a chemical synthesis for that ingredient. By isolating one ingredient and discarding the rest, and using a chemicalized form, they invite the side effects and toxicities that were prevented by using the whole natural plant. The reason for doing it this way, for making an artificial copy of something easily used whole, is money. Plants are substances found in nature, as are vitamins, and as such they are not patentable by United States law. An item that cannot be patented cannot be held to a controlled market, and a controlled market is the source of inflated prices and high profits. Where a bottle of herbal foxglove extract costs about $6, digitalis requiring a doctor's prescription costs much more. That plants are not patentable and that no one can make big bucks from them, is the source of their being disparaged or totally ignored by the medical system. The drug companies cannot control the supply or pricing of herbs, however much they would like to, and the FDA continually harasses herb sellers and the healthfood industry.

Herbs are used for healing in this book in several forms. They may be made into teas, infusions or decoctions, tinctures, capsules, poultices or compresses, douches, or as salves and oils. They are used internally and externally, and may be purchased (or picked) as raw plant matter, dried plant matter, or as already prepared capsules or extracts. When buying loose dried herbs, look for plant matter with good color and fragrance; if it is lifeless and grey it is useless. If there is mold in it, or it smells moldy, discard it. Keep dried plant matter in a dark place and for no longer than a year.

Prepared capsules are less susceptible to mold growth, and are potent for about a year also, except for roots which last longer. Herbal tinctures (extracts) prepared in an alcohol (or alcohol and glycerin) preservative base last almost indefinitely and never lose effectiveness, as long as kept in a cool dark place. They are usually sold in dark bottles. Those preserved in cider vinegar are less stable, but remain active for at least a year. In my opinion, the strongest and most effective use of herbs is in the alcohol-based tincture form.

Tissanes (or herbal teas) are most women's first use of herbs. They are made by pouring boiling water over dried herbs in a tea basket (or as teabags), and steeping for five to ten minutes. This is the least concentrated use of herbs, and is most often used for beverage teas and for chronic dis-eases where herbs are taken everyday longterm. Use a teaspoon or two or dried herbs to a cup of boiling water, or an ounce of herb matter to a pint of water in an eight-cup teapot. The water is boiled in a glass, enameled or stainless steel kettle on the stove (never aluminum), then taken away from the flame to pour over the herbs. Herbs become bitter when steeped longer than fifteen minutes, so lift the teabasket from the cup (or strain the pot) before that time. Cover against the light while cooling and steeping; put a saucer over the mouth of the cup. If your tap water is fluoridated or chemicalized, use spring water, bottled water or distilled water.

In acute healing much more herb for the amount of water is used. I like mine strong and use at least two tablespoons of herb in the strainer basket for a mug-sized cup, or at least half a cup of dried herb matter in an eight-cup teapot. When making a potful, strain each cup through the teabasket as it's poured or strain the whole pot into another container (not metal or plastic). Teas will keep overnight if they are strained and can be reheated; store in the refrigerator, but discard if it gets bitter or sour. Drink the tea at comfortable sipping temperatures. If using fresh plant matter instead of dried, use three times the amount. Take two to three cups of herbal tea a day.

An infusion is a stronger tea for acute dis-eases. This is made from dried herb also, but uses a pint of boiling water poured over an ounce of dried plant matter (or three ounces of fresh). Let steep for six to eight hours in a tightly covered glass jar and keep in a dark place. The finished infusion is poured through a strainer to fill half a cup and hot water is added to the top. This is Billie Potts' recipe (*Witches Heal: Lesbian Herbal Self-Sufficiency*, Hecuba's Daughters Press, 1981, now reprinted by DuReve Publications). Use two to three times daily.

A decoction is used for harder plants like stems, roots, barks or seeds; they are boiled directly to bring out their healing properties. Softer plant parts—leaves, flowers, and soft stems—are used in tissanes or infusions and are not boiled. To make a decoction, the herb is placed in water in a pot on the stove, brought to a boil, and simmered for one or two minutes. Some decoctions bring the water to a boil, then shut the flame, letting the herbs steep for a few minutes or until cool. Another way to make a decoction is to simmer a quart of water and two ounces of herb (valerian root or ginger root, for example) until the water boils down to half (a pint). Break up plant matter before putting it in the pot; even powder it in a mortar. A tissane boiled down to half its water amount is also a decoction; boil the strained tea, not the herb matter. To use, take a tablespoonful to half a cup, diluted in a cup of hot water for taste, a couple of times a day. These are more concentrated than tissanes or infusions.

Herbal tinctures (or extracts) are more concentrated yet, are taken by the drop, about twenty drops or a third to half eyedropperful three times a day. They are preserved in alcohol or cider vinegar, and though the taste of alcohol tinctures is bad, very little actual alcohol is ingested. To remove the alcohol, put the tincture drops in about a tablespoonful of hot water and it will evaporate. Taken straight from the dropper under the tongue, the herb goes into the body in the fastest way possible, bypassing the digestive system. Herbs taken in the alcohol tincture form are my highest recommendation. They are at their most powerful and most active, never deteriorate in storage, and work the fastest.

Tinctures may be bought at healthfood stores at prices varying from about six to fifteen dollars. The herbal antibiotics—goldenseal, echinacea and pau d'arco—are the expensive ones but are also used the least frequently. These are herbs to save for serious dis-eases, as the body builds a tolerance for them and it's best to use them only when really needed. Other tinctures cost much less, and since they are taken in such small amounts and usually for a short time, the one ounce bottles go a long way. Alcohol tinctures keep indefinitely so women can build up a medicine chest of them. Remember that cider-preserved tinctures last only about a year. Tinctures are reliably effective, more so than herbs taken in other forms.

To make an herbal tincture at home, place six to eight ounces of dried plant matter in a wide-mouthed quart jar and fill to the top with 60 proof/ 30 percent or higher alcohol (or apple cider vinegar). To make smaller amounts use a ratio of one part herb to four parts liquid. Let stand for three to six weeks (some sources say two weeks, shaking the bottle night and morning), then separate the liquid from the herbs, squeezing out the herbs before returning them to the earth. Store the liquid, which is the tincture, in brown glass bottles with glass (not plastic) eyedroppers. Plastic and metals react unfavorably with the herbs. Alcohol tinctures can be made to taste better by using a little vegetable glycerin as part of the preservative. While tinctures don't exactly taste good, they go down fast, and some taste better than others. It always amazes me how a very bad tasting herbal can taste fine to someone who needs it.

Capsules are another way to use herbs, and they can be bought prepared or made at home from dried loose herbs and gelatin capsules. Women who have digestive problems may find herbs less effective this way, as they are less easy to assimilate in capsule than in liquid form. In some parts of the country, however, it's the only way herbals are available. Some herbs also are too bad tasting—like goldenseal or cayenne—to taste going down, either as a tea or tincture. And some herbs taken specifically for the digestive tract—like slippery elm for indigestion, food poisoning or diarrhea—need to go through that system to soothe it. To use these, take two capsules, usually three times a day.

To fill your own capsules, place the loose herbs in a bowl and bring the halves of the capsule together through the mix. Both gelatin capsules and loose dried herbs are generally available at food co-ops, and encapsulators are available. Dust off the capsules before putting them away. It is easier to make a lot at one time and have them handy than to make a few. Store in the dark, in a dark container, and drink a lot of water with capsules. They are generally used when you have to take a lot of herbs, but tinctures and infusions are still more effective, though capsules may be more convenient. Herb roots remain fresh for a long time, but other dried herb parts (in or out of capsules) do not. When buying prepared capsules, it is hard to know if they are fresh. Also be aware that some women, though rarely, may be allergic to the gelatin/cellulose of capsules. Herbs to be sucked, as slippery elm lozenges (or zinc gluconate lozenges), both for sore throats, are also sold in healthfood stores.

These are all internal uses for herbs. Poultices or compresses (fomentations) are used externally. A compress is a cloth wet with the herb infusion liquid and used hot (but not burning hot) against the skin. A chamomile compress for boils is an example. A poultice is made with the tea dregs, the plant matter itself softened by boiling water poured over it, and wrapped in gauze. An onion and honey poultice for bronchitis or pneumonia is an example, or a plantain poultice for poison ivy or insect bites. Naturopathy uses poultices of various herbs, household items and foods; they soothe and draw out toxins. In most cases, use them hot and change the herbs as they cool.

Other women's uses for herbs are in douches, rinses and baths. Try a douche of goldenseal and myrrh, boiled as a decoction, strained, diluted, and cooled to body temperature for yeast infections and trichomonas vaginitis. Use three times a day while needed and for a day or two after. Women with hypoglycemia need to use goldenseal carefully, however, as it lowers blood sugar. Use a decoction of nettles, black walnut (for dark hair or rosemary for light) and yarrow as a hair rinse, made in the same way as above but poured over hair after washing. It makes hair shine, reduces dandruff and stops hair loss. Further uses for herbs are in baths for relaxing or detoxifying the body. Try a bath of valerian or lavender for insomnia— make a decoction or tea, and add it strained to the bath water.

Herbs used externally, for the skin, may be made into salves or oils. An infused oil is made by placing half to two pounds of dried herbs in a quart jar and filling the jar with olive oil, covering the herbs completely. Close tightly and store in a dark place for three to six weeks (some sources say two to three weeks). Pour off the oil and store it in dark glass bottles. These make wonderful liniments, massage oils and scented oils. Try dandelion flower massage oil to reduce body or back pain, or rose oil for relaxing and emotional healing.

For salves, place herbs covered with olive oil in a lidded oven casserole dish and bake at 200–250°F for two hours. Strain out the herbs and bring the oil to the top of the stove, add 1/8 to 1/4 ounce of beeswax to three or four ounces of herb oil. Warm until the wax has fully melted, pour onto a cool plate, and when hardened solid scrape into small widemouthed jars. (Or use already made herbal oil and add the beeswax, starting at the top of the stove.) A comfrey, plantain and goldenseal salve is a wonder for skin irritations and slow-healing sores. These recipes come primarily from Billie Potts' *Witches Heal*, an herbal I recommend highly for all women interested in using herbs.

Herbs in this book are used internally except where noted, and herb tinctures are the most recommended form. Poultices and fomentations are also used, as well as douches, and these require infused or decocted dried herbs. Herbs taken internally can also be used as teas, infusions or capsules, but the tinctures are the most powerful and fastest acting.

Where herbs are named, they are single herbs in most cases, with no more than three herbs used together. It becomes confusing and expensive to use the herb combinations some healers recommend that involve purchasing a dozen different items. And it is not necessary. While there may be several possibilities for healing, say menopause symptoms, I urge women to pick the one that seems the most positive for their needs, and only to go to another if the first does not work or is uncomfortable. Where two or three herbs are used together it is indicated, and where one choice is probably the most effective for the most women, it is also indicated. When using herbs for acute or infectious dis-eases, make sure to continue for at least a few days after symptoms disappear completely, particularly when using herbal antibiotics, to prevent the dis-ease from returning. When using echinacea, you must stay on it for at least ten days. As with vitamins in high doses, when no longer needed decrease amounts and frequency rather than stopping all at once. Avoid the following herbs when pregnant or nursing:

Goldenseal	Squawgrass or Cohosh
Valerian	Pennyroyal
Ginger	Sage
Cotton Root	Rue
Motherwort	Ginseng
Tansy	St. John's Wort[1]
Vervain	Aloe Vera (internally)
Couchgrass	

For more information on herbs for healing, try the herb chapter in *All Women Are Healers*, Billie Potts' *Witches Heal*, and Joy Gardner's *The New Healing Yourself* (The Crossing Press, 1989). These provide thorough information on preparing and using herbs for healing. The herbal remedies for this book come primarily from these sources, plus Dr. Ross Trattler, *Better Health Through Natural Healing* (McGraw-Hill Book Co., 1985), Mildred Jackson, ND, and Terri Teague, ND, DC, *The Handbook of Alternatives to Chemical Medicine* (Bookpeople, 1975, and Louise Tenney, MH's *Health Handbook* (Woodland Books, 1987). There were many other less major sources in addition; see the bibliography. Herbal healing is a primary method of this book.

---

[1]Cathryn Bauer, *Acupressure For Women* (Freedom, CA, The Crossing Press, 1987), p. 72.

Naturopathy

All healing happens in the body itself, and all healing is self-healing. If you cut your finger, your mother can kiss it and your lover can put a band-aid on it, but it must be your own body that regrows the cut skin. The purpose of healing is to support the body in this healing process, aiding it to return to its normal state, which is good health. The role of naturopathy is to return the body as simply as possible to wellness and to maintain it. A naturopath may use any or all of the methods of this book and more to do this. By the use of therapies that support but do not interfere with the healing process, blocks to good health are removed. Healing is supported, rather than dis-ease attacked. Naturopathy offers simple common sense methods for aiding the body to reject dis-ease and return to optimal well-being.

This sounds like the basic philosophy of holistic/women's healing, and it is. Naturopathy places the responsibility for wellness and healing on the individual, not as a means of blaming anyone for her dis-ease, but as a means of empowering her to heal herself and stay well. A healthy daily life is the foundation of well-being, with emphasis on rest, quality nutrition, sunlight and fresh air, exercise, cleanliness, positive thinking and living in a positive environment. Quality nutrition means a diet high in organic whole foods, as sugar- and additive-free as possible. A positive environment includes reducing stress, worry, anger and fear, and living and working in a beneficial setting.

In naturopathic theory, dis-ease is the result of unhealthful living habits, which deplete resistance and allow the accumulation of toxins. Dis-ease comes from within, not from an outside invasion of bacteria or "germs," and wellness also comes from within, from the body's inherent vitality and predisposition to well-being. The symptoms that standard medicine calls illness, naturopathy calls healing—recognizing them as an indication of the body's attempt to remove toxins and return to good health. The naturopathic concept of vitalism—that living Be-ings are comprised of structural, biochemical and emotional levels—is a reflection of the psychic healer's four bodies (physical, emotional, mental and spiritual). In both approaches, all the levels must be treated for healing to occur.

This healing process from within is not to be suppressed with drugs, but supported on all three levels to resolve the dis-ease, as long as the woman has the strength to do it. Children, elders and those who are debilitated are treated more aggressively. Their own vitality and abilities to heal from within are utilized as much as possible. In the case of chronic dis-ease, considered deeper dysfunction than acute illness, attempts are first made to stimulate the active dis-ease phase, sometimes causing an aggravation of symptoms (as in homeopathy) before the releasing and cure.[1]

Healing from the structural level means working with the skeletal system to remove spinal misalignments. This is done through osteopathic or chiropractic treatments. As anyone with a bad back or migraines knows, spinal subluxations can cause symptoms that seem totally unrelated to the back itself. Many dis-eases of all types can be helped significantly with musculo-skeletal work and massage, including injuries and stresses to the body, digestive problems, headaches and migraines, and heart and lung conditions.

Treating the biochemical level means primarily using adequate nourishment—quality foods with as few additives and pollutants as possible. Chemicals added to foods in growing, processing and preserving, along with pollutants in air, food and water, cause reduced nutrition and an accumulation of metabolic wastes and toxins in the body. These affect the body fluids, digestion and elimination, and reduce the functioning of all organs. Refined foods, dietary deficiencies, and harmful substances (alcohol, caffeine, smoking, medical or street drugs, junk foods, sugar and too much meat), all upset the body's balance at the biochemical level. A water or juice fast for a few days, followed by a change to a whole foods organic diet will help eliminate these toxins. In the case of dis-ease, the fast may be followed by a mono-food diet for a short time, where only one specific food is eaten until the body rebalances, and other foods are introduced slowly. Roast onions or peeled raw apples are sometimes used for this.

The emotional level is a factor that both holistic healing and standard medicine are considering more and more. Eighty-five percent of all dis-ease in the west is directly stress related. Naturopathy looks at this

---

[1]Michael Van Straten, ND, DO, *The Complete Natural Health Care Consultant* (New York, Prentice Hall, 1987), p. 90. Much of the naturopathic theory of this section comes from this source.

mechanistically, seeing stress as imbalancing the body's hormones, but women are aware of the political causes and implications as well. Stress depresses the immune system and produces an over-amount of adrenaline that builds up, creating body-level tensions. Too much of this causes adrenal exhaustion, nutrient and energy depletion, reduced resistance, and opens the way for dis-ease. Women's healing also believes that there is an emotional component to all dis-ease and that component must be released for full healing to occur. It goes beyond body mechanics to analyze the politics of stress for women under patriarchy.

There are two major forms of naturopathic treatment, one to break down toxins in the body (called catabolic), and the other to build up and regenerate (called anabolic). Catabolic treatment may include fasting, detoxification baths or sweats, hydrotherapy, or foods that cause break-down of harmful substances (such as apple cider vinegar and water to break down calcium buildups in osteoarthritis). It also uses cleansing herbs such as red clover and burdock or enemas of various sorts to eliminate toxins from the body. Anabolic treatment builds strength and resistance to dis-ease, boosting the immune system and supplementing nutrition where needed. Vitamins and herbs are used here, along with specific foods for the dis-ease, a nutritional program, and physical or breathing exercises. Since vitamins and herbs are discussed in separate sections, it is primarily fasts, foods and household remedies that are offered as naturopathic healing suggestions in this book. Women are urged to eat a healthy whole foods diet and eliminate as many contaminants from their bodies as possible.

Fasting is done to detoxify the body, rest the digestive system, and revitalize. It is usually done for a period of one to three days and does not mean no food. A water-only fast is less often used than a fruit juice fast, and only in specific illnesses. It should not be undertaken by the beginner or unsupervised. Do not fast when you are under mental or physical stress or when you are required to be very active and busy. Fasts should not be broken by a heavy meal. If you have a cold or flu or other dis-ease where your body is uninterested in eating anyway, a fruit juice fast can help you to fight infection, clear the skin, and heal wounds more rapidly.

Here is a fast suggested by naturopaths Mildred Jackson and Terri Teague, from their book *The Handbook of Alternatives to Chemical Medicine* (Bookpeople, 1975). It is a general cleansing fast to use from one day to one month, with no longer than three days recommended unsupervised. All of the juices used should be organic. Combine:

> 6 ounces papaya concentrate
> 4 ounces prune juice

4 ounces fresh pineapple juice
8 ounces orange juice
1 quart distilled water

Have another quart of distilled water handy. Once an hour, drink four ounces of the above mix and four ounces of the second quart's distilled water. This is a fast that should not result in hunger pains, dizziness, nausea or fatigue; it will cleanse the whole body and all the body's systems in three days.[2]

There may be detoxification symptoms during a fast, particularly after the first day. These can include bad breath, headaches, constipation or diarrhea (try an enema, not laxatives), and coated tongue. You may feel spacy by the second day and will wish to stay home and rest. Since no solid food is being taken, avoid taking vitamin pills or other supplements. A fast can be combined with a cleansing bath (do only one in the three days) and/ or an enema (try coffee enema) every other day. A good cleansing bath is one cup of sea salt and one cup of baking soda in a full hot tub; soak for twenty-five minutes, towel dry, then go to bed and sweat for about two hours. By the end of the fast you will feel well, revitalized, very clear and clean, and much healthier.

It is important how you break a fast. Too much food all at once will make you sick, and the wrong foods will negate the fast's cleansing. Mildred Jackson and Terri Teague suggest:

Day 1: Eat an apple, and a small bowl of vegetable
        broth or soup. Sip slowly, use no salt or spices.
Day 2: Repeat day one, and add a portion of mashed
        potatoes (no gravy), a glass of sour milk and
        some yoghurt.
Day 3: Increase the above portions, and add a small
        raw vegetable salad, some brown rice and
        some cottage cheese.
Day 4: Normal diet, snacks should be fruit only.

Continue to drink a lot of water and fruit juices during the change-over from fasting to normal eating.[3]

For less drastic fasting, try a ten-day diet of organic brown rice and fish, nothing else for that period. It will cleanse and detoxify, add minerals to the body, and rest and aid the spleen. Use a variety of types of fish and drink only distilled water. Another simple fast that includes food is to do

---

[2]Mildred Jackson, ND, and Terri Teague, ND, DC, *The Handbook of Alternatives to Chemical Medicine* (Berkeley, CA, Bookpeople, 1975), p. 134–135.
[3]*Ibid.*, p. 135.

a two-day fast of raw vegetables only, and drink three eight-ounce glasses of distilled water each day. This fast cleanses the body of toxins, metabolizes already-present carbohydrates, stimulates digestive enzymes and tones the digestive system. For any fasts more drastic or longer lasting than those given above, or if you are experiencing more than a minor disease or debility, seek expert supervision.

Most methods listed under naturopathy in this book use foods, juices, or household items to cleanse and detoxify, build the immune system or provide a needed nutrient. The baking soda and seasalt cleansing bath described above is an example and some others follow. Many of these are considered folk remedies and some were used and popularized by psychic healer/channeler Edgar Cayce. None can harm when used with common sense, and all have been proven by long use and tradition.

Bee Pollen is a whole food remedy, a miracle food that aids digestion and circulation, and boosts the immune system. It is a major remedy for women with allergies, sinusitis, hay fever or asthma and will reduce symptoms. It increases resistance to dis-ease and stress, boosts endurance, retards aging, speeds healing and helps regeneration after debilitating dis-ease. Pollen is the single richest source for vitamins, minerals and enzymes, and is the only non-meat source that contains all of the amino acids. It is a vegetable source of the B-complex, B-12, B-6, vitamin C, rutin (bioflavinoid), E and essential fatty acids. Bee pollen is a brain stimulant and reduces alcohol cravings, helps chronic constipation or diarrhea, benefits arteriosclerosis, aids anemia and migraines, is an antibacterial and an antioxidant.

For women's concerns in particular, bee pollen is important. It aids menstrual problems and promotes orgasm by balancing the reproductive system hormones. Bee pollen helps in pregnancy and milk production, and reduces menopause symptoms.[4] It may prevent or delay the appearance of malignant breast tumors and reduce tumor size of existing ones; it is a cancer preventive useful for all forms of cancer. Use from two tablets (chewable, tastes wonderful) to an ounce a day; the pollen used does not have to be local pollen. Other bee products have the same benefits. Try propolis, honey, royal jelly, and honeycomb. The only side effect I have found is that bee pollen may increase hunger. Expect to pay about six dollars for a hundred tablets.

Garlic is another remedy that falls under the category of naturopathic. It is recommended here in its odorless form, a product called *Kyolic*, since raw garlic can cause gas and a strong body odor. *Kyolic*/garlic is an antibacterial, antiviral and antifungal. It is an immune system booster that

---

[4]C. C. Pollen Co., "Is Honeybee Pollen the World's Only Perfect Food?" (Phoenix, AZ, C. C. Pollen Co., 1984), pamphlet, p. 4–10.

helps in lowering blood pressure, resisting dis-ease and is particularly important for women in healing systemic candida albicans, vaginal yeast infections and recurrent bladder infections (as well as any other recurrent infections from boils to tonsillitis to colds).

For women who have recurrent yeast vaginitis or systemic candida (yeast) over-run, take two tablets three times a day with meals to start, decreasing slowly after all symptoms have stopped. Stay on a maintenance amount of two tablets a day for at least three months longer, and increase again at any sign of a cold, infection or illness. After about a week on the tablets, you may experience a detox reaction consisting of diarrhea, flu-like symptoms, bowel movements of a strange color, nausea, weakness or dizziness that will last a few days. Drink a lot of water and stick with it; the sense of well-being once this ends makes it worth it. Once the detox takes place, many recurrent illnesses will stop altogether. I have had one cold in just about two years and no vaginal infections since starting *Kyolic* at only two tablets per day. Previously I had a vaginal infection monthly, and colds about every six weeks. There are no side effects other than the detox, and a slight body-odor change that is pleasant. It is a major immune system booster, particularly recommended for women under stress, and is essential for women with herpes or hypertension.

Apple Cider Vinegar is another naturopathic remedy of importance for women. Mix one teaspoon of this with one teaspoon of honey in a glass of warm or cold water and sip slowly, alone or with meals. It can also be used without the honey, but it must be apple cider vinegar rather than white vinegar. It tastes pleasant, and has the effect of remineralizing the body and replacing and balancing potassium. Use it for osteoarthritis, to break down calcium deposits in the joints and send the minerals to where they are needed in the bones. Use it as a preventive for osteoporosis. This combination is also positive for digestive upsets, poor assimilation, and to prevent or remedy food poisoning (if vomiting, take a small sip every five minutes), kidney and bladder infections, chronic fatigue, headaches and migraines, high blood pressure, dizziness, heat exhaustion, obesity, sinusitis and allergies, and for infertility. It is antibacterial, antifungal and boosts the immune system. For chronic dis-eases use daily one to three times a day. For acute illnesses use as needed or short-term. For sore throats, use a gargle of one teaspoon of apple cider vinegar in a glass of water.[5]

Castor Oil, another naturopathic remedy, was popularized by psychic Edgar Cayce. It is an herbal oil pressed from a bean, usually used externally in heated packs. This has been used to heal virtually every

[5]D. C. Jarvis, MD, *Folk Medicine* (New York, Fawcett Crest Books, 1958), p. 61–98.

external and internal dis-ease and is a miracle cure for many of them. Rub it on the skin nightly to dissolve warts and help arthritic knees or joints, and use it externally on skin cancer, acne, boils, bruises, wounds and sores, including mouth sores and herpes. Use it as an external pack for almost any internal ailment, including breast lumps and uterine or ovarian cysts, any tumors malignant or benign, gall bladder trouble, appendicitis, liver problems or detoxification, post-surgical complications, and for bowel dis-eases.

To make a castor oil pack, fold a washcloth or dishtowel several times and soak it in castor oil until it is wet but not dripping. Place the cloth on top of the body part that needs healing, and cover it with plastic, wrapping the body part in a plastic sheet (do not cover the head or restrict breathing, of course). Over that place a heating pad set on medium, and raise it to high if you can tolerate that comfortably. Wrap a towel around everything and relax with this for an hour to an hour and a half. Then remove it, using baking soda and water (two teaspoons to a quart of water) to wash the castor oil from the skin. Use this from one night a week to every night until the dis-ease is resolved. I have seen breast lumps disappear in a month with this treatment, but it may take longer. The pack can be reused—put it in a plastic container and add more castor oil if needed.[6] A disposable diaper makes a good pack, also. This is truly a heal-all.

Naturopathy uses a number of remedies of this sort. Use boric acid and water compresses for boils, infected cuts, and under-the-skin swellings, as well as an eyewash for conjunctivitis. Use clay in similar ways to castor oil packs. Various types of clay are used for various dis-eases, and clay is also taken internally (in water). Cranberry juice is a remedy for bladder infections, with cherry juice a good second choice, while beet juice will help lessen the side effects of cancer chemotherapy. Use lemon juice in water similarly to apple cider vinegar in water, and olive oil similarly to castor oil.

Apricots are good for relieving constipation and they clean the intestinal wall. Buttermilk helps to balance bowel flora and prevent vaginal infections after antibiotic use. Peroxide is an antibacterial that may be used by the drop internally for systemic infections; start with two drops a day in water and increase very slowly. Kelp (seaweed) tablets add all the necessary minerals to the body, balance the thyroid, help in obesity and fat metabolism, aid the heart and relieve angina, help in bone fracture healing and bone mineral dis-eases (osteoporosis), and are useful for restoring thin, falling or brittle hair.

These are only a few of the remedies used by naturopaths to help the

---

[6]William A. McGarey, MD, *The Edgar Cayce Remedies* (New York, Bantam Books, 1983), p. 50–51.

body heal itself. They are things often found around the house or in supermarkets, remedies of low expense and no toxicity. In many cases they are more effective than medical drugs and they are always positive to use. The healing suggestions of this book under naturopathy list a number of remedies of this type, but the full scope of naturopathic medicine includes the methods of the entire book plus further aspects untouched upon. All natural medicine is naturopathic.

My primary sources for this healing category are: Dr. Ross Trattler, *Better Health Through Natural Healing* (McGraw-Hill Book Co., 1985), Mildred Jackson, ND and Terri Teague, ND, DC, *The Handbook of Alternatives to Chemical Medicine* (Bookpeople), 1975), and Michael Van Straten, ND, DO, *The Complete Natural Health Consultant* (Prentice Hall Press, 1987).

Homeopathy and Cell Salts

Homeopathy is based on the concept of "like cures like," and the idea that only very minimal amounts of a substance are needed to boost the vital force into a self-cure. Homeopathic remedies start with an herb or other substance that in toxic doses can create in a well woman the symptoms it will later heal when homeopathically prepared. The substance is then made into a remedy by a process called potentization, a series of dilutions and succussions (agitating the remedy sharply). The more diluted it is, the more potent it becomes. The process of making and vitalizing the remedies is unique to homeopathic medicine. By the end of the process there may be no physical molecules left of the original substance, but the energy level of that substance remains. Homeopathic remedies work on a beyond-the-physical level, healing the body from the etheric, emotional, and mental layers of the aura.

The remedies are very precisely chosen, and highly specific to the symptoms they are used to cure. They are matched to the symptoms of the illness. The standard medical name of the dis-ease is irrelevant. Each remedy is tested (proven) for what combination of symptoms it will produce, and it is only that exact combination it will heal. There are thousands of remedies (about a hundred are most often used), and each woman's dis-ease has different symptoms. The homeopathic remedy that will stop one woman's migraines may have no effect at all on another woman's. The right choice of remedy will result in a rapid improvement or cure, sometimes within minutes for an acute dis-ease. The remedy may only need to be taken once. The challenge in homeopathy is to find the one remedy that will match and heal the symptoms. It takes work to learn it, but the results are gratifying. Since its discovery and implementation two hundred years ago, homeopathy has become a major healing system for women both in and out of medicine.

A guidebook called a *Materia Medica* directory is used to find the right remedy for the dis-ease. It contains what are called remedy pictures, and a way of cross-referencing symptoms with possible remedies. There are several versions in print—all of them outdated with sexist and racist language, and in serious need of revision. Other than the *Materia Medicas* (still essential for the serious user of homeopathy despite its problems), there are a number of how-to books available that will help women in many acute cases. The best of these is Stephen Cummings, FPN, and Dana Ullman, MPH, *Everybody's Guide to Homeopathic Medicines* (J. P. Tarcher, Inc., 1984). I also use a booklet put out by Boericke and Tafel, a maker of remedies, called *The Family Guide to Self-Medication (Homeopathic)*, (Boericke and Tafel, Inc., 1988).

If your city's healthfood stores do not carry homeopathic remedies and books, order them by phone from Boericke and Tafel at 1-800-272-2920 or from Beckett Apothecary at 1-800-727-8188. Both are in Philadelphia and there are other sources. For acute dis-eases in self-help, use remedies in the 6X to 30C potency; the higher numbers last longer and need to be repeated less often. A C designation is many times more potent than the same number followed by an X. Higher yet may be useful, but may require a doctor's prescription to order. A homeopathic physician can use extremely high potencies. At the turn of the century in the United States, over half of medical doctors were also homeopaths, and this is still true in many countries. Today there are far fewer here but numbers are increasing and many are women. They can be located by writing to the International Foundation of Homeopathy, 2366 Eastlake E., Seattle, WA 98102, (206) 324-8230. Many good homeopaths are not MD's, and many laywomen are developing strong expertise in this field of healing. However, only an MD can legally prescribe the remedies. It is becoming more difficult for laywomen to order remedies in the higher doses, thanks to FDA harassment.

The easiest way to find a remedy for your particular dis-ease is to look it up in one of the how-to books. A list of symptoms will be given; choose the remedy that most closely matches your own symptoms for that dis-ease. For example, if you have a cold, is it in the first stages with a sudden onset, and fever, cough, sore throat or stuffed nose? The remedy here is *Aconite*. Do you have a high fever with hot, red skin and flushed face? Use *Belladonna*. Is it a chest cold, with a dry painful cough and a thirst for cold drinks? The remedy is *Bryonia alba*. Are the closest symptoms sneezing, watery runny nose, rough dry throat, flu symptoms, chills and fever, headache and body aches? The remedy is *Gelsemium*.[1] There are many types of colds and several remedies to choose from.

---

[1]Boericke and Tafel, Inc., *The Family Guide to Self-Medication (Homeopathic)* (Philadelphia, PA, Boericke and Tafel, Inc., 1988), p. 13.

Once you have picked the remedy to use, buy it from a healthfood store. The cost of remedies is $3.50–$5.00 for a good amount. Women who use homeopathy regularly keep a medicine chest of them on hand and kits are available in various sizes. To take the remedy, shake a couple of the pellets into the bottle cap—do not touch them with your hands—and toss them under your tongue where they will melt. The remedies are placed on milk sugar pellets and taste sweet.

A number of things can antidote (cancel) these fragile remedies. First, you do not want to touch them with your hands and if a pellet drops on the floor, throw it away. Any strong fragrance may antidote a homeopathic remedy, including aromatherapy scents, camphor odors, and the strong smells of pine or disinfectant used in some floor cleaners. If you drink coffee, including decaffeinated coffee, do not use it during homeopathic treatment as this will usually antidote the remedies. Peppermint in any form, including peppermint toothpaste, may negate a remedy, or menthol. If a remedy has clearly acted and then clearly and abruptly stops acting, suspect antidote. If something in your environment cancels your remedy, stop the antidote and take the remedy again. Do not eat or drink for at least fifteen minutes before or after taking a remedy.

If you have used the correct remedy for your symptoms, there will be some response, usually within a few minutes. This may be a lessening of symptoms, but it can also be a temporary aggravation of the illness. The onset of an aggravation is considered positive proof that you have chosen the correct remedy. Stick it out; it doesn't last long, usually only a few minutes with a low potency remedy. Once the aggravation ends there will be a clear improvement in symptoms and in feelings of well-being. As long as there is improvement, no more of the remedy is needed. If you start to feel worse again, take another dose of the same remedy. If your symptoms change after using a remedy, you have peeled off a layer of the dis-ease and may now require a different one. Go back to the how-to book and compare symptoms again. In acute dis-eases, usually only one remedy is required, and a few doses of it will do the job. Use one remedy at a time; never mix them.

Take remedies no more than once an hour (there are some exceptions to this). If there has been no response from a remedy after taking it a couple of times, it is the wrong remedy. In this case, nothing will happen, as long as you stop taking it; it will neither heal nor harm. Finding the correct remedy to match your symptoms is the hardest part of homeopathy and can be frustrating. Using this method of healing requires study and intuition; a pendulum at times has guided me. Homeopathic suggestions in this book are from: *Everybody's Guide to Homeopathic Medicine* and *The Family Guide to Self-Medication (Homeopathic)*, as well as Moshe Olshevsky,

CA, PhD, *et. al.*, *The Manual of Natural Therapy* (Citadel Press, 1989), Michael Van Straten, ND, DO, *The Complete Natural Health Consultant*, (Prentice Hall, 1987), and John Clarke, MD, *The Prescriber* (Health Science Press, 1972). For more information, read these books, as well as *All Women Are Healers*. There are a number of other good sources available.

   Cell or Tissue Salts are a series of twelve homeopathically pre-pared remedies based on the chemical composition of the cells of the body. They are available at healthfood stores and where homeopathic remedies are sold, and are usually easy to find. The cell salts are nutrient supple-ments that balance the minute amounts of trace minerals. They direct the body to absorb more of a needed mineral or to release an excess of it. These remedies were first prepared by homeopath Wilhelm Schuessler of late nineteenth century Germany, who believed that all dis-ease was caused by a mineral deficiency in the cells' biochemistry, and that by supplementing these minerals all dis-ease could be healed.

   The cell salts have their place in women's healing for both physical and emotional dis-ease. The twelve salts each have specific indications. A combination of them, called Bioplasma or Combination Cell Salts, is a good immune system booster, energy balancer and general tonic. It is particularly good when recovering from dis-ease or debility. There is a response similar to that of other homeopathic remedies upon using tissue salts and they are gently and slowly effective. They cost about five dollars for a bottle of five hundred pellets. To use them, shake a few to half a teaspoonful into the bottle cap and toss them under the tongue to melt. For nutritional supplementation, use the 6X potency. 12X is considered best for healing dis-ease.

   Unlike other homeopathic remedies, more than one cell salt may be used at a time but they are not usually taken together (except in Bioplasma and a few combinations). Alternate them when using more than one. Take cell salts three times a day for chronic illness, and they can be used longterm. For acute healing, take them as often as every half hour for as long as needed. They are safe for children as well as adults, and like other homeopathic remedies, I have also used them on pets. The minerals are components of cell chemistry, and the homeopathic method of preparation makes them easy to assimilate. Taken on or under the tongue and allowed to melt there, they are not passed through the digestive system but go directly into the bloodstream.

   Each of the dis-eases discussed in the remedy section of this book is assigned a cell salt. The primary sources are the following list and the sources for homeopathy. Here is a run-down of the twelve Schuessler cell salts, and how to use them for healing dis-ease.

Schuessler Cell Salts[2]

1. *Calc. Flour.* (Calcium Fluoride)—Elastic Tissue Builder. For relaxed conditions of elastic fibers and blood vessels, muscular weakness, impaired circulation, piles, deficient enamel of teeth, cracks in the skin, bone bruises and varicose veins.

2. *Calc. Phos.* (Calcium Phosphate)—General Nutrient: Gastric, Bones and Teeth. For chilblains, simple anemia, impaired digestion, malassimilation, bone dis-eases, infant teething troubles. The ideal tonic after dis-ease, particularly good for elders.

3. *Calc. Sulph.* (Calcium Sulphate)—Blood Purifier. For minor skin ailments, acne, pimples during adolescence, slow skin healing, sore lips, chronic oozing ulcers.

4. *Ferr. Phos.* (Iron Phosphate)—Oxygen Carrier. Use for minor respiratory dis-eases, coughs, colds, chills, diarrhea, inflammations, congestion, fevers and headaches. Also for nosebleeds and heavy menstrual flows. The preeminent biochemic first aid.

5. *Kali Mur.* (Potassium Chloride)—Blood Conditioner, and minor respiratory disorders. For coughs, colds, chills, bronchitis, sinus and chest congestions, warts. Alternate with Ferr. Phos. The children's remedy.

6. *Kali. Phos.* (Potassium Phosphate)—Nerve Nutrient. Use for nervous exhaustion, nervous indigestion, nervous headaches and migraines. Relieves stress, worry, anxiety and insomnia.

7. *Kali. Sulph.* (Potassium Sulphate)—Oxygen Exchanger. For minor skin eruptions with scaling or sticky exhudation, pain in limbs, bronchial congestion, brittle nails, falling hair, evening aggravation of symptoms.

8. *Mag. Phos.* (Magnesium Phosphate)—Nerve Stabilizer. Soft tissues. Use for spasmodic darting pains, cramps, neuralgia, colic, flatulence, backaches and sciatica.

9. *Natrum Mur.* (Sodium Chloride)—Water Distributor. For dryness or excessive moisture in any part of the body, running watery colds, vaginitis with watery discharge, loss of smell or taste, salt cravings.

10. *Natrum Phos.* (Sodium Phosphate)—Acid Neutralizer. For over-acidity, digestive upsets, heartburn, rheumatic pains, jaundice, gastric ulcers.

11. *Natrum Sulph.* (Sodium Sulphate)—Excess Water Eliminator. Use for liver symptoms, gall bladder, biliousness, queasiness, influenza, watery infiltrations. The liver salt.

12. *Silica* (Silicic Oxide)—Cleanser. For impure blood, boils, pus formation, pimples, brittle nails with ridges, lackluster hair, ingrown nails, poor memory. Alternate with Kali. Sulph.

---

[2]This information is from the package insert that comes with the remedies.

Amino Acids

In women's bodies, the muscles, ligaments, tendons, organs, glands, nails, hair, body fluids, enzymes, hormones and genes are all comprised of protein, and protein is also essential for bone growth. Amino acids are the chemical components of which proteins are made. The twenty-nine known amino acids in various combinations create 50,000 different proteins and 20,000 enzymes in the body. The combinations are specific and cannot occur if even one amino acid is missing or in short supply. Amino acids are neurotransmitters or neurotransmitter precursors for the central nervous system and brain, allowing the brain to receive and send messages.[1] They comprise the nucleus of every cell. Obviously, amino acids are essential to human and mammalian life.

Of the twenty-nine known amino acids, the liver produces about eighty percent and the rest must come from diet. Essential amino acids are the ones that must be obtained from outside the body. The eight essential amino acids are: isoleucine, leucine, lysine, methionine, phenylalanine, threonine, tryptophan and valine. Cysteine and tyrosine are synthesized in the body from methionine and phenylalanine, respectively. Amino acids produced in the body from other sources are alanine, arginine, aspartic acid, glutamic acid, glutamine, histidine, glycine, ornithine, proline and serine. Amino acid supplements that come in the L (alpha) form are considered natural and are more compatible to women's body chemistry than those in the D form. The exception here is phenylalanine, which also comes as DL-phenylalanine.

The use of amino acids and proteins in the body is continuous, and a depletion or shortage of any of the essential amino acids leads rapidly to dis-ease. Deficiencies can occur from improper or imbalanced diet, longterm vegan vegetarianism, or inability to properly assimilate protein

[1]James F. Balch, MD, and Phyllis A. Balch, CNC, *Prescription for Nutritional Healing* (Garden City, NY, Avery Publishing Group, Inc., 1990), p. 27. The information for this section comes primarily from this source.

via the digestive system. Since vitamins and minerals require amino acids for their use in the body, and since protein comprises more of body weight than any other substance except water, amino acids require women's attention.

Much of my own lack of energy and too early exhaustion have been remedied by taking an amino acids combination supplement, and I believe that many more women can benefit from them. If you have any form of degenerative dis-ease, mental or nervous disorder, heart dis-ease, chronic fatigue syndrome, diabetes, epilepsy, anemia, are in recovery from alcohol or drugs, or are a longterm vegetarian who feels something missing, amino acids may be important for you. If you have herpes, you are probably already aware of L-lysine as a factor in preventing and reducing attacks.

Amino acids are available singly and in combinations. Twin Labs is a good brand. Combinations are sold as free-form amino acids, which are considered the purest and are made from a grain base. Free form amino acids combinations and single amino acids are taken alone on an empty stomach, rather than with meals. Combination amino acids are also sold as liver extract or predigested liver amino acids. Twin Labs makes this, as does Enzymatics Therapy. These may be taken with meals and cost about $10–13 for 100 capsules; take one or two a day. Free form amino acids are often found in the body building section of healthfood chains. The pictures of musclemen on the bottles may put you off, but they are fast acting and vegetarian. Some healthfood stores now have full sections of amino acid supplements, without the body builders.

Here is what each amino acid does; twenty-eight of them are listed here, and women will recognize their own needs immediately from the descriptions. Their uses are startling—why haven't we known about these before?—and important for many many women. The information is primarily from James F. Balch, MD, and Phyllis A. Balch, CNC, *Prescription for Nutritional Healing*, and *The Vitamin Herb Guide* (Global Health Ltd., 1990), plus some healthfood store handout sheets. Little information has been readily available on amino acids, but I feel they are highly important for women's well-being.

L-Alanine is important in glucose metabolism, and is useful for women who are diabetic, hypoglycemic or have fatigue or energy problems.

L-Arginine slows tumors and cancer growth, detoxifies the liver, regulates growth hormones, aids in kidney disorders, helps wound healing, and helps to maintain the immune system. It is used by body builders to increase muscle mass and reduce fat, and is important in healing or preventing cirrhosis of the liver and fatty liver disorders. Use it with l-lysine. Avoid arginine if pregnant or nursing, or if you have herpes.

L-Asparagine balances the central nervous system, preventing both hyper-nervousness and over-calming. Try it for mood swing disorders and hyperactivity in children or adults.

L-Aspartic Acid increases stamina and endurance, and prevents fatigue and exhaustion. Some forms of chronic fatigue syndrome may be aspartic acid deficiencies. It detoxifies and protects the central nervous system, liver and bloodstream, promotes RNA/DNA formation, and aids cell metabolism.

L-Carnitine prevents fat build-up in the body and arteries, helping in weight loss and prevention of heart dis-ease and atherosclerosis. It is helpful in reducing angina attacks, in heart healing, hypoglycemia, diabetes, kidney and liver dis-ease, in acclimation to cold temperatures, and in reducing ketosis (a serious acid blood condition). Carnitine converts fat to energy and enhances the antioxidant vitamins E and C. It helps in athletic performance. Vegetarians are more likely to be deficient in this than meat eaters, as well as in lysine. This is an essential nutrient for newborns.

L-Citrulline boosts the immune system, increases energy, and detoxifies ammonia (a damaging liver pollutant) in the body.

L-Cysteine is an antioxidant and free radical destroyer best used for this with selenium and vitamin E. It protects the cells from radiation, and protects the liver and brain from cigarette smoke and alcohol consumption. It breaks down mucus and is recommended in treatment of bronchitis, emphysema, tuberculosis and pneumonia. Cysteine is also recommended for rheumatoid arthritis, and detoxifies excess copper from the body. If you are having radiation therapy or are otherwise exposed to x-rays or radiation, this is a protection. If you are a smoker or exposed to secondary cigarette smoke, this amino acid is important. L-cysteine changes easily to L-cystine; they both do the same things.

L-Cystine also helps to detoxify the body of heavy metals and toxins, and helps in respiratory disorders. It is necessary for the healing of burns and wounds, for skin formation, and assists in the assimilation of insulin. Use it after surgery for faster healing, for diabetes, wound healing and to protect the body from radiation, alcohol and cigarettes.

Gamma-Aminobutyric Acid (GABA) is a fully natural tranquilizer, an addiction-free, non-prescription alternative to valium or librium. Use 750 mg per day with niacin/amide and inositol (the full B-complex is best) to reduce anxiety, stress and depression. The need for chemical tranquilizers can be much reduced or ended for many women with this amino acid available in healthfood stores.

L-Glutamic Acid (Glutamate) is a brain food and fuel that helps to correct personality disorders. It metabolizes sugars and fats.

L-Glutamine is converted to glutamic acid in the brain. It is important for reducing fatigue and depression, lessens alcohol and sugar cravings, and is helpful in epilepsy, senility, schizophrenia, mental retardation, peptic ulcers, digestive dis-eases, and for increasing intelligence. Its use increases the need for GABA. Do not substitute L-glutamine with glutamic acid for use in alcoholism; L-glutamine is more effective for this dis-ease.

L-Glutathione is an antioxidant that protects the body from damage by cigarette smoking and radiation. Use this to reduce the side effects of chemotherapy and cancer radiation treatments. It detoxifies heavy metals, drugs and alcohol poisoning, and is used in liver and blood detoxification and dis-eases.

L-Glycine prevents central nervous system and muscular degeneration. It helps prevent epileptic seizures, boosts the pituitary and immune system, and is used to treat bipolar depression. Too much can cause fatigue; the right amount increases energy. Use glycine for muscular dystrophy, multiple sclerosis and other degenerative dis-eases.

L-Histidine is used to heal gastric ulcers, hyperacidity, digestive dis-eases, allergies, rheumatoid arthritis and anemia. It is important for tissue growth and repair, and for red and white blood cell production.

L-Isoleucine is another amino acid for regulating blood sugar and energy levels. This one is important particularly for women who are hypoglycemic. Balanced amounts of valine and leucine are needed with isoleucine, and this amino acid is also important in blood formation.

L-Leucine lowers blood sugar levels, in balance with valine and isoleucine. Use leucine for diabetes and post-surgical recovery; it is a factor in the healing of bones, skin and muscles. Too much may aggravate hypoglycemia.

L-Lysine helps calcium absorption in adults and is required for bone development and normal growth in children. Women with herpes and cold sores know this amino acid's value is healing and prevention. Lysine helps post-surgical recovery by aiding tissue and muscle regrowth, aids in antibody, hormone and enzyme production, and in collagen formation for wound healing. It lowers serum triglycerides in the blood, a factor in heart dis-ease. Deficiency symptoms include low energy, lack of alertness and concentration, irritability, bloodshot eyes, anemia, hair loss, retarded growth and reproductive disorders.

L-Methionine is important in treating toxemia of pregnancy, rheumatic fever, allergies, chemical sensitivities, chronic fatigue and osteoporosis. It is a detoxifier that helps to break down fats in the liver and arteries, aids digestion and muscle weakness, and helps in cases of brittle hair and nails. Methionine is used by the body to create choline, and must be obtained from food. Use it for atherosclerosis, high cholesterol levels, edema, fat metabolism and schizophrenia.

L-Ornithine converts fat into muscle and energy, in combination with L-arginine and L-carnitine, and is needed in immune system and liver function. It promotes wound healing and tissue growth, and detoxifies ammonia from the body. Because it releases a growth hormone, it is not for use by children without expert direction.

L-Phenylalanine controls hunger, aids in memory and learning ability, and enhances sexual arousal. It is a mood raiser useful for depression and decreases physical pain, especially in migraines, menstruation and arthritis. Do not use phenylalanine if you are pregnant or have high blood pressure, phenylketonuria (PKU), or if you have preexisting pigmented melanoma cancer.

DL-Phenylalanine works in the same ways as L-phenylalanine. Use it for chronic pain, arthritis, and Parkinson's dis-ease. It suppresses appetite, aids mental alertness, and is a strong nonaddictive antidepressant. It should be avoided by the same women that are contraindicated in the L form.

L-Proline heals and strengthens cartilage, joints, tendons, the heart, and the texture of the skin.

L-Serine is important for the immune system in the production of antibodies and immunoglobulins. It is needed for metabolism of fats and fatty acids, and for muscle growth. If you have recurrent colds or infections, a depleted immune system, or atherosclerosis, serine is indicated.

L-Taurine heals heart dis-ease, atherosclerosis, high blood pressure, hypoglycemia, and edema. Use it for epilepsy, anxiety, hyperactivity and poor brain function, as well as for the central nervous system, muscular system, the white blood cells, and bile. It aids in the digestion and assimilation of fats and fat soluble vitamins, and is important for multiple sclerosis and other degenerative dis-eases.

L-Threonine helps to prevent and control epileptic seizures. It is important in skin formation and in the functioning of the liver, central nervous system and heart.

L-Tryptophan is converted to niacin (vitamin B-3) in the body. Find it in amino acids combinations; it is no longer available singly. A blood disorder called EMS (eosinophilia-myalgia syndrome) surfaced in 1989 and was linked by the FDA to L-tryptophan supplements made in New Mexico. It seems to have come from a tampered-with or contaminated batch. L-tryptophan was taken off the market—all of it—and is now found only in amino acids combinations, some of which substitute niacin for it.

A full inquiry into EMS and its real cause was never made. Nutritionists feel that L-tryptophan will be back on the market eventually. The FDA is dragging its feet, as usual.

This amino acid is a mood stabilizer, antidepressant and stress reducer. It helps insomnia and hyperactivity, promotes children's growth, lowers pain sensitivity and helps in reducing alcohol and food cravings. A warm glass of milk before bed helps insomnia because of milk's tryptophan content.

L-Tyrosine is an antidepressant and anxiety reducer; it aids fatigue and exhaustion, and alleviates withdrawal symptoms for those coming off cocaine and other drugs. It is useful in allergies, headaches, irritability, mood disorders, and hypothyroidism. It helps to reduce body fat and suppress appetite, aids in skin and hair pigment production (for premature greying, for vitiligo and age spots), and in adrenal, thyroid and pituitary gland function. Tyrosine deficiency results in deficiency in the hormone norepinephrine, causing depression and mood swings.

L-Valine is a natural stimulant. Use it with leucine and isoleucine for muscle and tissue repair.

Obviously, amino acids are more than minor healing agents for women's dis-eases. They have been promoted in the health market for men's body building, but have far more serious uses that may be lifesaving for many women. They are substances that women need to know about and use. The primary sources for amino acids in this book are James F. Balch, MD, and Phyllis A. Balch, CNC, *Prescription for Nutritional Healing* (Avery Publishing Group, 1990), and Louise Tenney, MH, *Health Handbook* (Woodland Books, 1987).

Acupressure

Acupressure is also known as reflexology, and consists of using finger pressure on the body, hands, ears or feet to release energy blocks. Specific points for specific organs and dis-eases relieve pain and symptoms. This form of healing comes from China, and is one of the most ancient healing systems. It was known in Asia by 4000 BCE and in Egypt by 2330 BCE. It predates acupuncture, the use of needles inserted into the pressure or reflex points, by thousands of years. The Chinese Nei Jing, dated at about 300 BCE, is the oldest known written book of medicine, and contains information on acupressure, acupuncture and herbal healing. The system of meridians—the map of energy lines and pressure points on the body—is detailed in the Nei Jing, and is still used today. While acupuncture is done by a trained technician or Chinese doctor, acupressure is a good tool for women's self-healing.

The totality of Be-ing, and the attainment of harmony and balance within are the central ideas in Asian healing. Health is harmony and balance; dis-ease is imbalance or the blockage of free energy flow. The physical and aura bodies are taken as a whole, and acupressure (by balancing meridian points and removing energy blocks) affects both physical and auric bodies. By applying pressure to or massaging the reflex points that are involved in a dis-ease, excess and deficiency of energy are both eliminated. With restoration of a free flow of energy, dis-ease is removed and the body returns to its natural balance and wellness.

The meridians are the energy channels of the body's organs, pathways that carry energy to and from them. There are fourteen major meridians used in pairs of yin and yang that include the five Chinese elements (water, wood, fire, earth and metal). Yin and yang are the Chinese words for receptive and active, energy out and energy in. They are intrinsic flows that have nothing to do with gender. There are 365 classic acupuncture/acupressure points, 150 of which are standardly used. In addition there are over 2000 possible reflex massage points, used singly and multiply, that are used in acupressure to relieve dis-ease and return the body to balance. A student acupuncturist learns the meridian points and acupressure first, before using needles. Acupressure was the healing tool of laywomen and wisewomen in early China and still today.

From the meridians, energy (in China called Qi or C'hi) branches into the nadis, the multitude of tiny nerve endings in the skin. These have also been mapped in modern times by electrical means. The meridians and nadis are the electrical flows of the body. The meridian endings, where all the pathways come together, are in the ears, hands and feet and are the basis for ear reflexology and ear acupuncture, and hand and foot reflexology. All are a part of the same system of energy flows. The skin of the ears, the palms of the hands and the soles of the feet each contain a complete energy map of the body. Every organ is represented, and pressure points on these body parts can affect healing in every part of the body and every organ. Acupressure massage of the fleshy parts of the ear, whole hand or whole foot is a powerful tool for women's over-all well-being.

In this book, acupressure points are identified for each of the dis-eases in the remedy section. Use them along with other forms of healing to bring the energy flows into harmony and promote good health. Maps of the ears, hands, feet and body reflex points are included in the next few pages, as well. They provide a basis for acupressure/reflexology anatomy, and a beginning of pressure point healing for every dis-ease. For some of the dis-eases in the remedy section, acupressure points are on the hands or feet. Remember that each reflex system has a full body map, and if points are shown for the feet, there are also hand, ear and body meridian points as well. Pressure points shown on the body are usually along the lines of the meridians, while those on hands and feet are on the seiketsu, or meridian endings. Seiketsu is a Japanese word.

To do this form of healing, use a finger, thumb or the whole hand to apply pressure to the designated points. Even using both hands or a blunt object like a crystal to press with is valid. Use whatever is comfortable and provides the most even pressure. Pressure is firm but without force, and may include a massaging motion. Excessive pressure that causes pain or uses undue strength is not necessary or positive. Look for the correct point to apply the pressure to. You will recognize it by the strange tingling, sometimes sharp sensation that occurs when you make contact. There is a slight depression in the skin at acupressure points which you will learn to feel in time. When you apply pressure directly to the correct reflex point, much can be accomplished with little actual pressure. In a few moments time, you will feel the tension under your fingers relax, and at that point the reflex is released. A released acupressure point pulses slightly under your fingers. One that needs releasing has a heavier, slower pulse and tighter feeling. You will soon recognize the difference.

Body Reflexology

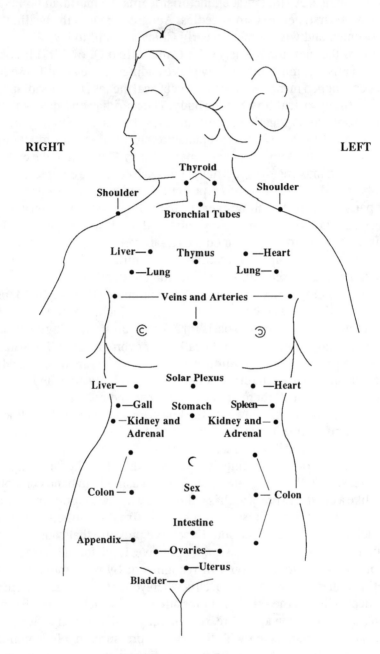

Mildred Carter, *Body Reflexology* (W. Nyack, NY, Parker Publishing Co., 1983), p. 38.

Foot Reflexology Body Map

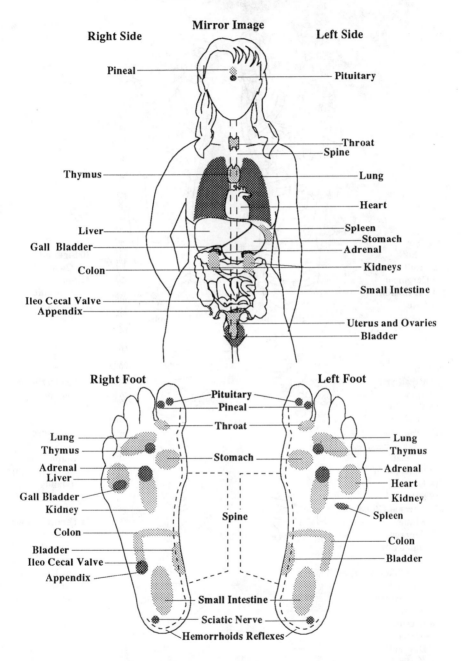

Mildred Carter, *Body Reflexology* (W. Nyack, NY, Parker Publishing Co., 1983), p. 33.

Foot Reflexology Body Map

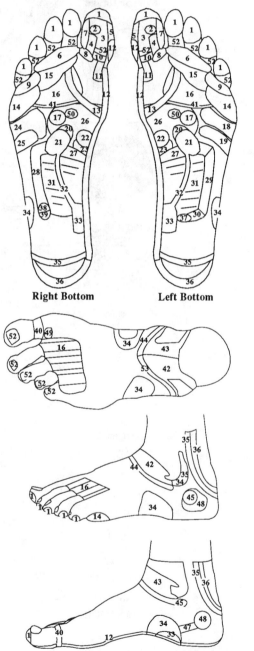

Right Bottom   **Left Bottom**

1 Sinus
2 Pituitary
3 Cerebrum
4 Cerebellum
5 Nose
6 Eye
7 Temple
8 Neck
9 Ear
10 Throat
11 Parathyroid
12 Spine
13 Thyroid
14 Shoulder
15 Trapezius
16 Lung, Chest, Breast
17 Solar Plexus
18 Heart
19 Spleen
20 Adrenal Gland
21 Kidney
22 Pancreas
23 Duodenum
24 Liver
25 Gall Bladder
26 Stomach
27 Transverse Colon
28 Ascending Colon
29 Descending Colon

30 Sigmoid Colon
31 Small Intestine
32 Urinary Tract
33 Bladder
34 Leg, Knee, Hip, Lower Back
35 Sciatic
36 Hemorrhoids
37 Rectum
38 Ileo Cecal Valve
39 Appendix
40 Jaws
41 Diaphragm
42 Upper Lymph Glands
43 Lower Lymph Glands
44 Uterine Tube
45 Ovary
46 Uterus
47 Vagina
48 Sex Hormones
49 Tonsils
50 Thymus
51 Cranial Nerves
52 Hair Problems
53 Groin

Moshe Olshevsky, CA, PhD., *et. al.*, *The Manual of Natural Therapy* (New York, Citadel Press, 1989), p. 7 and 11.

Hand Reflexology Body Map

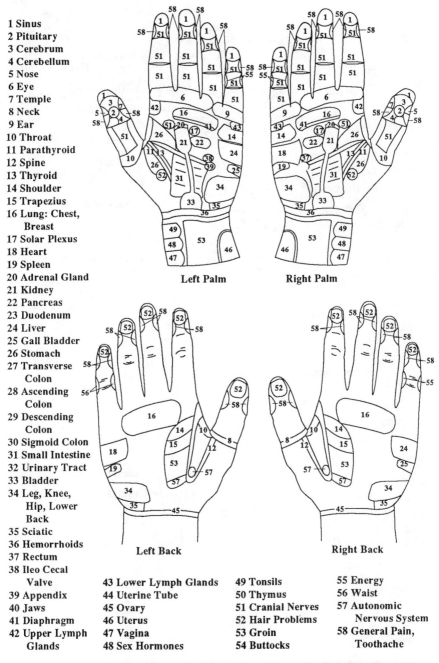

1 Sinus
2 Pituitary
3 Cerebrum
4 Cerebellum
5 Nose
6 Eye
7 Temple
8 Neck
9 Ear
10 Throat
11 Parathyroid
12 Spine
13 Thyroid
14 Shoulder
15 Trapezius
16 Lung: Chest,
   Breast
17 Solar Plexus
18 Heart
19 Spleen
20 Adrenal Gland
21 Kidney
22 Pancreas
23 Duodenum
24 Liver
25 Gall Bladder
26 Stomach
27 Transverse
   Colon
28 Ascending
   Colon
29 Descending
   Colon
30 Sigmoid Colon
31 Small Intestine
32 Urinary Tract
33 Bladder
34 Leg, Knee,
   Hip, Lower
   Back
35 Sciatic
36 Hemorrhoids
37 Rectum
38 Ileo Cecal
   Valve
39 Appendix
40 Jaws
41 Diaphragm
42 Upper Lymph
   Glands

Left Palm   Right Palm

Left Back   Right Back

43 Lower Lymph Glands	49 Tonsils	55 Energy
44 Uterine Tube	50 Thymus	56 Waist
45 Ovary	51 Cranial Nerves	57 Autonomic
46 Uterus	52 Hair Problems	Nervous System
47 Vagina	53 Groin	58 General Pain,
48 Sex Hormones	54 Buttocks	Toothache

Moshe Olshevsky, CA, PhD., *et. al.*, *The Manual of Natural Therapy* (New York, Citadel Press, 1989), p. 7 and 9-10.

Acupressure for the Ear

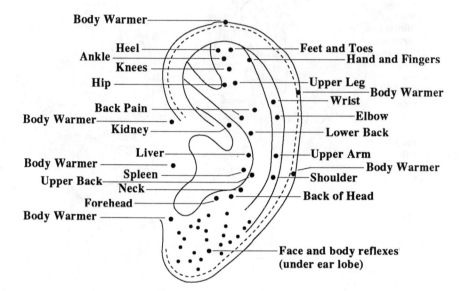

- Body Warmer
- Heel
- Ankle
- Knees
- Hip
- Back Pain
- Body Warmer
- Kidney
- Liver
- Body Warmer
- Upper Back
- Spleen
- Neck
- Forehead
- Body Warmer
- Feet and Toes
- Hand and Fingers
- Upper Leg
- Body Warmer
- Wrist
- Elbow
- Lower Back
- Upper Arm
- Body Warmer
- Shoulder
- Back of Head
- Face and body reflexes (under ear lobe)

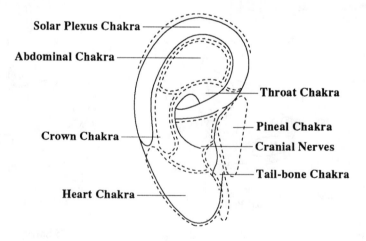

- Solar Plexus Chakra
- Abdominal Chakra
- Crown Chakra
- Heart Chakra
- Throat Chakra
- Pineal Chakra
- Cranial Nerves
- Tail-bone Chakra

Mildred Carter, *Body Reflexology* (W. Nyack,NY, Parker Publishing Co., 1983), p. 46.

Acupressure for the Ears

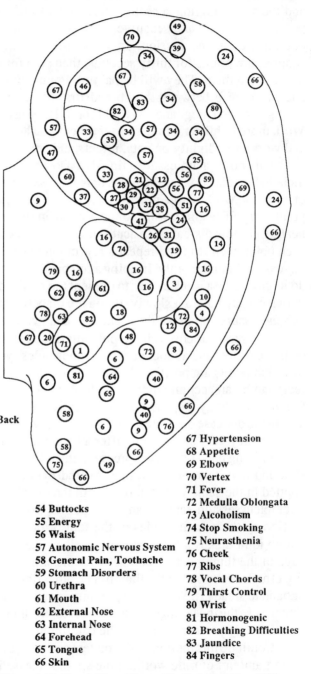

1 Sinus
2 Pituitary
3 Cerebrum
4 Cerebellum
5 Nose
6 Eye
7 Temple
8 Neck
9 Ear
10 Throat
11 Parathyroid
12 Spine
13 Thyroid
14 Shoulder
15 Trapezius
16 Lung: Chest, Breast
17 Solar Plexus
18 Heart
19 Spleen
20 Adrenal Gland
21 Kidney
22 Pancreas
23 Duodenum
24 Liver
25 Gall Bladder
26 Stomach
27 Transverse Colon
28 Ascending Colon
29 Descending Colon
30 Sigmoid Colon
31 Small Intestine
32 Urinary Tract
33 Bladder
34 Leg, Knee, Hip, Lower Back
35 Sciatic
36 Hemorrhoids
37 Rectum
38 Ileo Cecal Valve
39 Appendix
40 Jaws
41 Diaphragm
42 Upper Lymph Glands
43 Lower Lymph Glands
44 Uterine Tube
45 Ovary
46 Uterus
47 Vagina
48 Sex Hormones
49 Tonsils
50 Thymus
51 Cranial Nerves
52 Hair Problems
53 Groin

54 Buttocks
55 Energy
56 Waist
57 Autonomic Nervous System
58 General Pain, Toothache
59 Stomach Disorders
60 Urethra
61 Mouth
62 External Nose
63 Internal Nose
64 Forehead
65 Tongue
66 Skin

67 Hypertension
68 Appetite
69 Elbow
70 Vertex
71 Fever
72 Medulla Oblongata
73 Alcoholism
74 Stop Smoking
75 Neurasthenia
76 Cheek
77 Ribs
78 Vocal Chords
79 Thirst Control
80 Wrist
81 Hormonogenic
82 Breathing Difficulties
83 Jaundice
84 Fingers

Moshe Olshevsky, CA, PhD., *et. al.*, *The Manual of Natural Therapy* (New York, Citadel Press, 1989), p. 7-8.

Most points are held for about a minute, and can be massaged rather than using steady pressure. The points will be sensitive before releasing, and the sharp tingling sensation disappears from a released point. If the point is very tense and sensitive, know when to stop—years of pain may not release in one session. In acute pain, as in migraine, work the acupressure points for thirty seconds, then stop for thirty seconds before returning to them. They will be painful. Points for the abdomen and legs, and in the web between thumb and first finger, should not be pressed during a wanted pregnancy. Avoid foot reflexology in pregnancy, as well. Work more lightly and for a shorter time if you are debilitated or an elder, and work more lightly on pets, infants and children.

Full body acupressure (Jin Shin Do or shiatsu) sessions are not included in this book, as the focus here is on self-healing and they require one-on-one work with a practitioner. In using acupressure on individual points for self-healing, work for no more than five minutes twice a day in healing chronic dis-eases. In acute situations, work for a minute or two on each point, then stop and repeat a few minute later if needed; most acute dis-eases respond rapidly. In doing a full hand or foot acupressure session, do it only twice a week at first to prevent too much toxin release. Build up to twice a day but do it slowly. If you are diabetic, monitor insulin levels, as acupressure can make these change, and avoid pressure points on the legs if you have varicose veins or phlebitis (blood clots). Avoid acupressure on the legs, feet and abdomen in pregnancy unless you are knowledgeable of which points are positive. Whole hand or foot acupressure (especially feet) can be an accurate diagnostic tool for sensitive healers. Pain spots found on the body map are highly indicative, and a pain spot may appear before the dis-ease does. Be aware that every woman's body is unique and the map may vary slightly on different women's hands and feet.

In using hand or foot acupressure, the reflex points are under tougher skin and may take more probing to find than on the body. Pressure is applied in the same way, but only with the thumb or index finger. To do a complete session, rather than single points, work the thumb in a creeping motion up the sole and sides of the foot or palm. The movement of the thumb joint makes a forward motion, like a caterpillar walk. The inside edge of the thumb makes contact with the skin of the sole or palm—not fingernails or the ball of the thumb. The other fingers wrap around the foot or hand to steady it. Where less pressure is needed, as around the toes and fingers, use the index finger in the same creeping motion. Body acupressure uses a steady pressure, without the caterpillar movement.

Continue this motion until you feel a sensitive or sore spot and spend a short amount of time working the spot to release it. Then go on. Use a hooking motion of the thumb on tougher places, as where the skin on the feet is thick, and for small or hard-to-reach areas. For tender areas on the lower half of the foot or hand, use reflex rotation. This is done by holding your thumb on the pain spot and using your other hand to rotate the foot or palm gently against it until the painful point is released. Each located pain spot has its correspondence to a body part or organ, and will have other pain spots on the hand (or foot if working on the hand), ear and body. When doing a full foot or full hand acupressure treatment, make sure to do both feet or both hands. More accurate diagnosing and healing can probably be accomplished on the feet.

The acupressure points used in this book are single points, with often a number of points illustrated for each dis-ease. Make sure you have located the point before applying pressure, and press gradually and steadily until you feel the point release. You will feel a difference in well-being immediately. Combine acupressure with other methods of healing for dis-eases discussed in this book.

The primary acupressure references are: Cathryn Bauer, *Acupressure For Women* (The Crossing Press, 1987); three books by Mildred Carter, *Body Reflexology, Hand Reflexology, Key to Perfect Health*, and *Helping Yourself with Foot Reflexology* (all from Parker Publishing Co., 1983, 1975 and 1969); Iona Marsaa Teeguarden, *Acupressure Way of Health* (Japan Publications, 1978); and Moshe Olshevsky, CA, PhD., et. al., *The Manual of Natural Therapy* (Citadel Press, 1989). Also see the chapters on acupressure and reflexology in *All Women Are Healers*.

Aromatherapy

The human sense of smell is 10,000 times as powerful as the sense of taste, yet it is the least understood and least utilized of the senses. Aromatherapy is the use of essential oils as fragrances to heal. An ancient therapy, traditionally traced to Atlantis and Mu, fragrances for healing have been found—still fresh—in the Egyptian tombs. Fragrance is a way of healing that operates on physical, emotional, mental and spiritual levels. It works on the subtle bodies and on the physical body to stimulate and calm, alter mental states, boost the immune system, relieve pain, stimulate spiritual oneness, and balance body functions. Essential oils are the hormones of plants, and the concentrated active ingredients of herbs. Modern aromatherapy began in France at the turn of the last century, and has now begun to reach women here. It opens up a whole new era in reclaiming women's ancient heritage as healers.

Essential oils are more than perfumes; they have profound effects on wellness. They are germicidal and antiviral, are antidepressants, aphrodisiacs, hormonal balancers, detoxificants, anticarcinogenics, mental stimulants, fever and blood pressure reducers, and more. Because they work on a level of the brain that is nonverbal (or preverbal), they have a profound effect that goes beyond cognitive knowledge or memory, even working on cellular levels. They go deeper as healing agents than has yet been analyzed or researched. Aromas work on the level of the subconscious mind that is the entrance to the nonphysical bodies, to the aura and the soul.

Different fragrances, like the different herbs and plants they are derived from, do different things, and each has its own healing attributes. The oils may be perceived as pleasant or unpleasant odors; some are highly astringent in fragrance, while others are lighter, and some have a green or woodsy smell. Some seem familiar and others do not, and women's perception of various scents becomes more acute by using them.

The scents may be used singly or in combinations. They may be diluted and placed directly on the skin, put into massage oils or baths, added to creams or lotions, used in a steam vaporizer, sprayed in the air, put on lightbulbs or in candle lamps to heat, used in diffusers, or just sniffed from the bottle.

Only natural essential oils (not synthetic replicas) are healers. Some are contraindicated in pregnancy, epilepsy or high blood pressure, and some can be skin irritants (see pages 72-73). Anyone can also be allergic to anything, so test them diluted on your inside elbow for sensitivity. Essential oils range in price from about $2.50 to hundreds of dollars, and anything expensive can usually be substituted for with something equally effective and cheaper. Essential oils come in very small bottles, but they are used in single drop amounts and keep indefinitely; a very little goes a long, long way. Aromatherapy oils are sold frequently in healthfood stores and food co-ops, as well as in aroma shops and the more sophisticated beauty parlors. Make sure that the oils you buy for healing are natural oils and are absolutely pure.

Some aromatherapy fragrances are familiar to women as kitchen herbs, with surprising uses in fragrance form. *Basil* treats respiratory problems and indigestion, rehabilitates after the flu, and is good for stress, depression and insomnia. *Cinnamon* is a stimulant for warding off colds and flu; it is warm and invigorating. *Fennel* helps cystitis, removes toxins from the skin, and dispels nausea and indigestion. *Ginger* is a warming tonic, good for cramps, indigestion and motion sickness. *Lemon* stops bleeding, is a lymphatic stimulant, and is used to treat obesity, water retention, excess acid and cellulite. *Marjoram* is a sedative and womb remedy, but is not for use in pregnancy. *Rosemary* strengthens the central nervous system, aids circulation, acts as a skin and hair tonic, and is used for arthritis and rheumatism.

Still other familiar herbs are used as essential oil fragrances. *Chamomile* is helpful for children's colic, as well as for internal inflammation, and menstrual tension and pain. *Eucalyptus* is for congested lungs and is an antiseptic, and *Geranium* is a hormone balancer that boosts the immune system. *Jasmine* heals women's reproductive dis-eases, and aids anxiety and depression. *Juniper* is a detoxifier. *Lavender*, one of the most familiar fragrances for women, is used as a nerve tonic, antiseptic and calmative. It reduces stress and heals headaches and migraines.

Aromatherapy Chart

Aniseed: Flatulence, migraine, tachycardia (overly fast irregular heartbeat).

Basil: Stress, intellectual overwork, nervous insomnia, depression, rehabilitation after flu, stomach and intestinal cramps.

Bergamot: General antiseptic, blenorrhoea, herpes (in combination with Eucalyptus and Geranium), psoriasis, scabies, intestinal parasites, cramps.
• External application: 5 drops essence of Bergamot mixed into 1 oz. of Sweet Almond oil.
• In fragrance compositions it provides a fresh fruity and floral top note.

Cajeput: Neuralgic, tooth and earaches.
• 2 drops put on cotton puff and rubbed on teeth and gums.
• Dilute 5 drops in 1 oz. of vegetable (Sweet Almond, Olive) oil for use on ears and jaws.

Chamomile: Skin/mucous membrane/genital infections and inflammations, gastritis, conjunctivitis. Very universal, consult literature.
• External application: 1 drop of essence in 1 oz. of Sweet Almond oil.
• (Septic) wounds: mix 1 drop and 3 drops Lavender.

Clary Sage: Centering, nervousness, depression, weakness, can be mildly intoxicating.
• One drop rubbed on temples results in light euphoria. Used in perfumery for its fragrance reminiscent of ambergris.

Cypress: Balances the nervous system, influenza, asthma, irritability, hemorrhoids.
• External application: 5–10 drops in 1 oz. of Sweet Almond oil.
• Inhalations: 5 drops for one large bowl of hot water.

Eucalyptus: Respiratory tract infections, herpes, influenza, combine with equal parts Rosemary and Lavender for sore muscles, strains, athlete's foot, parasites, fleas, universal.
• External application: 10 drops of Eucalyptus, Rosemary, Lavender mix in 1 oz. of Sweet Almond oil.
• Inhalations.
• Use in diffusers for air disinfection.

Geranium: Stops bleeding, astringent, fatigue (adrenal deficiency), anxiety, glossitis, dry eczema, herpes, skin diseases, diarrhea.
• External application: combines well with many essences, non-irritating, 10 drops of essence or more can be used per ounce of oil or cream.

Hyssop: Hay fever, asthma, chronic bronchitis.
• For relief of hay fever symptoms, take equal amounts of hyssop/cypress in the mornings and rub 4 drops of the mix on palms of hands during the day and inhale. Procedures can be repeated frequently.

Juniper: Diuretic, eliminates toxins, slow digestion, kidney and bladder disorders, arthritis, asteriosclerosis, hemorrhoids.
• Combination for kidney/bladder infections: 2 Lavender, 2 Eucalyptus, 2 Juniper, 1 Thyme.

Lavender: Antiseptic, anti-inflammative, respiratory diseases, migraine, vertigo, diarrhea.
• External application: 10 drops in one oz. of vegetable oil or cream.
• Can be put neat on wounds and burns for antiseptic conditions and quick healing.
• Neat on insect stings, mosquito bites. Should be used as often as possible in skin preparations and cosmetics.

Aromatherapy Chart

It is rejuvenating for the skin. Frequent use has an excellent preventive effect against infections. Very universal, consult literature.

Lemon: Infections, stomach over-acidity, arteriosclerosis, weak blood vessels.

Marjoram Sauvage: Sedative, warming, anxiety, stress, insomnia, high blood pressure, "plant tranquilizer."

Niaouli: Chronic bronchitis, rhinitis, sinusitis, kidney/bladder infections.

Peppermint: Nausea, irritable colon, flatulence, cramps, painful period, scabies.
• Refreshing and cooling in baths
• External application: 5 drops mixed into 1 oz. of oil or cream.

Rosemary: Stimulant, fatigue, slow digestion, low blood pressure, liver disorders. External application—see Eucalyptus.

Sage: Nerve and adrenal stimulant, restores the energies of the whole organism, lymphatic disorders, stomatitis.
• Gargle 2 drops in a cup of water.

Sandalwood: Specific antiseptic for urinary tract infections (cystitis), depression, classic choice in all cosmetic preparations for dry skin. Very mild and non-irritating.

Tarragon: Slow digestion, intestinal parasites, balances the nervous system.

Thyme: Strong antiseptic, stimulant, colds, influenza, fatigue, yeast and fungus infections (candida albicans, etc.).
• External application: 5 drops to 1 oz. of Sweet Almond Oil. Mix carefully. Undiluted essence of Thyme can cause considerable, but nonhazardous, irritation.

Ylang-Ylang: Anxiety, high blood pressure, tachycardia. Best used very sparingly because of its intensely sweet fragrance.
• One drop to a big bowl of water for a facial wash will have a considerably relaxing effect.

Taking essential oils orally

Internal application: Essential oils provide much freedom in terms of dosage, so that personal intuition may be followed without the danger of overdose. For all the oils listed on the chart, 2–3 drops 3 times a day is the dosage recommended by the mentioned authors. Essences can be taken on sugar, mixed into honey, in a glass of sweetened water, or with fresh fruit.

Purity

For use in Aromatherapy, essential oils must be absolutely pure. Adulterated or synthetic essences will result in no or adverse effects. Only use essences guaranteed to be of "Aromatherapy quality."

This chart is not a prescription. Its mere purpose is to summarize the views of the mentioned authorities in the field of Aromatherapy. This chart does not intend to replace the service of a physician. See a physician for severe problems.

This is an aromatherapy chart of the healing power and uses of essential oils as described by Dr. Jean Valnet and Robert Tisserand. It was provided by Sylla Sheppard-Hangar, Atlantic Institute of Aromatherapy, handout sheet.

Here are a few more oils and their uses. *Myrrh* is an anti-inflammatory, often used for mouth abscesses and gum dis-ease, and is a cleanser
for the aura bodies. *Patchouli*, another women's favorite, is an antiseptic,
antifungal and decongestant, and is used in skin dis-eases for cell regeneration. *Peppermint* freshens the breath and aids in indigestion, nausea
and fevers; it also helps singers bring clarity and tone to the voice. *Rose*
is known as the women's remedy and is used for healing the reproductive
system. It is also a skin toner and anti-inflammatory, and is used in
meditation. *Tea-Tree* oil is an anti-fungal and immune system stimulant,
used as an inhalant for sinus congestion, coughs and the chest. *Vanilla* is
a female aphrodisiac, and *Ylang Ylang* is both aphrodisiac and sedative. It
is used for nervous tension, hyperactivity and insomnia, and to slow
overly rapid heart and breathing rates.[2]

These are only a beginning of the aromatherapy fragrances and their
uses in healing, and there are a number of ways to apply them. The simplest
use is to open the bottle of an oil and sniff it. I had my first experience with
aromatherapy in this way. I was in a healthfood store with a beginning
migraine, and saw a display of aroma combinations. I picked up the one
marked "headaches" and took a deep sniff. The pain lifted immediately.
The combination, made by Tiferet-Lifetree, contains lavender, marjoram,
aniseed, niaouli, peppermint and basil. The same company makes combinations for relaxing, pain relief, joint pain, respiratory, digestive, moon
time, circulation, everyday balancing, cellulite, dry skin and invigorating.
They cost ten dollars each and can be ordered from Tiferet-Lifetree, 210
Crest Dr., Eugene, OR 97405.

Another way to use the oils is to place a few drops on the skin, on the
chakras, pulse points or under the nose. They can be placed on slightly
dampened cottonballs and held close, or put a drop on your pillow. The
goal is to breathe in the fragrance. Only a few drops are needed, the scents
are penetrating and a little goes a long way. When I do this at night, the
scent is still strong the next morning.

Essential oils are also made into massage oils by adding four to ten
drops of aromatherapy scent per ounce of carrier oil. Some carrier oils are
almond, peanut, avocado or jojoba. Peanut oil is an especially good carrier
base for use on women with painful joints, and dandelion essential oil
added to a carrier oil is especially good for back or body pain. Jasmine or
yarrow in massage blend helps heal the aura bodies, and yarrow is
especially good for protecting healers from others' pain. Essential oils can
be made into skin creams by adding three to six drops of aromatherapy oil

---

[2]Patricia Kaminski, "Aromatherapy as a Healing Art" (Nevada City, CA, Flower Essence Society,
1989), p. 9–16. Pamphlet.

to two ounces of skin cream. For the cream base, use Nivea, Eucerin, vitamin E cream, or an herbal blend.

Add essential oils to a hot bath for another way to use these oils in healing. Use six to eight drops of aromatherapy oil, and add it while the water is running at full force. Swish your arm through the water vigorously for a few minutes to make sure the oil mixes, then soak in the bath for at least twenty minutes. Pat the skin dry afterwards and relax in bed for at least a half an hour. Wait until the next day before rinsing the oils off; let them go into the skin. Women with dry or sensitive skin can mix the essential oil with an ounce of a carrier oil before putting it into the bath. When using oils in the tub, be careful not to slip. A lavender oil bath at the end of a hard day makes for a relaxing, full night's sleep.

Oils can be put into the air to breathe with misting bottles, which are spray bottles that use a combination of water with a few drops of an essential oil. Oils should be stored in glass, rather than plastic bottles, and when mixed with water will remain active for only a couple of months. Spray the mist on the face, hair or over all the body, or spray it into the air. I have found that the plastic misting bottles available in healthfood stores don't last long. The sprayers break. Glass perfume bottles are better. Electrical full-room diffusers are available, and are wonderful, but they are a small appliance and somewhat of an investment. Lotus oil in a diffuser makes a wonderful atmosphere for meditation.

Other ways to disperse essential oils through a room are to put a few drops on a lightbulb, then turn the lamp on. The heating oil will radiate fragrance through the room. Lightbulb rings are sold for this and are inexpensive. Essential oils can also be placed in a little water in a candle lantern/potpourri lamp; the candle warming the water and fragrance causes the scent to disperse.

When using aromatherapy for respiratory healing, add essential oil drops to the water of a steam vaporizer, or add them to a boiling pot of water and inhale the steam. Oils for flu, colds, coughs and sinus, as well as for headaches, the skin or depression work very well this way. Another way of doing this is to pour hot (almost boiling) water into a large bowl. After thirty seconds, add the drops of essential oil. Cover your head and the bowl with a towel to make a tent, and inhale the vapors.

Occasionally essential oils are used internally, a single drop placed on a sugar cube and ingested. This is recommended only under expert direction as some oils are toxic and others have contraindications. It is recommended only rarely for the uses of this book. Essential oils are used here primarily by breathing their fragrances in, or taken through the skin in baths or massage oils. If you are pregnant, avoid the following oils: basil, clary sage, hyssop, juniper, marjoram, myrrh and sage. If you have high blood pressure, do not use hyssop, rosemary, sage or thyme oils. If you are epileptic, avoid using sweet fennel, hyssop, origanum, sage or wormwood. The following oils may be skin irritants: basil, cinnamon leaf, fennel, fir seed, lemon, lemongrass, parsley seed, peppermint, pimento leaf, thyme and tea-tree.[3] Only lavender oil may be used undiluted on the skin without risk of irritation.

Aromatherapy opens a new world for women's healing, and a very powerful and positive one. As in other healing methods, it is best used in the earliest stages of dis-ease, and as a way of enhancing and maintaining wellness. Aromatherapy oils will antidote (cancel) homeopathic remedies, but may be used with any other healing methods. The remedy suggestions for essential oils in this book come primarily from: Marcel Lavabre, *Aromatherapy Workbook* (Healing Arts Press, 1990), and Moshe Olshevsky, CA, PhD., et. al., *The Manual of Natural Therapy* (Citadel Press, 1989).

[3]Information from Sylla Sheppard-Hangar, Atlantic Institute of Aromatherapy, handout sheet.

Flower Essences

Flower essences contain the etheric imprint of plant energy, and are very different from essential oils, which are highly concentrated physical plant matter. There is no aroma to flower essences, and no plant parts are contained in them. Except for the alcohol preservative, there is no taste. Flower essences (and gemstone essences) are closest in description to homeopathic remedies, in that they contain the life force essence rather than the physical substance of the flower. It is this life force essence that is the active component and has effect on women's bodies. By working at the rapid vibration rate of the aura, flower essences create healing on the nonphysical levels that will later manifest to body level healing. Healing in this mode works primarily on the mental and emotional aura body levels, with some flower essence remedies extending to the physical or spiritual. In metaphysical healing, the four bodies are the physical, emotional, mental and spiritual, and healing must happen on the faster vibrating aura levels before the physical body is changed.

The field of vibrational medicine, of working with energy and the bodies-beyond-the-physical to manifest physical wellness, is the most advanced science of today's medical technologies. From CAT scans to MRI (Magnetic Resonance Imaging) to electrotherapy for healing bone fractures, nonphysical vibration is entering into standard medicine. The explanations of matter and Be-ing that physics offers today put etheric healing into scientifically acceptable language, making these vibrational technologies possible.

Vibrational healing—in the form of flower essences, gemstones and crystals, aromatherapy, the acupuncture/acupressure meridian system, and all forms of color work, aura work and psychic healing—has been known on earth for as long as human souls have incarnated here. They may be the original forms of women's healing. Tradition states that flower essences were used on Mu and Atlantis and were probably brought here as a system from other planets. India has used energy healing, in the form of gemstones, for thousands of years, and every early culture had its forms of nonphysical healing. Homeopathy is a more recent subtle body healing method, but is over two hundred years old. Modern physics and medicine boast of new discoveries, but vibrational healing has always been known to healers.

Richard Gerber, MD, in his fascinating book *Vibrational Medicine* (Bear and Co., 1988) describes the difference between physical and subtle (nonphysical) matter:

> When we speak of vibration, we are merely using another synonym for frequency. Different frequencies of energy reflect varying rates of vibration. We know that matter and energy are two different manifestations of the same primary energetic substance of which everything in the universe is composed, including our physical and subtle bodies....Matter which vibrates at a very slow frequency is referred to as physical matter. That which vibrates at speeds exceeding light velocity is known as subtle matter. Subtle matter is as real as dense matter; its vibratory rate is simply faster. In order to therapeutically alter our subtle bodies, we must administer energy that vibrates at frequencies beyond the physical plane. Vibrational medicines contain such high-frequency subtle energies.[1]

Among the methods that heal on the subtle level are flower essences, which vibrate at frequencies beyond the physical plane.

Flower essences were rediscovered by Edward Bach, an English homeopath and physician, in the 1930's, and most women who know flower essences are familiar with the Bach Flower Remedies. Bach researched the healing properties of thirty-eight flowers and the method of preparing and preserving the elixirs or essences. His work was with flowers for emotional healing, rather than for healing physical dis-eases. For more information, see the chapter on flower essences in *All Women Are Healers*.

Bach was aware that there were many more flowers to study and that much more work was needed. He was a highly sensitive psychic, able to discern a plant's healing properties by placing it in his mouth. His work on flower essences is currently being continued in the United States by channelers Kevin Ryerson and John Fox, whose information is compiled and published by Gurudas. Gurudas' comprehensive *Flower Essences and Vibrational Healing* (Cassandra Press, 1983, revised 1989) is a primary source for the flower essence remedies suggested in this book.

[1]Richard Gerber, MD, *Vibrational Medicine: New Choices for Healing Ourselves* (Santa Fe, NM, Bear and Co., 1988), p. 241–242.

Bach
Flower Remedies

Agrimony For those not wishing to burden others with their troubles and who cover up their suffering behind a cheerful facade. They are distressed by argument or quarrel, and may seek escape from pain and worry through the use of drugs and alcohol.

Aspen For those who experience vague fears and anxieties of unknown origin, they are often apprehensive.

Beech For those who while desiring perfection easily find fault with people and things. Critical and at times intolerant, they may overreact to small annoyances or idiosyncracies of others.

Centaury For those who are over-anxious to please, often weak willed and easily exploited or dominated by others. As a result they may neglect their own particular interests.

Cerato For those who lack confidence in their own judgment and decisions. They constantly seek the advice of others and may often be misguided.

Cherry Plum For fear of losing mental and physical control, of doing something desperate. May have impulses to do things thought or known to be wrong.

Chestnut Bud For those who fail to learn from experience, repeating the same patterns or mistakes again and again.

Chicory For those who are overfull of care for others and need to direct and control those close to them. Always finding something to correct or put right.

Clematis For those who tend to live in the future, lack concentration, are daydreamers, drowsy or spacey and have a half-hearted interest in their present circumstances.

Crab Apple For those who may feel something is not quite clean about themselves, or have a fear of being contaminated. For feelings of shame or poor self image. For example, thinking oneself not attractive for one reason or another. When necessary, may be taken to assist in detoxification, for example, during a cold or while fasting.

Elm For those who at times may experience momentary feelings of inadequacy, being overwhelmed by their responsibilities.

Gentian For those who become easily discouraged by small delays or hindrances. This may cause self-doubt.

Gorse For feelings of hopelessness and futility. When there is little hope of relief.

Heather For those who seek the companionship of anyone who will listen to their troubles. They are generally not good listeners and have difficulty being alone for any length of time.

Holly To be used when troubled by negative feelings such as envy, jealousy, suspicion, revenge. Vexations of the heart, states indicating a need for more love.

Honeysuckle For those dwelling in the past, nostalgia, homesickness, always talking about the good old days, when things were better.

Hornbeam For the Monday morning feeling of not being able to face the day. For those feeling some part of the body or mind needs strengthening. Constant fatigue, tiredness.

Impatiens For those quick in thought and action, who require all things to be done without delay. They are impatient with people who are slow and often prefer to work alone.

Larch For those who, despite being capable, lack self confidence or feel inferior. Anticipating failure, they often refuse to make a real effort to succeed.

Mimulus For fear of known things, such as heights, water, the dark, other people, of being alone, etc.

Bach
Flower Remedies

Mustard For deep gloom which comes on for no known reason, sudden melancholia or heavy sadness. Will lift just as suddenly.

Oak For those who struggle on despite despondency from hardships, even when ill and overworked, they never give up.

Olive For mental and physical exhaustion, sapped vitality with no reserve. This may come on after an illness or personal ordeal.

Pine For those who feel they should do or should have done better, who are self-reproachful or blame themselves for the mistakes of others. Hardworking people who suffer much from the faults they attach to themselves, they are never satisfied with their success.

Red Chestnut For those who find it difficult not to be overly concerned or anxious for others, always fearing something wrong may happen to those they care for.

Rock Rose For those who experience states of terror, panic and hysteria; also when troubled by nightmares.

Rock Water For those who are very strict with themselves in their daily living. They are hard masters to themselves struggling toward some ideal or to set an example for others. This would include strict adherence to a living style or to religious, personal or social disciplines.

Scleranthus For those unable to decide between two things, first one seeming right then the other. Often presenting extreme variations in energy or mood swings.

Star of Bethlehem For grief, trauma, loss. For the mental and emotional effect during and after a trauma.

Sweet Chestnut For those who feel they have reached the limits of their endurance. For those moments of deep despair when the anguish seems to be unbearable.

Vervain For those who have strong opinions and who usually need to have the last word, always teaching or philosophizing. When taken to an extreme they can be argumentative and overbearing.

Vine For those who are strong willed. Leaders in their own right who are unquestionably in charge. However, when taken to an extreme they may become dictatorial.

Walnut Assists in stabilizing emotional upsets during transition periods, such as puberty, adolescence, menopause. Also helps to break past links and emotionally adjust to new beginnings such as moving, changing or taking a new job, beginning or ending a relationship.

Water Violet For those who are gentle, independent, aloof and self-reliant, who do not interfere in the affairs of others, and when ill or in trouble prefer to bear their difficulties alone.

White Chestnut For constant and persistent unwanted thoughts, such as mental arguments, worries or repetitious thoughts that prevent peace of mind, and disrupt concentration.

Wild Oat For the dissatisfaction with not having succeeded in one's career or life goal. When there is unfulfilled ambition, career uncertainty or boredom with one's present postition or station in life.

Wild Rose For those, who for no apparent reason, have resigned themselves to their circumstances. Having become indifferent, little effort is made to improve things or find joy.

Willow For those who have suffered some circumstance or misfortune, which they feel was unfair or unjust. As a result they become resentful and bitter toward life or toward those who they feel were at fault.

Bach Centre USA, *The Bach Flower Remedies* (Windemere, NY, Bach Centre USA, 1983), pp. 8–9.

The Flower Essence Society (POB 1769, Nevada City, CA 95959), was founded by Richard Katz in 1979, to further the work of Edward Bach and to experiment with flowers native to the United States. Both Gurudas (Pegasus Products, POB 228, Boulder, CO 80306) and FES (Flower Essence Society) now prepare and sell these essences, and continue to research them. The primary emphasis has continued to be on emotional and mental level healing.

Gurudas' book contains healing information on 112 flowers, as well as detailed material on the origins of flower essence healing, the connections of this healing method with homeopathy, the subtle bodies, detailed instructions for the healer, dis-ease charts, and methods for preparing the remedies. Healing information is given on several levels, and information is given for using the remedies with animals. Gurudas is the only source so far that offers healing information for physical level dis-eases with flower essence remedies. It is these physical level essences that are emphasized in the remedy section here.

The remedies can be made at home, at little cost, or purchased from Pegasus Products or the Flower Essence Society. If the flowers are available, making your own is empowering, but they are inexpensive to buy. (FES remedies are $3 for a dram, $8 an ounce; they are used by the drop.) Supplies needed for making your own include primarily a clear glass or crystal bowl with no design on it that holds at least twelve ounces of liquid, and distilled or pure spring water. You will also need storage bottles, a funnel (glass rather than plastic), and labels for the bottles. These items should be new. Sterilize the glassware in hot water in an enamel, glass or stainless steel pot for about ten minutes before using. The remedies require 25%–50% brandy in storage bottles as a preservative; bacteria may form in the bottles otherwise. Cider vinegar or vegetable glycerin may also be used, but are less stable. A copper pyramid is beneficial to place the bottles under: it will clear them of any contaminants and increase the purity and healing ability of the remedies. Mine cost eight dollars at a gemshow; it is invaluable also for clearing gemstones.

It is best to prepare flower essences early in the morning on cloudless sunny days, preferably in the spring or summer. Choose flowers growing away from polluted areas and roads if possible. Use a meditative state and intuition in choosing which blooms to pick; you may become aware of plant devas and ask them to assist. Place the bowl on the ground (not on concrete) near the plants and fill it with distilled water. Pick the healthiest blooms from several plants and put them on top of the water, touching them as little as possible, and covering the whole water surface if there are enough plants. A single bloom will make an essence, if that's all you have. Leave the bowl and flowers in the sun for three hours, longer on a day with clouds or if you start later than early morning.

After three hours, fill up to half of each storage bottle with a good quality brandy. Remove the flowers from the water (without touching it if possible), and use a crystal or a leaf to remove any debris that may have fallen into the liquid. Pour the water through a funnel into the bottles, and label the bottles. If you are making more than one essence at a time, wash your hands before handling another bowl. Place the filled bottles under the copper pyramid for two more hours to finish the process, keeping different essences separate from each other, even after bottling.[3] Night-blooming flowers should be prepared in the evening, and any flower essence will have more connection with the Goddess and female energy when prepared under the waxing or full moon. Clean the utensils in hot water again before using them to prepare other essences.

The water upon which the flowers were placed is called the Mother Essence. When the Mother Essence is placed into storage bottles it may be potentized homeopathically by shaking, tapping or striking the bottle sharply against your hand fifteen to twenty times. This is called succussion. Then a Stock Bottle is made by placing two drops of the potentized Mother Essence in a one ounce dropper bottle filled with 25% -50% brandy and the rest pure water, and potentizing it again. This is how the remedies are sold, in Stock Bottle potency, and they can be used directly from the Stock Bottle if you wish.

Next the Dosage Bottle, the third potentization, is made by placing two drops from the Stock Bottle in a one ounce bottle of pure water and about a teaspoon of brandy. Amber or blue colored eyedropper bottles are recommended here. If you are using more than one flower essence, the drops from more than one may be made into the Dosage Bottle. Potentize the Dosage Bottle before each use. The essences are taken under the tongue, four drops four times a day from the Dosage Bottle, more frequently in acute situations. Like essential oils, they can also be added to baths or massage oils, or applied directly to the skin. Each dilution and potentization, as in homeopathic remedies, makes the essence stronger, and each potentization raises the vibration rate further into the subtle/auric/energy bodies.

Flowers are the reproductive organs of plants, and are powerful female symbols usually used to represent vulvas. They are the highest concentration of the plant's life force energy. Flower essences are the electromagnetic beyond-physical imprints of the flower's lifeforce; they do not contain the plant itself (as do essential oils) but only the nonphysical vibration and vitality. Used for healing, this vibration transfers to the

[3]Gurudas, *Flower Essences and Vibrational Healing* (San Rafael, CA, Cassandra Press, 1989), p. 17–20.

woman who takes the essence, helping her own nonphysical vibrations to normalize. Only a few drops are needed of the highly diluted and potentized essence, but take them frequently and consistently.

Flower essences work gently and at varying rates of speed. They cause changes in attitude or thought pattern, and changes in physical wellness that may happen rapidly, or slowly and almost imperceptibly. Follow your intuition for how long to use a particular remedy, or use a pendulum to assist you. The changes always happen in natural ways, and happen from the nonphysical levels to the physical. Essences taken for their emotional or mental attributes may create shifts in physical wellness as a side benefit. Flower essences work well with essential oils, and may work synergistically with a homeopathic remedy or gemstone essence. Too many types of remedies together, however, can block each other's actions, so proceed carefully in using flower essences with other modes of healing. The more psychically sensitive you are, and the more your physical body is cleared of toxins and contaminants, the more effective flower essences will be for body healing.

For more information on using and making flower essences, read Gurudas' *Flower Essences and Vibrational Healing* (Cassandra Press, 1989), and send for the Flower Essence Society catalog. The flower essences suggested in the remedy section of this book are from these sources. Refer to the reference chart of flower essence emotional healing qualities. Essences for physical dis-eases are listed with each dis-ease.

Flower Essence Descriptions

Allspice—Promotes Memory
Almond—Maturation/Rejuvenation
Aloe Vera—Personal Survival
Amaranthus—Immune System
Amaryllis—Crown Chakra
Angelica—Urban Stress
Angel's Trumpet—Stimulates Visions
Apricot—Gaiety & Lightness
Banana—Male Sexuality
Beech—Greater Acceptance
Birch—Female-Interpersonal Relationships
Birch—Male-Interpersonal Relationships
Black-Eyed Susan—Improves Self-Esteem
Bleeding Heart—Peace & Harmony
California Bay Laurel—Flexibility/Wisdom
California Poppy—Psychic/Spiritual Balance
Carob—Empathy/Group Interaction
Cedar—Cleansing/Stress
Celandine—Communication
Cerato—Self-Reliance
Chervil—Spiritual Identity
Cinnamon—Emotional Expression
Clematis—Enthusiasm/Stability
Coffee—Decisiveness
Comfrey—Telepathy
Corn-Sweet—Urban Dwellers
Crab Apple—Mental Cleansing
Cyclamen—Channeling
Dog Rose—Enthusiasm
Elm—Strength/Confidence
Eucalyptus—Breath/Grief
Eyebright—Psychic Perception
Fig—Mental Clarity
Fireweed—Transmuting Karma
Fuchsia—Childhood Issues
Garlic—Eases Anxiety
Ginseng—Mental Clarity
Goldenrod—Spiritual Inspiration
Goldenseal—Emotional Scars
Green Rose—Psychic Balance
Heather—Self-Confidence
Hibiscus—Female Sexuality
Jimson Weed—Stimulates Dreams
Jojoba—Massage Therapy
Kidney Bean—Hidden Fears
Koenign Van Daenmark—Left/Right Brain
Lemon—Mental Activity
Lima Bean—Grounding
Live Forever—Higher Guidance
Lotus—Emotional/Spiritual Harmony

Luffa—Cleansing
Macademia—Friendship/Bonding
Mango—Energizer
Maple—Yin/Yang
Milkmaids—Self-Esteem
Nectarine—Psycho-Spiritual Balance
Nutmeg—Past Life Therapy
Oak—Perseverance
Onion—Emotional Cleansing
Orange—Psychological Counseling
Orchid—Dream Clarification
Papaya—Higher Self-Assimilation
Passion Flower—Christ Consciousness
Pennyroyal—Psychic Protection
Peony—Honest Communication
Periwinkle—Higher Spiritual Concepts
Pineapple—Chakra Amplification
Plum Tree—Inspiration/New Ideas
Pomegranate—Nurturing
Potato—Dimensional Exploration
Purple Nightshade—Soothing Calm
Quinoa—Kundalini Opening & Grounding
Raspberry—Self-Expression
Rosa Banksla—Divine Intellect
Rosa Beggeriana—Increases Intuition
Rosa Chinensis Mutabilis—Creative Forces
Rosa Gallica Officinalis—Spiritual Rejuvenation
Rosa Macrophylla—Greater Love
Rosa Sinowlisonii—Clairaudience
Rosa Webbiana—Earth & Angelic Attunement
Rosemary—Inner Peace
Sandalwood—Aroma Therapy
Self Heal—Fasting Assistance
Sensitive Plant—Shyness
Shooting Star—Astrological Awareness
Silversword—Spiritual Awakening
Skullcap—Massage/Psychic Healing
Solomon's Seal—Psychic Grace
Squash-Zucchini—Youthfulness
Strawberry—Stimulates Visions
Tree of Life—Upliftment
Tree Tobacco—Smoke-Free
Vanilla—Balanced Weight Loss
Watermelon—Emotions of Pregnancy
Wintergreen—Past Life Therapy
Witch Hazel—Spiritual Healing
Yarrow-White—Psychic Healing
Ylang Ylang—Earth Attunement
Yucca—Transforms Anger
Zinnia—Laughter

Pegasus Products, Inc., POB 228, Boulder, CO 80306.

Gemstones and Gemstone Essences

Gemstones and crystals have been used for healing by women from every culture and every age of the world. They are part of the legends of Atlantis and Mu, and their use, like so many other traditions, probably began off-planet. The legends state that people were brought to earth, we did not evolve here, and many of the healing methods were brought with us. Gemstone healing is known from Africa to Native America, from South America to China and Europe. Clear crystal is known universally, while other available stones may change from place to place. Texts on gemstone healing exist that are hundreds of years old. In the past fifteen years, gemstones and crystals have come into wide notice in the Women's Spirituality and metaphysical communities, and much lost knowledge about gemstone healing has been reclaimed. Women have learned it by intuition and channeling, and through experience and direct work. A number of good books on the subject and workshops at the women's music festivals and at metaphysical bookstores have helped to share and extend the knowledge. Today's women are discovering what women worldwide and throughout herstory have always known, that gemstones and crystals are powerful tools for healing.

Like flower essences and homeopathy, gemstones operate at a faster vibration than the physical. They work on the nonphysical levels of the subtle bodies. Crystals resonate with the vibration of the aura, and "tune" the body part the specific gemstone harmonizes with. A woman who has never seen a particular type of gemstone, but who is attracted to it visually or kinesthetically, will choose it to heal some part of herself that needs this vibratory retuning. She may not know what the stone is, what it does or why she needs it, but if she is attracted to its resonance, that resonance will match something she needs for her healing.

Color is also a factor in gemstone healing, and color itself is vibrational frequency. The light spectrum, used in the east and west to delineate the chakra system, is also a system to differentiate what gemstones do. There are ten basic colors used in the aura system, and each color (and gemstones of that color) resonates with a specific body system. Here is a brief and simplified overview. *Black* is used for grounding and connecting with the earth, for calming and protection. *Red* is for survival, red blood and the life force, the womb and menstruation. *Orange* is for the blood cleansing organs, for the ovaries, for sexuality, and for holding or releasing pictures from the past. *Yellow* is for the digestive organs, for assimilating energy and intelligence, and for self-confidence. *Green* is for the thymus (immune system), for healing and regeneration, infectious diseases, cleansing the blood and for the heart muscle. *Pink* (an alternate for green) is for the emotional heart, for love and self-love, universal love, and for coming to terms with one's feelings.

Blue is for the throat and hearing, for expressing emotions and creativity, for giving and receiving. *Indigo* is for vision (physical and psychic), for healing the lymphatic and endocrine systems, and for the spine and central nervous system. *Violet* is women's connection with their spiritual selves, and for healing the head, skull and brain. *Clear* or *white* is for all-aura healing, the vibratory and electrical systems of the body, and for receiving divine guidance, women's connection with the universe/Goddess. Gemstones of these colors resonate with these systems.

Gemstones vibrationally function in the middle spectrum of nonphysical healing. Flower essences are faster moving vibrations, and homeopathic remedies are slower and closer to the physical. (Vitamins and herbs work entirely on the physical body level.) Flower essences work primarily on the emotional and mental bodies, and homeopathic remedies work most often on the physical body. Gemstones, being crystalline, work with the body's crystalline structures, the formations of cells, bones and organs. They have healing effects on all levels, and are used as often for physical healing as for emotional, mental or spiritual. By making gemstones into essences similar to flower essences, the energy is the most refined and fastest assimilated into the subtle and physical bodies.

To use gemstones for healing, they can be held in the aura or taken into the body. To hold them in the aura means to simply hold them in the hand, wear them as jewelry, or carry them in a pocket. They can be placed under a pillow while sleeping. I have had my best uses of gemstones and crystals over the years by holding them in my hand while I sleep. Within a night or two, or sooner, I will know what effect that stone has on the body, or at least on my own body, emotions and mental states. In ancient times gemstones were crushed and made into gemstone elixirs to be ingested. Today's gemstone essences are made by placing the undamaged stone in water in the sun or under the full moon; the water becomes a powerful healing drink. The gemstone remains intact and may be reused any number of times.

In any use of gemstones, it is essential that they be cleared frequently. Both crystals and gems absorb vibrations and retain them until they are removed. A crystal may be used to draw off pain or a dis-ease, but that dis-ease remains in the gemstone until it is cleared. Uncleared, it will return dis-ease energy to the next user, or the stone itself will eventually shatter or disappear. To remove these vibrations, the stones need to be cleared after every healing, and if carried in a pocket or worn, they can be cleared weekly or even nightly. This is done in a number of ways: place them in dry seasalt overnight or for at least a couple of hours, place them in the sun or under moonlight, smudge them with incense smoke or sage smoke, wash them in running water or seawater, or bury them in the earth for a short time. The method I use that has worked the best for me is to place them under a pyramid, nightly if possible. This is the same pyramid that is used in cleansing and raising the healing vibrations of flower essences.

To make a gemstone elixir or essence, the process is the same as making a flower essence. Take a small piece of gemstone (half-inch will do) and clear it thoroughly under a pyramid, then place it in a clear bowl of distilled water in the sun of the early day. Leave it for about three hours, then bottle and use in the same ways as the directions for the flower essences. The gemstone can be rough, cut or tumbled, and should be as high a quality as possible. Some porous gemstones can be toxic, so if using malachite, chrysocolla, or any other highly porous stone, pick a piece that is tumbled or cut. A tumbled or polished piece will release less gemstone matter into the water. Leave these stones that may be toxic in the water for no more than half an hour. For chrysocolla, use it in the gem silica form that does not dissolve.

To make gemstone essences for immediate use, place the piece of gemstone in a ceramic cup or clear glass on the windowsill for an hour on a sunny day. For cloudy days, it can take several hours. Then drink the water, leaving the stone; refill it and put the glass back on the windowsill to recharge. If you are attuned to Reiki or use touch healing and are familiar with the healing energy, place your hands around the glass of water and gemstone to charge it also. I have used these secondary methods with very little fuss or precautions to make highly effective gemstone essences, even using tap water in the glass. Essences made this way will not keep and must be used immediately. Without preservative or bottling, the water will lose the charge quickly once the gemstone is removed. Gemstone essences work more rapidly than carrying the whole stones in the aura, and they work on a higher level of the nonphysical bodies.

Says Gurudas on gemstone essences:

> Gems influence specific organs in the physical body, while homeopathic remedies have a wider impact on the entire physical body. Gems carry the pattern of a crystalline structure, which focuses the physical body's mineral and crystalline structures on the biomolecular levels; therefore, gems work more closely with the biomolecular structure to integrate the life force into the body.[1]

Gem essences have greatest impact on the etheric level of the body, the energy double of the physical body; flower essences reach the mental and emotional bodies and homeopathic remedies primarily affect the physical. Gemstones operate in between. Where flower essences "hold the pattern of consciousness," gem essences and gemstones "amplify consciousness."[2]

A woman attracted to a specific gemstone will feel a sense of well-being almost as soon as she picks it up. The feelings result from a change in emotional state or mental mindset, and lead fairly quickly to physical changes. If she puts the stone down, the effects disappear, but if she holds the stone longer they will stay. If she keeps the stone in her aura for as long as she needs it (making sure it is cleared frequently), the physical, emotional and mental changes become permanent. The time for this varies from woman to woman; it may take an hour or years. At that point, she will either lose the stone, lose interest in it, or give it away—it's done its job and is ready to be used elsewhere.

In using gemstone essences, the changes happen rapidly. One glass of an essence made on the windowsill, or one dose of preserved essence from the eyedropper, may be enough for permanent change. Usually it takes longer, and this time varies with the individual. Use a gemstone essence three or four times a day to start, and use them every day, until intuition tells you that it's no longer needed. A pendulum will help with this. If you find yourself forgetting it when you've been taking it faithfully, you're probably ready to use it less often or stop.

The "book indications" used for various gemstones are a good beginning for how to use them in gemstone essences. They are only a beginning, however, as the essences go further into the nonphysical bodies than other ways to use gemstones. The stone affects more as an essence. If you are drawn to a particular stone and want to use it in an essence, or

---

[1]Gurudas, *Flower Essences and Vibrational Healing*, p. 33.
[2]Ibid.

drawn to a particular description of a gemstone essence, there is a reason. If its vibrations harmonize with yours, you will like the essence or stone and want to continue using it. This will only be the case if the essence/ gemstone has something for your well-being. If the books indicate a stone that should be good for you, but you are not drawn to it or have aversion to it, it is not your stone and will not be beneficial. Go with gut feelings on this one. A pendulum will also help you to pick the gemstone or gem essence that is the most beneficial.

Within types of stones, individual stones are also not alike. You may be in love with kunzite, as I am, but find one piece attractive and a second one not. If you feel that a particular type of stone would make a good essence for you, make it from a piece of that stone that you are highly attracted to, rather than one you are indifferent to or don't like at all. If your intuition says you need kunzite, but the piece you have doesn't interest you for a gemstone essence, find another piece and see what happens. You may be also attracted to a gemstone mined in one country, rather than another. Canadian amethyst may attract you more than Brazilian or Mexican—the minerals in each country are slightly different and there may be something in the Canadian amethyst that the others lack.

The stone that the books say will heal your dis-ease may not be your stone. Another stone may heal that dis-ease for you, and you'll be attracted to it. No two auras vibrate alike, and no two women are alike. Always go with your own feelings. Only you know what you need, and your aura will respond to it. A book can give you herstorical and traditional uses for a stone, or what resonates for the author, but your own needs may be very different. If you have a pendulum, it can be very helpful in picking the correct stone or gemstone essence. If in any doubt, go with the stone (or bottle) you just can't put down.

Healing in standard medicine works with the physical body only, while vibrational healing methods (flower essences, homeopathy, essential oils, gemstones) work from nonphysical levels down to the physical. The theory here is that dis-ease manifests on the physical level last, and develops in the energy bodies long before it reaches the physical. The energy bodies are the template, the blueprint, for the physical body and by healing them you not only heal the physical dis-ease, but the body's propensity for dis-ease. Changes only on the physical level are not permanent changes; the medical system cuts out a tumor and it appears somewhere else. Vibrational level healing heals the template that programs that body; when cancer is healed on the vibrational level, the tumor is no longer part of the blueprint. It doesn't appear again somewhere else. Healing done with vibrational methods has the ability to change the

Gem Elixir Descriptions

Agate-fire—Color Therapy
Alexandrite—Self-esteem/Centering
Amber—Spiritualizes Intellect
Amethyst—Well-being
Apophyllite—Creative Joy
Aquamarine—Stimulates Healing
Azurite-Malachite—Clairvoyance
Boji Stone—Attunement to Nature
Bloodstone—Vitality/Courage
Celestite—Recognizing Potential
Chalcedony—Inspiration
Chrysocolla—Emotional Balance
Copper—Self-confidence
Coral-red/white—Emotional Calm
Diamond-white—Higher Self-alignment
Dioptase—Loving Change
Electrum—Mental Balance
Emerald—Balance
Fluorite—Life Force
Garnet-Hessonite—Earth Attunement
Gem Silica—Psychic Comfort
Gold—Greater Love
Herkimer Diamond—Balances Personality
Ivory—Inner Discipline
Jade—Higher Love/Talents
Jasper-green—Healing Attributes
Jasper-picture—Past Life Recall
Kunzite—Self-esteem
Labradorite—Childhood Issues

Lapis Lazuli—Communication
Lepidolite—Mood Enhancer
Lodestone-neg./pos.—Yin/Yang Balance
Malachite—Opens Heart
Manganocalcite—Spiritualizes Emotions
Meteorite—Cosmic Awareness
Moldavite—Telepathy/Clairvoyance
Moonstone—Feminine Balance
Opal-dark—Sensitizes Emotions
Opal-light—Mystical Experiences
Pearl-dark/light—Emotional Balance
Peridot—Creative Visualization
Platinum—Calms Stress
Quartz-black (smoky)—Kundalini Energy
Quartz-citrine—Clear Thinking
Quart-rose—Opens Heart
Rhodochrosite—Self-identity
Rubellite—Will Power
Ruby—Spiritual Balance
Silver—Eases Tension/Stress
Star Sapphire—Higher Inspiration
Staurolite—Earth Attunement
Sugilite—Crown Chakra
Sulfur—Spiritualizes Intellect
Topaz—Spiritual Rebirth
Tourmaline-black—Protection
Tourmaline-watermelon—Heart Alignment
Turquoise—Master Healer

Pegasus Products, Inc., P.O. Box 228, Boulder, CO 80306.

cellular structure of the body; the cells grow back healthy instead of as cancer cells. Dis-ease is changed to wellness which is the propensity of the body as a whole.

Says Gurudas again:

> Based upon these principles, disease within the body physical, although it may first seem to be on the anatomical level, has been traced by the scientists to the cellular level and eventually to the level of the biomolecular system, contained perhaps within the very genetic structure in its own right. In the final analysis, the body physical is healed through energy, energy upon the biomolecular level, not even upon the level of chemical reactions but more so upon molecular structures. Real healing extends from the biomolecular to the cellular level, and eventually to the anatomical level, where it is brought into harmony with other levels of the body physical. This is because the biochemical properties of the body physical in their final element are based upon vibration.[4]

Vibrational healing, known to women's healing since the beginnings of the earth, will be the healing methods of the future. Gemstones, along with several other methods of women's healing, already work with that nonphysical level to create permanent changes in women's health. Where physical-only healing methods remedy symptoms but not sources, subtle body healing goes to the source of the dis-ease, changing the template for wellness. Gemstones are one method of this, a method women have worked with for a number of years. Gemstone essences take that familiarity a step further, into a vibrational level not easily reached with the gemstone used physically (on the body instead of inside it). The power of gemstone essences has barely been tapped, and the possibilities of it for healing are only beginning. With other forms of vibrational healing, gemstone essences are a new field, a way of going beyond physical level healing for real change.

For more information on using gemstone essences and gemstones for healing, see Gurudas, *Gem Elixers and Vibrational Healing, Vol. I* (Cassandra Press, 1985), and Diane Stein, *All Women Are Healers* (The Crossing Press, 1990)—the chapters on laying on of stones and gemstone essences. The *Women's Book of Healing* (Diane Stein, Llewellyn Publications, 1987), is also a resource for information on colors, the aura and the chakras, and on psychic and direct metaphysical healing. Gem essence suggestions for this book are made primarily from these sources and from my own longtime gemstone experience. Gemstones are a form of healing I recommend highly to all women.

[4]Gurudas, *Gem Elixers and Vibrational Healing, Vol. I* (Boulder, CO, Cassandra Press, 1985), p. 3.

Emotional Healing

Emotional healing is not a remedy to eat, sniff or swallow in a capsule or tincture; it builds well-being by healing thought patterns and life's pain. Emotional healing is a factor in healing all dis-ease and much of any healer's skill is based upon awareness of it. The most intangible and hardest to touch of remedy systems, it is perhaps the most important remedy of all, and certainly the most complex. Flower and gemstone essences, homeopathy, and to some extent aromatherapy are the beginning of emotional level healing.

Women's bodies do not stop at the skin, and the body is actually four bodies, the physical, emotional, mental and spiritual. The dense physical body, what can be seen and touched, is what the medical system treats, and what woman's healing treats by physical level methods (using herbs, nutrition or vitamins). These methods directly affect the body; their biochemical ingredients make changes in the biochemical components of physiology. When a bone is broken, the physical body is where we put the splint or cast. But what is it that causes the broken bone to knit, to form new bone so that the injured area becomes stronger than before the break? What directs the rebuilding process? Why is it that humans cannot regrow limbs, but lizards can? And what is it that sometimes causes a fractured bone to not knit and rebuild? The human body contains sixty trillion cells; what directs some of them to be skin cells, while others are bone, organ, blood or lymph cells? Why is a bone cell not a hair cell? And why do normal cells sometimes become cancerous?

The answers lie beyond the physical body level, in the unseen energy levels, called the four subtle or vibrational bodies in most metaphysical traditions. These are where the dense physical body is designed and directed. Health or dis-ease begin in the vibrational energy levels, and healing that is permanent must also treat these levels. The lack of success in standard medicine, with its need to cut out, burn out or drug out symptoms instead of healing disease, comes from its inability to accept the energy bodies or to treat them. Physical level healing alone is not a cure, or to put it in another way, what the medical system calls cures is not healing.

The four bodies—physical, emotional, mental and spiritual—are present in the seven layers of the aura. Many women can see these bodies visually, or see some of them, and many more who have experience as healers are able to sense or touch them. Women who receive information psychically are given instructions as healers on how to work with these bodies. When I do healing, I put my hands down in the Reiki positions, and my guides work through my hands to reshape and rebuild the nonphysical aura levels and bodies. I may or may not be consciously aware of what is taking place, but I know that I work on more than physical levels. This work results in vibrational changes that become physical ones.

The first of the energy bodies, moving at a frequency rate that is closest to the physical body, is the etheric double or physical body aura. This is an energy mirror twin of the physical body, and often dis-ease can be seen or sensed at this level before it physically manifests. For healing to take place, dis-ease must be removed from this energy level and replaced with wellness. Blocks or shadows in the etheric double become dis-ease, and a psychic works to remove these. A block, spot, shadow or tear on this level that is healed causes the physical dis-ease to heal soon after, usually within three days. The chakras, energy centers that bring vibrations from the unseen bodies to the physical, are also located on this level. Work with gemstones and colors is work with the chakras for etheric body (and often beyond) healing.

Women who meditate can learn to visualize their etheric bodies and chakras, and to clear blockages from them before they result in physical dis-ease. In the meditative state, visualize each chakra in turn and fill it with its designated color (the colors of the gemstones— read my *Women's Book of Healing* or Barbara Ann Brennan's *Hands of Light* [Bantam Books, 1988] for much more on the aura and chakras). If any center seems dull, tarnished, out of position or torn, create imagery to repair it—use metaphors like polishing cloths and Goddess tape. Remember also, that imagery does not have to be visual, but can involve any of the senses. Fill each chakra with light, then go to the aura surrounding the body and all of the chakras. Clear it in the same way, and fill it with all the chakra colors in turn or with golden light. Imagine light/energy flowing through the aura, first entering at the head and leaving at the feet, then entering at the feet and leaving through the crown of the head. Use light in all the chakra colors in series or pick the color you feel you most need. All of the colors, including black, are positive but for this use blue, clear or golden light.

In an example, if you have a sore throat, visualize the chakras and aura as a whole first, and light up each chakra with its color. Perhaps the throat center looks less healthy—it may have speckles of red in it, be dull in color, look muddy or cracked. Use your visualized healing fingers to take the bits of red out and put them into an imagined purifying fire. Use astral "Windex" to wash and polish the chakra, and then fill it with blue light. If it doesn't hold the healing, repeat it, trying different ways to clear and energize the center. Ask yourself, "What is there that I need to say, but feel I can't? What words am I swallowing? Who am I angry at and need to confront?" Say it now while alone and watch the chakra clear. The next morning your sore throat will also be gone, if you have released all that needed to be said. This is an example of healing from the nonphysical bodies, and of emotional healing. By releasing the withheld emotion (often anger in this center), the dis-ease energy is released from the vibrational field, and physical healing can now happen.

The faster-moving vibrational body next to the etheric double/physical body aura is the emotional body. And since bodies and aura layers carry energy in specific order (from spiritual to mental, mental to emotional, and emotional to physical or the other way from the physical, moving through the emotional, then mental to spiritual), every dis-ease moves through the emotional body. As you might expect, the emotional body is where emotions form and are processed—or are held and need to be processed. Spiritual and mental energy pass through the emotional body before they reach the etheric double or the dense body itself. With all of that traffic, the emotions are obviously important to women's health. Women who see auras see the emotional body as changing colors; the colors reflect the woman's changing emotions.

Here's an example of how the emotional body works. A child is having a very hard time with her third grade teacher, and because of it she doesn't want to go to school. She tells her mother, who says she has to go anyway. One day the child comes home from school with a stomach ache, and since she has a slight fever, her mother lets her stay home the next day. When things get tough at school, the child develops another stomach ache and she gets another day off. Suddenly this child is having a whole string of illnesses, physically real, and neither the child nor her mother may be aware that they are emotionally caused. The next term, with a better teacher, the child feels good about school and has fewer illnesses. It would have been better had she been able to change teachers; none of the illnesses would have happened. If she couldn't change teachers, emotional support from her mother or others would have helped. Understand that the child was not faking, nor was she causing the dis-eases intentionally.

There are adults who do similar things, probably not consciously (the emotional body is also the subconscious mind). If an adult woman feels her life is hopeless or too difficult and painful to want to live through she can go so far as to manifest terminal dis-eases. Instead of dying, why not change the things that aren't working in one's life? Sometimes change is harder to go through than death. In cases like these, the healer's role is to ask questions that lead her friend into consciousness of her process. It is not up to the healer to blame, accuse or judge her in any way. Every choice is valid, including the choice to die, but do it with understanding. Any healer or doctor can tell you that if someone wants to die, they can die of something very minor, and if they choose to live, really want to live, they will heal their bodies of seemingly hopeless dis-eases. By understanding the emotional roots of a dis-ease, many women become those who heal despite all odds. The emotional body operates this way for all dis-ease, major and minor. It does not have to be life threatening.

Next is the mental body, and women who see auras visually may see this body as flashing colors that move in and out of the emotional body aura. The mental body filters through the emotional before it reaches the etheric double and dense physical body. In the mental body, women can create what they want for their lives and healing, but they must do so very carefully. Here's another example: a woman discovers a lump in her breast and makes an appointment to have it biopsied. She can visualize mentally in two different ways. In the positive way, she can realize that eighty percent of breast lumps are benign (if this one isn't, she has caught it early). She can see herself emerging from the biopsy with the information that this is only a cyst, or visualize that by the time she goes for the biopsy, the lump has disappeared by itself (and it probably will, if she makes that image and concentrates on it often enough). She can begin holistic therapies of her choice immediately, to go along with the visualization.

The other way to visualize is the negative way. She can see herself dying horribly of cancer, her body mutilated by the medical system's surgeries, radiation and chemotherapy. She can imagine herself in the hospital looking awful and even see her own funeral. If she continues on that track, she can manifest what she sees, and is much less likely to leave the biopsy appointment with a clean bill of health. What we create in our minds/mental bodies, aided by the emotions the thoughts raise, have direct repercussions on what happens in the physical body. The woman who visualizes positively is much likelier to have a positive outcome than the woman who allows her fears to run wild. Negative thought patterns, many of them so habitual as to be no longer conscious for examining, have great effect in creating women's dis-eases. By changing the negative thought patterns, no matter how well-rooted, women change their bodies' reactions from dis-ease to health. Emotional healing uncovers the negative patterns, allowing women to change their thoughts, emotions and bodies—if they choose to work that way.

The spiritual level is the fastest vibrating of the four bodies, and more and more women who see or sense psychically are able to reach and work with it. This is the level that guided healings often work from and the level from which healing psychically has the most profound results. This is also the level where the body template exists, the blueprint that says a particular cell is a liver cell instead of a fingernail cell, and that your hair will grow in brown instead of red. It is the level that directs a cell to grow in healthy or nonhealthy ways, to knit a broken bone or not. This is also the level from which women connect with divinity (in whatever name they choose), and with their own purpose for this incarnation. There is a connection between the two: women who have knowledge of who they are in the universe, that they are here for a reason and are part of a universal plan, are women who will manifest less physical, emotional or mental disease in their lives.

Women who are able to feel themselves as part of Goddess (or whatever they call source energy), are women who will have happier, more fulfilled, and healthier lives. That connection with purpose and reason for Be-ing is all-important in how the body manifests dis-ease or wellness. Healing this level involves a healing direction from Goddess to the physical body (through the mental and emotional bodies), so that change manifests in the spiritual/template body. This kind of healing is profound indeed, involving miraculous cures and new patterns on every level of awareness. Such miracles happen daily in women's healing.

Healing that begins with the physical body (i.e., herbs for an infection) changes the etheric double/physical body aura. The next layer is the emotional body. Here the woman looks at her emotions around the infection—what made her immune system low? Did she have the infection because she is working too hard and needs a dis-ease to give her permission to stop? Did she have the infection because there is an infected emotion (anger, resentment, hate) that needs cleaning out? Once she has a handle on the cause of the infection in the emotional sense, she uses her conscious mind to create solutions to heal the emotion.

In one example, her dis-ease-causing emotion is about her boss, and she chooses to change it. Instead of holding her resentment for him inside and developing infections in her body, she decides to find another job. She writes her boss a nastygram, telling him all the things she would like to say and releasing the emotions by saying it. She doesn't mail the letter, but starts job hunting. These are constructive uses of the mental body to solve an emotional level feeling. (The emotions feel, and the mental body defines the feelings.) On the spiritual level, she reaffirms her connection with Goddess and her own place in the universe, understands that "You are Goddess" means her, and perhaps does a Self-Blessing. Her infection is healed by the next day and does not recur, as long as she follows through with her decision to work elsewhere. She finds a more positive job and the emotions are resolved.

Every dis-ease, from the trivial to the terminal, has an emotional body co-ordinate, and releasing the emotion releases the physical dis-ease. This has been the work of healer Louise Hay, and she teaches it in her books and workshops. In her theory, every negative experience in life, every dis-ease, is the result of an unreleased emotion that becomes a negative thought pattern. By discovering what these patterns are and changing the thinking, the negative is changed to positive well-being. By working through the emotion, by taking action that resolves the situation or by forgiving and letting go, dis-ease is changed to health.

The issue here is awareness and responsibility, never blame. Coming to terms with an emotion and changing the connecting thought pattern go a long way toward releasing dis-ease and creating positive change in one's life. This means that with awareness, women can take more responsibility for their healing, do more for themselves, take more of their own power. What it does not mean is, "You created the dis-ease, so you can go and heal it." The emotional causes of dis-ease are not conscious and therefore are not in women's conscious control. Awareness of the contributing thought patterns gives a beginning of where to look for self-healing. Remember also that women in a patriarchal society have inherited many conditions beyond our choosing—we did not ask to be second class citizens (or if poor, nonwhite or disabled, less than second class). We know our own worth, but are not the ones running the world—yet.

There is also the concept of karma that says we have each aspect of our lives for a reason. Our dis-eases are there not because we "deserve" them, but because there is something for us to learn in having them. That learning may be in developing the awareness and growth to change old emotions and thoughtforms to effect the healing. When this happens, not only is the dis-ease healed, but women's lives are healed and become more positive in other ways. Says Louise Hay on this:

> I have learned that for every condition in our lives there is a NEED FOR IT, otherwise we would not have it. This symptom is only an outer effect. We must go within to dissolve the mental cause. This is why Will Power and Discipline do not work. They are only battling the outer effect. It is like cutting down the weed

instead of getting the root out. So...work on the WILLING-
NESS TO RELEASE THE NEED for the cigarettes, or the
headache, or...whatever. When the need is gone the outer effect
must die. No plant can live if the root is cut away.[1]

The emotional healing co-ordinates to dis-eases in this book are
offered as a beginning in hunting for the negative emotion or thought
pattern. They are based on the work of Louise Hay, in *Heal Your Body* and
You Can Heal Your Life (Hay House, 1982 and 1984) and Alice Steadman
in *Who's the Matter With Me?* (ESP Inc., 1966), as well as on my own work
in self-healing and as a healer. Where there is political awareness, it is my
own. To use these comments or co-ordinates, look at them and ask
yourself, "Is this true for me?" It may be, or something else may be
operating. If the comment misses the mark, ask yourself, "If this doesn't
work for me, what does? What is the real cause?" Once you have defined
for your own needs and life the emotional reason behind your illness, ask
yourself next, "What can I do to change it?" Then follow through.

Sometimes the awareness is enough. Looking back on the emotional
pain that caused the situation to begin with may release it. Sometimes you
will need help to release the emotion, especially if it is a deep one or
originated when you were very young.Talking it out with someone else,
or even therapy may be beneficial. In other instances direct action is
needed, as in finding a new job or new lover.

Sometimes a thought pattern was positive in childhood, but now is
ineffective or negative and needs changing. In that case, watch for
situations to arise where that thoughtform kicks in. As soon as you
recognize it, stop and say "No" and replace the thinking with the positive
alternatives or affirmations you have chosen. (Choose carefully.) In many
or all cases, women have work to do in healing their self-image; we have
been trained to give up our power and have to retrain ourselves in self-
love. Goddess women can remember the Craft law, "You are Goddess,"
and meditate on what that means. The Self-Blessing ritual is powerful for
changing negative thought patterns to women's empowerment. Find more
on these in my book, *Casting the Circle: A Women's Book of Ritual* (The
Crossing Press, 1990).

Emotional healing, the comments and co-ordinates that tell you
where to start in healing the life pain that causes dis-ease, may be the most
important remedy suggestions in this book.

---

[1]Louise Hay, *Heal Your Body* (Santa Monica, CA, Hay House, 1982), p. 5. Emphasized words are Hay's.

Remedies

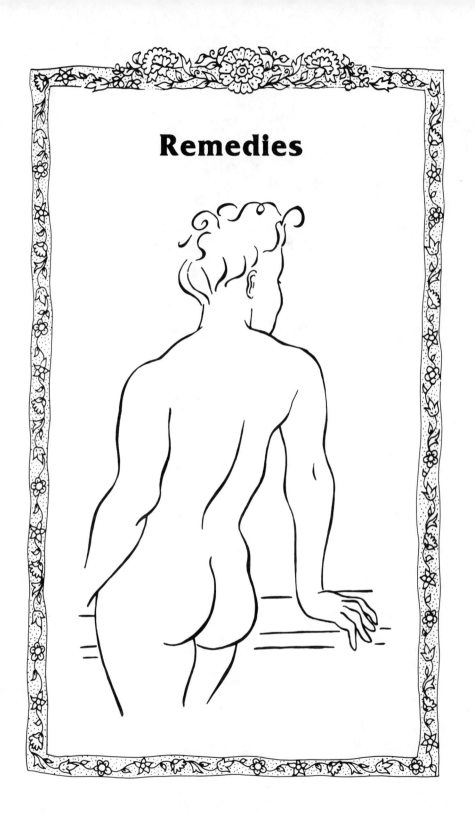

will provide a higher quality of life while life remains than the medical system can now offer.

Vitamins and Minerals: Holistic treatment for AIDS and HIV-positive people focuses on building the immune system. Along with a healthy lifestyle—quality food, enough sleep and exercise, reducing stress and avoiding harmful substances—the following vitamin regime is important. I have used this on HIV-positive gay men and watched their blood values normalize as long as they stayed on it. Two became HIV-negative after less than a year on the vitamins and better diet, with no other treatment. Use a high quality daily multiple vitamin and mineral supplement and double the standard dose. If you are using Schiff's Single Day, for example, use it twice a day with meals. Along with this add a B-complex-50 or -100 two or three times a day, and vitamin C to bowel tolerance. Use at least 10,000 mg (10 g) of C with bioflavinoids a day, and it can go far higher. These are essentials.

Dr. Robert Cathcart in California has ample evidence of HIV remission and total disappearance on megadoses of intravenous vitamin C, using 200–500 grams a day.[3] For C by mouth, use calcium ascorbate powder (nonacid form), 1/2–3/4 teaspoon taken in water six times a day. Use a straw to bypass the teeth (this is strong enough to eventually dissolve tooth enamel), and rinse your mouth with water after each use. Take a B-complex or calcium/magnesium tablet with it at least a few times a day to prevent kidney stones from the high dose of C.

Take 50,000–75,000 IU of beta-carotene per day, 100 mg of zinc, and 400–800 IU of vitamin E with 200 mcg of selenium. Supplement folic acid to about 400 mcg, B-6 to 250–500 mg, extra B-12 to 2000 mcg (injections are even better), extra biotin to 500 mcg, and 500–2000 mg of B-5 (pantothenic acid). B-15, pangamic acid, may be helpful in reducing nausea. If stopping any of these large amounts, decrease them slowly. Zinc should not exceed 100 mg total per day.

Minerals besides zinc include: copper (3 mg), manganese (10–20 mg), magnesium (500–1000 mg with double calcium), molybdenum (100 mcg), and chromium (500 mcg).[4] Germanium (200 mg), S.O.D. (an enzyme—super oxide dismutase), or coenzyme Q10 are highly recommended antioxidants. Use iron if needed. If you are on AZT, the above amounts should replace what the drug drains from the body and help in diarrhea and side effects. Egg lecithin (20 g) on an empty stomach divided through the day is also recommended, as well as essential fatty acids (evening primrose oil or black currant oil).

---

[3]Tom O'Connor, *Living With AIDS* (San Francisco, Corwin Publishers, 1987), p. 324–338.
[4]Lawrence Badgley, MD, *Healing AIDS Naturally* (San Bruno, CA, Human Energy Press, 1987), p. 114–133. Much of the remedy information is from Badgley.

Herbs: Use cayenne in water daily to prevent opportunistic infections of AIDS. Take a teaspoon of dried cayenne flowers to half a gallon of water and boil for one or two minutes before shutting off the flame. Cool and strain and place in a covered bottle in the refrigerator. Build up an ability to tolerate this—it's HOT. Start with a teaspoonful a day and work up to a juiceglass full. It may irritate the stomach.[2]

Use the herbal antibiotics, echinacea, yellow dock, goldenseal, chaparral or pau d'arco. Use blood cleansing herbs, particularly red clover with blue violet, and particularly with AIDS-related cancers. Silymarin, milk thistle extract, protects and repairs the liver and is needed if you are using doctor's medications and AIDS drugs. Dandelion also cleanses the liver. Ginseng, mullein, gingko biloba (for the brain), St. John's wort (hypericum), or Jason Winter's Tea (chaparral) are all positive. For medication side effects: use slippery elm for indigestion and diarrhea; catnip tea, chamomile, spearmint, raspberry leaf or peppermint for nausea, diarrhea and indigestion. Slippery elm can also be used as a food if nothing else will stay down, and alfalfa is an essential nutrient. For stress or insomnia, try scullcap, hops, catnip or passion flower, and for pain use valerian. Take your pick among these herbs and try one or two—do not use them all.

Naturopathy: The AIDS diet is an immune building and cleansing diet, using about 75% raw fruits and vegetables, with whole grains. If you are a meat-eater, use organic meat and poultry only. Totally avoid junk foods, sugar and refined flour products, saturated fats, smoking, recreational drugs, sweets, alcohol and soft drinks. Use wheatgrass, chlorophyll, sun chlorella, spirulina, Kyo-green or other "green drinks" and vegetable juices (carrot, beet, celery, etc.). Kelp tablets or Edgar Cayce's Atomidine are useful. There are several antiviral mushrooms, among them somastatin, shiitake, suma and ganoderma. Aloe vera juice is recommended as an immune builder and cleanser, as well as raw glandular extracts (thymus, spleen, or multiglandular combination), and RNA/DNA. Again, pick from among these, not all of them.

Garlic, in the form of odorless Kyolic tablets, is highly recommended (or raw garlic if you can stand it). It is antiviral, antibacterial and antifungal and an important immune builder, and is particularly indicated if you have candida albicans (thrush) infections. Use two tablets three times a day with meals. Bee propolis or pollen is good for bacterial infections of the mouth, lungs, throat and mucous membranes and is an immune builder. Acidophilus, in the form of Maxidophilus, Megadophilus or Superdophilus, returns friendly bacterial balance to the intestines and is important if there is diarrhea or candida.

[2] I want to thank Laurel Steinhice for this cayenne water recipe.

Homeopathy and Cell Salts: Because homeopathy is based on the user's own vital force, homeopathic remedies for AIDS may work best while the immune system is not deeply impaired. A homeopathic physician is recommended here, except in working with some of the lesser related symptoms. Nosodes of *Typhoidinum* and *Cyclosporin* have been tried with positive results. For lesser symptoms—diarrhea, indigestion, nausea, fever, etc.—see the sections on these in this book and match your symptoms as closely to the described remedies as possible. A good homeopathy how-to guide, like Cummings and Ullman's *Everybody's Guide to Homeopathic Medicine*, would be helpful.

Amino Acids: Use a free-form amino acids combination; it offers high nutrition and immune building, plus B-complex vitamins that are badly needed, and is an antioxidant besides. Single aminos include l-carnitine, cysteine, methionine and ornithine; take on an empty stomach with 500 mg vitamin C and 50 mg of B-6 (or B-complex).

Acupressure: Use full foot reflexology working gradually up to twice a day to stimulate the entire immune system. Pay particular attention to working the endocrine gland reflexes and the lymph glands (see these illustrated under Immune System Dis-eases). Anywhere you find a tender spot, use pressure or massage to gently work it until the pain releases. Also pay attention to the spleen, liver, kidneys, lungs, gall bladder, and stomach on the body map. See the illustration for points on the body (page 103), and the acupressure foot, hand and body maps in the acupressure methods section (pages 60-65). Massage the whole ear well—it is another body map of all the organs.

Aromatherapy: Use aromas in baths, massage oils, diffusers or placed on the body just to smell. If in bed, put a drop or two on your pillow. Immune building essential oils include tea-tree, lemon, geranium, juniper, St. John's wort, yarrow, lavender, cypress, eucalyptus, peppermint, cardamom, niaoli or lemon thyme.

Flower Essences: Amaranthus is for immune boosting and repels viral and bacterial dis-eases; chaparral cleanses the endocrine and immune systems and helps with blood toxicity; pansy focalizes the energy to destroy viruses, including HIV/AIDS. Use Saguaro if you are HIV positive with no symptoms, or for AIDS dementia. Lotus boosts other essences, for assimilation of all forms of healing.

Gemstones and Gem Essences: For immune system boosting, use any of the following in essence: emerald, jade, picture jasper, amethyst, blue quartz, citrine, rutile, ruby, blue tourmaline or pink tourmaline. The tourmalines, ruby and rutile are the most recommended. Hold or wear lapis lazuli, sugilite or pink tourmaline.

Acupressure for AIDS

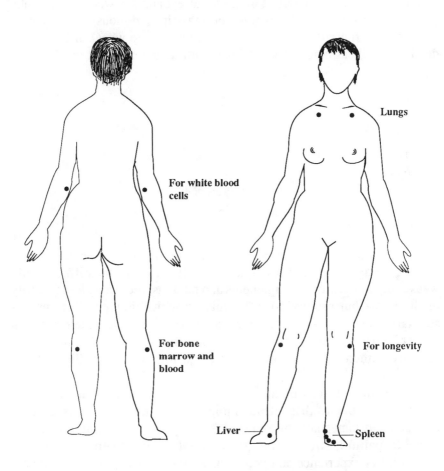

Lawrence Badgley, MD, *Healing AIDS Naturally* (San Bruno, CA Human Energy Press, 1987), p. 213.

Emotional Healing: Many people are leaving the planet now, an effect of the earth changes we are part of. Those that are leaving are unable to face the pain of watching the changes (and the deteriorating world that leads up to them), or the pain of making difficult internal changes in themselves. The first question, if you have HIV, is do you want to live? There is no judgment on those unable to continue. If deep in your heart, you *do* want to remain, put healing into effect and see where it may take you. If you do *not*, that is also a choice, but make it a conscious understanding. Life and death are both part of the same wheel, the wheel of birth, life, death and reincarnation. The soul is immortal and does not die.

Arthritis

Osteoarthritis is a degenerative joint dis-ease that involves deterioration of the cartilage at the ends of bones. It results in pain and stiffness, with weakening of the muscles, ligaments and tendons; there may be deformity of the joints but usually no inflammation with this type. The onset is sudden or gradual, and most frequent after age forty, unless there has been earlier injury, excessive joint stress, or deformity from birth. Three times as many women as men suffer osteoarthritis, totaling 15.8 million Americans.

Rheumatoid arthritis and juvenile rheumatoid arthritis attack the synovial membranes that surround joint lubricating fluids, causing them to become inflamed and thickened. Affected joints deteriorate, becoming unstable, painful, swollen and greatly misshapen; women with rheumatoid arthritis experience an over-all unwellness, weakness, feverishness and tiredness. The onset occurs in children and before age forty in adults. Stress, poor nutrition and bacterial infections can be onset factors. 2.1 million American adults and 71,000 children, mostly female, have rheumatoid arthritis. There are over two hundred types of arthritis but these are the most frequent ones. The following remedies are for both types unless indicated.

Vitamins and Minerals: Use a daily multiple vitamin and mineral supplement with vitamin C to bowel tolerance. Add a B-complex-50 to -

100 two or three times a day with meals, and extra B-3, B-5 and B-6 (100 mg each up to three times a day; 500 mg of B-5); PABA reduces swelling. Take 800–1200 IU of vitamin E (with selenium is best, 50–200 mcg), and 25,000–50,000 IU of vitamin A as beta-carotene. A calcium/magnesium supplement (1000 mg calcium, 500 mg magnesium) is important to prevent bone loss. Zinc (50 mg), manganese, copper, and iodine (as kelp tablets, six to eight per day) are helpful, as well as the antioxidant pain relievers coenzyme Q10 (60 mg), germanium (200 mg) or S.O.D. Do not take supplemental iron.

Herbs: An infusion of alfalfa, burdock and white willow bark helps pain, reduces inflammation and brings nutrients to the bones. It also detoxifies and it tastes good; drink as much as you can. Try feverfew tincture for pain and to reduce inflammation, or celery seed and parsley tea to remove toxins. White willow is a safe aspirin substitute, and devil's claw is anti-inflammatory and analgesic. Wintergreen oil or St. John's wort oil are used topically. Other herbs include chaparral, yucca (six to eight tablets daily), corn silk, white sage or ginseng. Try external poultices of valerian or comfrey. Dandelion or red clover are liver and blood cleansers.

Naturopathy: Start with a raw vegetable juice fast (carrot or celery juice), including spirulina, alfalfa, and watercress, celery or parsley juices. Return to solid foods slowly, watching for food allergy reactions, and begin a vegetarian whole foods diet primarily of raw vegetables. Avoid milk products, meat, sugar, citrus, wheat, nightshade foods (green peppers, eggplant, tomatoes, potatoes, peppers and tobacco), refined flour, salt, alcohol, junk foods and soft drinks. Do not drink liquids with meals; it dilutes the digestive enzymes.

Take epsom salt baths, use castor oil packs, and cabbage leaf poultices when pain is acute; massage with peanut oil, olive oil or castor oil. Take olive oil internally, six tablespoons per day for three weeks, then decrease slowly until a maintenance dose is determined. Essential fatty acids—black currant oil, salmon oil, fish lipid oils, wheat germ, or evening primrose oil—can have amazing results in reducing pain and inflammation, and freeing joint movement. They are highly recommended.

To break down mineral deposits in the joints and aid digestion, place a teaspoon of apple cider vinegar and a teaspoon of honey in a glass of warm or cold water; drink this with meals three times a day, the only exception to no liquids with meals. Hydrochloric acid tablets, betaine or bromelain are other versions of the same thing. Eat red or blue berries—cherries, hawthorne or blueberries—and use honey instead of sugar to help replace collagen. Carrots, avocados, bananas and papaya are also positive foods.

Check for candida albicans; it can aggravate or even mimic arthritis symptoms. Take Kyolic (odorless garlic), two capsules or tablets three times a day with meals to reduce inflammation and candida; decrease to two a day as a preventive when attacks cease. Eat lots of raw garlic and onions, as well. Bee pollen is also positive.

Homeopathy and Cell Salts: Triflora Analgesic Gel can be used topically. Try *Arnica montana* when joints feel bruised, pain is aggravated by movement, you have a sore back or shoulders and are afraid of being touched. For inflammation and edema (as if by a bee-sting) try *Apis. Bryonia* is used when every muscle aches, there is pain in back and limbs, swollen hot red joints, and the least movement aggravates the pain. The woman wants to be left alone and to immobilize the affected area. Try *Colocynthis* when touch aggravates the pain but pressure helps, warmth relieves it, and movement worsens it. *Rhus tox.* is the remedy when pain is increased by rest, is worse in the morning, worse in damp, cold weather, and is relieved by continual motion. The joints are weak, swollen and red, with loss of strength in the arms and the fingers.

Cell Salts: Use *Ferrum phos.* when one joint after another is affected, joints are puffy and slightly red, and movement aggravates. *Silica* is for rheumatic pain in the limbs, and *Natrum Sulph.* is for pain in hips, limbs and knees, made worse by damp, cold weather. *Kali mur.* is used when pain occurs at night and is worse for bed warmth, and pain is worse or only felt in motion.

Amino Acids: A combination free-form amino acids is highly recommended to ease pain and rebuild tissue. Take it between meals. Single aminos include histidine, methionine, DL-phenylalanine and cystine. Tryptophan will be available again eventually.

Acupressure: Look for sore reflex points in the following areas and use pressure to release them. For leg and hip pain, find them at the outer edge of the buttocks (back); there may be several. For sciatica, look for sore spots in the heel pad (back of foot); they may take pressing with a crystal or blunt object to locate. Look for meridian points around the area of the leg where the hip socket moves on the sides. For knee pain, use the thumb and middle finger like pincers to find reflexes about two inches above the kneecaps, and also about two inches below. Never use pressure on the knees themselves or on any swollen, painful or inflamed joints.

For neck, arm, shoulder and finger pain, there are points on the backs of the shoulders, between the neck and arm. These may be very tender. General arthritis meridian points are located on the tops of the feet, and on the back of the feet just above the heels. See the illustration.

Aromatherapy: Essential oils for arthritis include birch, bergamot,

Acupressure Points for Arthritis

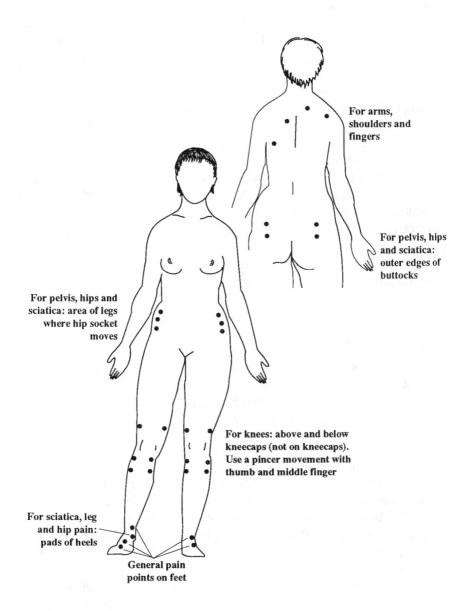

For arms, shoulders and fingers

For pelvis, hips and sciatica: outer edges of buttocks

For pelvis, hips and sciatica: area of legs where hip socket moves

For knees: above and below kneecaps (not on kneecaps). Use a pincer movement with thumb and middle finger

For sciatica, leg and hip pain: pads of heels

General pain points on feet

Mildred Carter, *Body Reflexology* (W. Nyack, NY, Parker Publishing Co., 1983), p. 112-115.

lavender, rosemary, chamomile, marjoram, ginger or cardamom. Use these particularly in baths and massage oils. Make a massage oil with pine and sassafras in an olive oil or peanut oil base. Tiferet-Lifetree has a Deep Joint Reliever combination.

Flower Essences: Redwood is for endocrine balancing, eliminating toxins, cell regeneration and the emotional aspects of the dis-ease. Dill is for inflammations, stress, and digestive assimilation, and hellebore is for rejuvenating.

Gemstones and Gem Essences: Use in essence azurite, chrysocolla, kunzite, chalcedony, peridot, sulfur or tourmaline quartz, or the metals silver, gold or copper. Hold or wear orange gems like coral or carnelian for osteoarthritis; where there is swelling and inflammation, try chrysocolla, amazonite or lapis.

Emotional Healing: People of strong unbending will who are in-flexible to change are prone to arthritis and rheumatism. Women who feel unloved are candidates, and women who give or receive over-amounts of criticism. Work on releasing anger and resentment, and on going with the flow. Arthritis in the hands comes with a feeling of being victimized and a desire to punish. Arthritic knees are need for flexibility, and a fear of moving forward on one's path.

Asthma

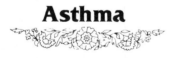

Asthma is recurring episodes of wheezing, breathing difficulties and breathlessness in varying degrees including life-threatening. Breathing out is obstructed, caused by spasms in the muscles surrounding the bronchi and bronchioles (airways to the lungs). Symptoms include chok-ing sensations, chest tightness, rapid breathing, distress and coughing with increased mucus secretion. Attacks usually end by expectoration. They most often occur at night, during exercise or at times of emotional stress, and are worse lying down. The muscle spasms that precipitate attacks are brought on by over-reaction of the body's immune system, often to various allergens. These may be sensitivities to the Typical American Diet, to food contaminants and additives or to chemicals, pollutants or tobacco fumes in the air. The "typical" asthmatic is hypoglycemic, has spinal misalignments, was weaned too early onto cow's milk and starch, and was given suppressive treatments (like cortisone) early.

In children asthma often begins with eczema and hay fever. Homeopaths believe that suppression of these with steroids will result in asthma. Food allergies are another cause, with dairy, eggs, yeast, wheat, fish and sulfite additives common sensitivities. In adult-onset asthma, allergies are less usually causes; extended emotional stress and anxiety can begin it. Causes of attacks in adults include chest infections, environmental irritants (chemicals, paint fumes, tobacco smoke, auto exhausts), sensitivity to food additives or preservatives, sudden changes in temperature or breathing patterns, or sudden vigorous exercise in sensitive individuals. Chiropractic, osteopathic or neuromuscular massage can often help greatly.

Vitamins and Minerals: Along with a multiple vitamin and mineral supplement, use vitamin A (15,000–25,000 IU daily) in dry form for the lungs and immune system. Use a B-complex-50 or -100 two or three times a day; important individual B-vitamins include B-6 (50–250 mg total), B-5, which is a natural antihistamine and anti-stress factor (500–2000 mg daily), and sublingual B-12. Use vitamin C with bioflavinoids to bowel tolerance or at *least* 3000 mg per day, and vitamin E with selenium up to 1200 IU per day. Minerals are even more important, and a calcium/magnesium tablet taken every half hour can lessen or stop attacks. For daily use take 1500 mg calcium to 750 mg magnesium in a complete calcium supplement—deficiencies in these may be the cause of asthma. Zinc for immune support can be supplemented at about 50 mg per day, and 5 mg of manganese taken twice a week. Coenzyme Q10 helps lessen the body's histamine reaction and oxygenates the blood. Germanium is also an oxygenator and immune builder, or Bromelin with Quercetin C. For children, give half the amounts.

Herbs: Blue violet leaf taken longterm helps to dry the moisture in the lungs that activates attacks; masterwort or honeysuckle stimulate the lungs, and prickly ash helps to remove obstructions. Nettles or mullein dry mucus, and nettles cleans the blood. Joy Gardner in *The New Healing Yourself* (The Crossing Press, 1989) recommends comfrey and lobelia tea: boil three cups of water and add two teaspoons of comfrey leaves. Simmer for ten minutes, then add two teaspoons each of lobelia herb and peppermint. Cover and steep for five minutes, and drink a cup every other day to strengthen the lungs. This is also good for bronchitis. Lobelia tincture, using a single dose of 30 drops during an attack or smaller doses of 15–20 drops three times a day is one of the major herbals for asthma and lung problems. Don't overdo the dose, as too much causes vomiting; it can also cause you to expectorate the phlegm from the lungs (which is positive and will end the attack). Ephedra (Ma-huang) is a powerful bronchodilator but also increases heart-rate; monitor this and also combine it with catnip to lessen the effect. Other asthma herbs include skunk cabbage, gingko biloba, asthma weed, licorice (can raise blood pressure), grindelia or sundew. Use Icelandic moss for children. Coltsfoot and mullein may be taken into the lungs by smoking.

Naturopathy: Children or adults with asthma need to have a diet that is as free of additives, chemicals, dyes and pollutants as possible. Start with a three-day fruit juice or vegetable juice fast, followed by a carrot mono diet (drinking only carrot juice and eating only raw carrots between meals, and meals of 3/4 cooked carrots and 1/4 cooked onions). Reintroduce other foods slowly, watching for allergy reactions and eliminate totally from the diet any foods that cause attacks. Watch for allergies to wheat/gluten, milk products, eggs, etc. The diet should totally exclude sugar, refined flour products, additives, alcohol, caffeine, smoking, and very hot or very cold foods. If the woman or child is hypoglycemic, more protein is needed than otherwise.

Bee pollen or raw comb honey is a major preventive of asthma attacks; start with a few granules and work up to a teaspoon a day. Some sources say that the pollen needs to be local and others do not. Chlorophyll, green drinks, wheatgrass juice or Kyo-green help to detoxify the body and are important. Aid calcium and mineral absorption by taking a glass of water containing a teaspoon of apple cider vinegar and a teaspoon of honey two or three times a day. Kelp adds minerals and iodine or try Atomidine. Glandular raw thymus and/or adrenal extract are helpful. Sources disagree on what foods or vegetables to use or avoid, and allergens vary from woman to woman. Try castor oil packs on the chest at night.

Homeopathy and Cell Salts: Use *Aconite* for attacks that occur after exposure to cold wind and that involve great fear. *Arsenicum album is* the remedy for attacks that improve with heat or warmth, come with great restlessness, anxiety and exhaustion, and usually between midnight and 2 AM. *Phosphorus* is the remedy when breathing is labored and wheezy. If there is a loud rattling cough and nausea or vomiting with attacks use *Ipecac. Kali carb.* is for attacks that occur between 3 and 5 AM. Homeopathic *Lobelia inflata* (6X) can also stop attacks in some women.

Cell Salts: Alternate *Ferrum phos.* and *Mag. phos.* every fifteen minutes to half hour during attacks and for three days after. Then use *Natrum sulph.* twice a day for four weeks, then *Calc. phos.* for another month. Use for children or adults, and particularly when weather changes bring on attacks.

Amino Acids: Take 500 mg of l-methionine with vitamins B-6 (50 mg) and C (500 mg) twice a day on an empty stomach.

Acupressure for Asthma
Points to Stop an Attack

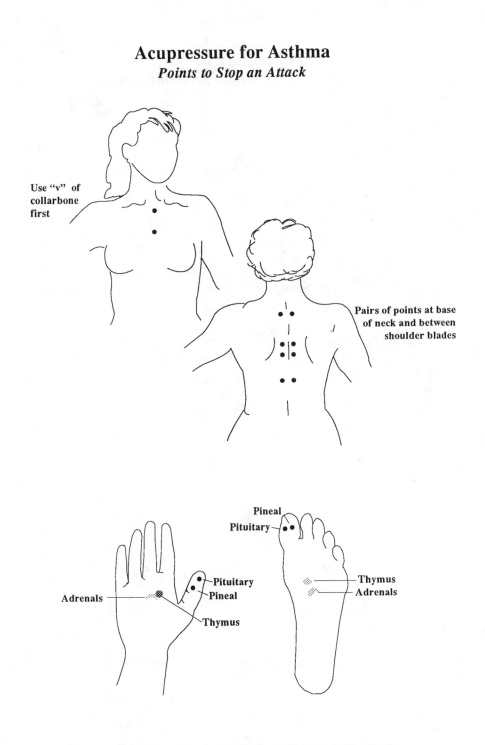

Use "v" of collarbone first

Pairs of points at base of neck and between shoulder blades

Pineal
Pituitary

Pituitary
Pineal

Adrenals

Thymus

Pineal
Pituitary

Thymus
Adrenals

Mildred Carter, *Body Reflexology* (W. Nyack, NY, Parker Publishing Co., 1983), p. 182-185.

Acupressure for Asthma
Points Used in Deep Breathing Release

Base of Thumbs

These points are in pairs, on both sides of the body.

Iona Marsaa Teeguarden, *Acupressure Way of Health: Jin Shin Do* (New York, Japan Publishing Co., 1978), p. 132.

Acupressure: Mildred Carter in *Body Reflexology* (Parker Publishing Co., 1983, p. 183) uses reflex points to stop most asthma attacks. The first is located in the V of the collarbone; place a finger there and pull down while pressing inward. Other points along the spine will be sore—look for them on the back between the spine and shoulder blades—but massaged and released will also stop an attack. She suggests they can be done alone by pressing your body against a doorframe. Next use the reflexes on the face (see illustration). There are acupressure points for the adrenal glands located in the centers of the palms and foot soles, and at the back of the hand behind the little finger and top of the foot and toe toward the wrist/ankle. Also work the pineal and pituitary gland points in the center pads of the thumbs and big toes.

For recurrent asthma, to prevent attacks, try the Jin Shin Do Deep Breathing Release from Iona Marsaa Teeguarden. See illustrations.

Aromatherapy: Use essential oils in baths, massage oils, compresses, diffusers or to directly inhale. Aromas include eucalyptus, cajeput, cypress, frankincense, lavender, myrrh, peppermint, rosemary, spruce, tea-tree or benzoin.

Flower Essences: Eucalyptus is for the connection between the lungs and emotions and useful for any breathing problems. Stinging nettles is a tonic for the lungs and nervous system, mineral assimilation, and emotional stress. Daisy helps shallow breathing.

Gemstones and Gem Essences: Opal or sulfur in essence heal the adrenals, and lapis lazuli, pyrite or blue tourmaline help the lungs. Hold or wear blue tourmaline, chrysocolla, turquoise or citrine.

Emotional Healing: You have not been allowed to express your feelings or emotions, and you feel stifled and smothered particularly by a parent. You need to cry, to express yourself in your own way, to come to terms with your real and individual emotional self. The fear may be of living; do you want to be here? Trust the process of life, and come out of childhood to your independent Be-ing.

Athlete's Foot
Fungus

This is a fungus infection that commonly appears on feet, scalp or around the fingernails, but can appear on other parts of the body, including genitals and skin folds. The symptoms are itching, burning, inflammation, blisters and scaling on top of calluses or dry patches of skin. Ringworm is a form of this, appearing as red round patches, usually on the scalp. Fungus thrives in warm wet places on the body or in the environment. It is contagious, and often brought home from swimming pool changing rooms. It also thrives in women who have taken a recent course of antibiotics, medicinal drugs or radiation therapy that destroy beneficial bacteria.[1]

Fungus-affected areas of the skin need to be kept very dry, even dried with a hair dryer after showers. Wear rubber gloves when washing dishes if hands are affected. For athlete's foot, wear sandals as much as possible to expose the feet to the air, and put a bit of cotton between the toes at night. When wearing closed shoes, wear socks with them and change them often. Wear shoes in public areas to prevent contagion to yourself and others.

Women who have fungal skin infections may also have systemic candida albicans. Read the information in that section.

Vitamins and Minerals: Adele Davis says that these infections are a direct result of B-complex deficiency, so along with a daily multiple vitamin and mineral supplement, try a B-complex-50 or -100 taken three times a day with meals. To replace healthy bowel flora, use acidophilus in the Megadophilus or Maxidophilus form, a teaspoon in water taken on an empty stomach twice daily. Zinc (50 mg daily) helps to clear the skin, aids healing and boosts the immune system. Vitamins A (25,000 IU) and E (400–800 IU per day) may also help, and dust vitamin C powder directly on the affected areas. If vitamin deficiencies are longterm, it may take some time to see results.

Herbs: Try one of these. Apply black walnut tincture directly to the fungus patches, and drink a tea of green crushed walnut hulls for fungus anywhere in the body. Use a strong tea of pau d'arco to drink and add

[1]James F. Balch, MD, and Phyllis A. Balch, CNC, *Prescription for Nutritional Healing* (Garden City Park, NY, Avery Publishing Group, 1990), p. 100.

twenty drops of Aerobic 07 (an oxygenator that functions as an antiseptic) to it for use externally. Use white oak bark, buchu tincture or tea-tree oil topically. Boil one cup of fresh clover blossoms with water until it thickens; when cool, dab it on affected areas nightly. For internal use, also try chaparral or the blood purifying herbs: burdock and red clover, sage, or raspberry. Use herbs internally and externally at the same time.

Naturopathy: Diet is important for clearing fungi of all types from the system. See the section on Candida Albicans in this book. The following remedies are probably the easiest and simplest and they work. Garlic is featured: take two Kyolic tablets three times a day internally, decreasing to two per day when all the infections are healed. With this, apply a raw crushed garlic clove to the affected area and leave it on for half an hour daily; dilute it with water if it burns. Dust your feet and shoes with garlic powder. Or:

Dab the affected areas with white vinegar two or three times a day; dilute with water if it burns. Also wash your socks in vinegar and let dry before wearing, and use vinegar to wipe the insides of your shoes. The acid kills fungus and bacteria.

If you are brave enough, urinate on your feet in the shower for athlete's foot. Or urinate into a jar and dilute by half with wine or white vinegar and apply with a cottonball. Antibodies are found in urine, a sterile liquid, that are individually made for fighting bacteria or fungus in your own body. Rinse with clear water afterwards. This method has a high success rate.

Onion juice can also be applied externally two or three times a day, or castor oil.

Homeopathy and Cell Salts: For simple fungus infection, with scaly patches that are dry or brownish, and with itching that turns to burning when scratched, *Sepia* is the remedy. *Arsenicum* is used when the skin is cracked or raw, and has a watery fluid that inflames what it touches. Try *Graphites* where the skin is dry, rough and cracked, or raw and crusted with a sticky honey-colored ooze. Use *Sulfur* if there is much itching, worsened by warmth, a first choice for athlete's foot.

Cell Salts: *Kali Mur.* 12X powder can be used alone or mixed with other dry remedies (like garlic powder) and dusted on the feet or body. Mix with carbolated vaseline or vegetable oil (try castor oil) for use on the scalp; rub on for twenty minutes, then wash hair and apply *Kali Mur.* powder when dry. Use internally as well.

Amino Acids: Use combination amino acids for rebuilding skin tissue and the immune system. Single aminos include cystine, leucine, isoleucine, valine or proline for the skin.

Acupressure for Athlete's Foot
Endocrine Balancing

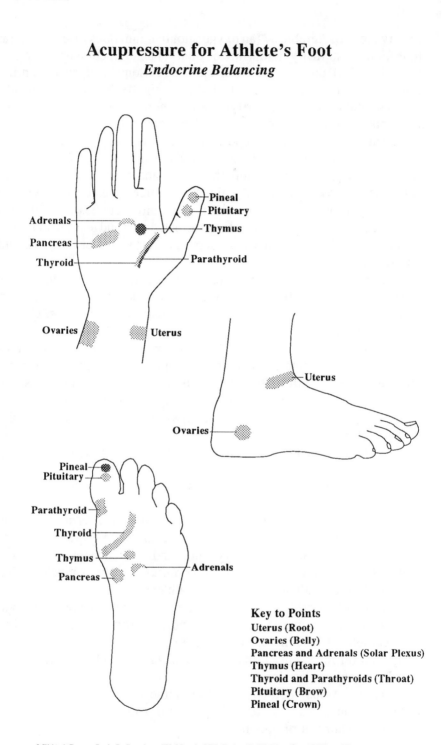

Adrenals
Pancreas
Thyroid

Pineal
Pituitary
Thymus
Parathyroid

Ovaries
Uterus

Uterus
Ovaries

Pineal
Pituitary
Parathyroid
Thyroid
Thymus
Pancreas
Adrenals

Key to Points
Uterus (Root)
Ovaries (Belly)
Pancreas and Adrenals (Solar Plexus)
Thymus (Heart)
Thyroid and Parathyroids (Throat)
Pituitary (Brow)
Pineal (Crown)

Mildred Carter, *Body Reflexology* (W. Nyack, NY, Parker Publishing Co., 1983), p. 30.

Acupressure: Do a full foot or hand acupressure massage session twice a week to stimulate the immune and endocrine systems; release any sore spots that you find. The endocrine glands correspond to the chakras. Do not press on broken, sore or cracked skin areas. Pay particular attention to the pituitary, thymus and solar plexus reflexes. Also use the Great Eliminator (LI 4) meridian point, in the webs between thumbs and first fingers of the hands (not for use in pregnancy). This balances the large intestine and helps the body to detoxify.

Aromatherapy: Use geranium essential oil in an olive oil base to massage the affected skin daily. For fungi around the nails, use crushed garlic in an olive oil base, fifty percent garlic. Dab tea-tree essential oil directly on the affected areas, or cedarwood or patchouli oils in olive oil.

Flower Essences: A flower essence of self-heal is used to cleanse the skin of toxins and regenerate skin tissue. Use it for external and internal wounds, bacterial or fungal infections, and to aid nutritional assimilation when wounds are healing.

Gemstones and Gem Essences: Use citrine in essence as well as held or worn. It is an antifungal and antibacterial and cleanses the body of toxins. Also hold or wear bloodstone.

Emotional Healing: Anything with the feet or legs is an inability to move forward, or to move forward easily or fast enough. With athlete's foot there is also frustration at not being accepted or understood. Try to be more understanding of yourself and others.

Back Pain

Half of all women experience back trouble at some time in their lives and one in ten lives with it chronically. Back problems come from injuries as children or adults, birth defects or birth traumas, car accidents, improper lifting, poor posture, high heeled shoes, arthritis or rheumatism, too soft mattresses, sports stresses or curvatures of the spine. Osteoporosis is discussed separately, and many more women are involved. Back pain can come from damaged or eroded discs, pressure on a nerve, subluxed or misaligned vertebrae, degenerative bone dis-eases, inflamed joints or muscle spasms. It can also be a sign of pelvic, kidney or bladder dis-ease, gallstones, gynecological disorders, or (rarely) cancer. Stress and the emotions play their part.

Manipulative therapies are the most successful for treating dis-eases of the spine. Osteopaths and chiropractors work wonders, and there are several types of gentle chiropractic therapies (applied kinesiology and directional nonforce chiropractic). Acupuncture works wonders, as does yoga and exercise tailored for the individual. Shiatsu, a form of acupressure massage, is highly helpful, along with neuromuscular massage. The remedies in this section are designed to work with manipulative therapies to relax muscles, reduce pain and stress, and rebuild the structures of the body from the inside.

Vitamins and Minerals are highly important in reducing back pain. With a multiple vitamin and mineral supplement, use a B-complex-50 to -100 twice a day and sublingual vitamin B-12 (2000 mcg) daily. Minerals are essential: take a complete calcium/magnesium supplement (200 mg calcium to 100 mg magnesium daily). A complete calcium will have small amounts with it of vitamins C, D, and A and zinc. You need 50 mg daily (total) of zinc and 3 mg of boron (stop boron when healed, unless over age fifty). Manganese helps in healing cartilage in the neck and back. Use at least 3000 mg (three grams) of vitamin C daily to ease pain and for tissue repair. Vitamins A, D and E are also important. Use germanium for pain (calcium/magnesium is also a pain reliever and muscle relaxant). For disc problems, vitamin C is important, along with vitamin E and a high protein (amino acids) diet. For sciatica, the focus is on B-complex and protein.

Herbs: Horsetail grass is an herb that aids in calcium uptake and contains silicon. Alfalfa is also important as a nutrient for minerals. Several herbs are helpful for pain relief, including feverfew, scullcap, valerian or hops. Make a tea of scullcap, valerian and catnip, or use tinctures of feverfew and scullcap together. These are relaxants to use before sleep. The mix for arthritis is also helpful—alfalfa, burdock and white willow—or try a tea of boston ivy or elderberry two or three times a day.

Naturopathy: Drink potato juice or celery juice for sciatica, and make sure you are drinking at least three glasses of water a day plus other beverages. Use a poultice of horseradish or bacon fat (but avoid eating meat), or castor oil packs, and rub castor oil on pain areas. Moist wet heat, from a thermaphore, hydroculator (commercially available wet-heat aids), or hot washcloth can help immensely, as can hot baths with epsom salts.

Homeopathy and Cell Salts: Arnica Gel used externally is helpful (as are Tiger Balm or Sunbreeze ointments, but these will antidote homeopathic remedies). Internally, use *Arnica montana* for pain resulting

AIDS

Acquired Immune Deficiency Syndrome ~ HIV

AIDS or HIV (Human Immune Deficiency Virus) is the dis-ease that no one wants to talk about in the American mainstream. Once called the "gay plague" here, in other nations it has primarily been a dis-ease of women and children and is rapidly becoming so in the United States. There is almost no point in printing statistics—the numbers are increasing at frightening speeds, but whole populations in Africa, Asia and India are being wiped out by AIDS[1], and the dis-ease is a real threat for depopulating much of the earth. AIDS is the tragedy of our time, with politicians fighting over research money and patients desperate for the (maybe) life-saving drugs the FDA doesn't want to release or allow into this country. Many people who need AIDS medications or hospitalizations can't afford them, and there is shamefully little home help for AIDS patients too debilitated to care for themselves or AIDS infants whose mothers have died. That the women and children infected with AIDS are primarily nonwhite has added to the neglect. That many of the women were partners of intravenous drug-users or users themselves has left them alone in "moral" America.

Where AIDS came from to begin with is still under controversy or coverup. That AIDS came through—it did not come from—the gay male population in this country has added to the unnecessary and painful homophobia of an increasingly right-wing nation, and has complicated efforts to do research and provide care for AIDS sufferers. That the next AIDS populations were drug-users did little to change that attitude, and now the greatest increases have been among women and children— another population the patriarchy systemically ignores, particularly when nonwhite. AIDS treatment in this country is also a mixed blessing, involving drugs that are highly toxic and cause as much misery as they purport to alleviate. Holistic methods may or may not cure AIDS, but they

[1]There will be 15,000,000 HIV adults by 1995 worldwide, says National Public Radio News (June 22, 1991).

from bruises, blows or overexertion. *Bryonia alba* is used for pain and stiffness at the nape of the neck or small of the back. *Cocculus indicus* is used at the start of lower back trouble, where there is paralytic pain and shoulders and arms feel bruised. *Colocynthis* is for drawing, tearing sciatic pain on the left side, made worse by gentle touch but better by pressure and heat. Use *Rhus tox.* for pain while sitting or lying down, as if bruised. The pain is relieved by lying on a hard surface, by warmth and exercise, and made worse by night and by cold, damp weather. This is especially good for sciatica.

Cell Salts: The major one here is *Mag. phos.*, for shooting, boring and cramping pains, involving muscles, bones or nerves. *Silica* is for pain in the limbs and coccyx, weak backs, and irritation after spinal injury. Some women with the symptoms of shifting pains in the legs will respond to *Kali sulph.* See also the cell salt remedies for Arthritis.

Amino Acids: Protein is important for relieving back pain, so use a combination amino acids, either free-form or liver-based. Individual aminos include DL-phenylalanine, tryptophan and methionine. Methionine is particularly important for disc problems, phenylalanine is an analgesic for pain, and tryptophan is a relaxant.

Acupressure can be extremely helpful for pain relief and releasing muscle spasms. See the acupressure positions for sciatica and knee pain under Arthritis, as well as the positions for arms and shoulders there. In foot reflexology, the inner edges of both feet running from the big toes to the heels contain the seiketsu for the spinal column. If your back pain is at the shoulders or neck, the tender spots will be closer to the big toe; if your pain is in the lower back or sciatica, the tender points will be low toward or in the heels. Acupressure points for the sciatic nerve are located at the heels of the feet on the bottoms and in the pads at the back. Sore spots along the spinal map can be very sore; don't try to release years of pain in one session, but work for a few moments on each spot, then go to the next one. Work twice a week at first, then daily if you go gently.

On the body map, use the positions for arthritis, as well as those pictured. Feel along the meridians for tender spots, and use pressure to release them. Also, see the Neck Release sequence in *All Women Are Healers* (p. 94). Do not press directly on the spine—the points are beside it, in muscle.

Aromatherapy for back pain includes using a poultice of thyme essence for sciatica, or marjoram and thyme in olive oil as a liniment. Also try lavender or chamomile. Dandelion in olive oil makes a wonderful pain-relieving massage oil, and is highly   recommended. Use rosemary, marjoram, chamomile, birch, clove, nutmeg or bay in compresses, baths

Acupressure Points for Back Pain

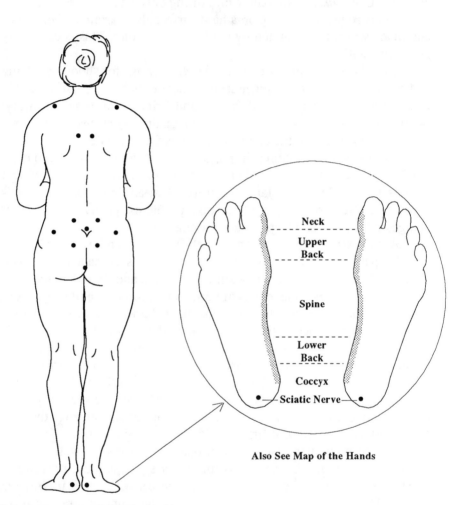

Neck

Upper
Back

Spine

Lower
Back

Coccyx

Sciatic Nerve

Also See Map of the Hands

Body Acupressure (from the back)

Mildred Carter, *Body Reflexology* (W. Nyack, NY, Parker Publishing Co., 1983), p. 33, 112-115; Cathryn Bauer, *Acupressure for Women* (Freedom, CA, The Crossing Press, 1987), p. 65.

or massage oils. Tiferet-Lifetree has aroma combinations for deep joint relief and for pain.

Flower Essences: Lilac is for spinal column inflammations, spinal fluid and nerves, and for vertebrae alignment. Dandelion essence is for pain, a muscle relaxant, and aids mineral absorption, and comfrey is for muscular and nerve regeneration. Also use ginseng, grapefruit, squash, hyssop, peach, pear or blackberry blossom.

Gemstones and Gem Essences: Try chrysocolla, lapis lazuli, carnelian, rose quartz, black tourmaline or emerald in gem essence. Hold or wear amazonite for the skeletal system and for mineral absorption, and kunzite or boji stone for pain.

Emotional Healing: The spine is the foundation of the body. If it is weak, perhaps your foundations are weak. How's your relationship? Are you moving forward in your life purpose? Is your homelife stable? Upper back pain is from feeling unloved or holding back on giving love, and a lack of emotional support. Middle back pain is guilt, or things you have put behind you that need processing and releasing. What (or who) do you need to get off your back? Lower back trouble can be financial support issues, and for women is often nonsupportive or broken relationships, even old ones long over. Try to be less of a perfectionist, and stop carrying the world or other people on your shoulders. Neck pain is flexibility issues, or something (or someone) that's a pain in the neck.

Blood Cleansing

Naturopaths believe that dis-ease results from toxins that build up in the body, in organs, blood, tissues and cells. These come from poor nutrition, junk foods, pollutants, refined sugar or flour, stress, and harmful substances like alcohol, caffeine, smoking, and medical or street drugs, as well as from unhealthful living habits such as not enough sleep or exercise. Underactive glands can also cause a toxin buildup and sluggish digestion or elimination. The kidneys and bladder, liver, spleen, lungs, skin and intestines are organs of toxin elimination that sometimes need stimulation. If you experience recurrent infections or colds, boils, skin eruptions or skin dis-eases, sinus problems, herpes, bad breath or body odor, blood cleansing methods are indicated. If you have bladder infections, frequent constipation, or menstrual or menopause difficulties, you may also benefit. Toxin accumulation can be a factor in mental and nervous disorder as well, particularly in depression.

A blood cleansing program usually starts with a three-day (or longer supervised) fruit juice fast using one of the red juices (cherry, cranberry, beet, grape, blackberry or red cabbage), or a vegetable juice or raw vegetable fast. Enemas are used to help the bowels remove the releasing toxins quickly and to prevent or remedy constipation. Constipation itself is a major cause of toxin buildup. Almost any dis-ease can benefit from blood cleansing herbs or methods. Blood cleansing differs from liver detoxification in that liver detox focuses on chemical or heavy metal pollution or poisoning, and recovery from alcohol or drug abuse, as well as quitting smoking. Liver detox aids in withdrawal and speeds up the recovery process.

Vitamins and Minerals: These for blood cleansing take a back seat to herbs and fasts. Along with a multiple vitamin and mineral supplement, try megadoses of vitamin C, 3000–10,000 mg per day or to bowel tolerance. Vitamins A and E are antioxidants and helpful here, about 25,000 IU of A and 800 IU of vitamin E. Zinc is important, up to a total of 100 mg (not over) per day. Use a calcium/magnesium supplement.

Herbs: Burdock and red clover together, or other red clover cleansing combinations are primary, but can sometimes be harsh. More blood cleansing herbs include nettles, sage, elder flowers, alfalfa, Oregon grape root or devil's claw. Most blood cleansing programs include at least one herbal antibiotic—echinacea, pau d'arco, yellow dock (for the liver), chaparral or goldenseal. Teas of parsley, chamomile, dandelion or yarrow are also positive.

Naturopathy: Begin with a three-day fast, and daily enemas. Use a coffee enema on the first day, a dandelion enema on the second day, and a clear water enema on the third day. Here are Joy Gardner's recipes for coffee and dandelion enemas (from *The New Healing Yourself*, p. 239–241). For a coffee enema, bring three cups of water to a boil and add three heaping tablespoons of drip grind (not instant) caffeinated coffee. Boil for three minutes, then simmer for fifteen minutes. Strain, add enough cool water to bring it up to a quart of liquid, and place it in the enema bag. For a dandelion root enema, bring a quart to water of a boil, add four teaspoons of dandelion root and simmer for twenty minutes. Strain, and pour into the enema bag. Colonics are also helpful, during or outside of fasting.

After the fruit or vegetable juice fast, gradually return to solid food with a raw vegetable diet, using vegetables, vegetable juices, seaweed, sprouts, seeds and grains, and some fruit. When the condition is cleared, broaden the diet but still avoid sugar, salt, refined flour, dairy products, saturated fats, meat, junk foods, caffeine, alcohol and smoking.

Baths containing a cup of baking soda and a cup of sea salt make good cleansers. Use the water as hot as you can be comfortable in, cover as much of yourself as possible, and stay in the water for twenty-five minutes. You may feel ill for a few minutes as toxins release, but stay in the bath. It will pass. The clear water will turn cloudy or grey. At the end of the time, pat dry (no need to rinse off), and go to bed for an hour or two to sweat off the rest of the toxins. You will feel drained when you leave the tub, but clear, exhilarated and good an hour later.

Garlic, kelp and alfalfa are important aids to any detox or blood cleansing program. Use four to six Kyolic tablets a day, four alfalfa tablets, and six to eight kelp tablets with meals. Do not take tablets or capsules while fasting.

Homeopathy and Cell Salts: Check the remedies for your individual dis-ease (colds, sinus, boils, skin problems, etc.). See Cummings and Ullman, *Everybody's Guide to Homeopathic Medicines* (J. P. Tarcher's, 1984) or Boericke and Tafel's, *Family Guide to Self-Medication* (Homeopathic).

Cell Salts: *Silica* is for blood, skin, hair, nails and mucous membranes, for poor assimilation of food, acne, boils, brittle nails, and excessive perspiration with offensive odor. Use *Kali sulph.* for eczema, dandruff and itchy, scaly skin. Use *Calc. sulph.* for skin eruptions, boils, pimples, and eczema. *Natrum mur.* is the choice for colds, constipation or runny diarrhea. *Combination Cell Salts* (Bioplasma) is positive to cleanse, balance and nutritionalize all the systems of the body.

Amino Acids: These are helpful in blood cleansing because of their sulfur content and action as antioxidants. Use a combination free-form amino acids, or cysteine by itself. Methionine and arginine are also positive. Arginine is used only with lysine, and should not be used at all by women with herpes.

Acupressure: Concentrate on immune building and endocrine balancing pressure points. Do a full foot acupressure massage twice a week to balance all the glands and systems, increasing the frequency of sessions gradually to twice a day. Use a foot massage roller for this, if you wish, building up to ten minutes twice a day gradually. See the endocrine pressure points for hands and feet under Athlete's Foot or Immune System Dis-eases. Also work the lymphatic points at the tops and sides of the feet and sides of the hands. Work the Great Eliminator reflex in the webs between thumbs and first fingers (not in pregnancy). It stimulates the autonomic nervous system.

Acupressure for Blood Cleansing

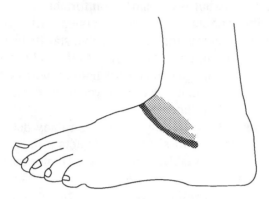

Lymph Glands on both feet

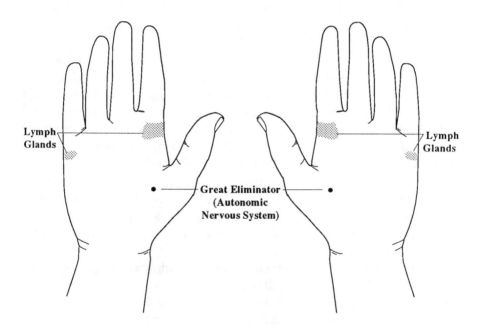

Lymph
Glands

Lymph
Glands

Great Eliminator
(Autonomic
Nervous System)

Also see endocrine gland positions under Athletes Foot

Moshe Olshevsky, CA, PhD., *et. al.*, *The Manual of Natural Therapy* (New York, Citadel Press, 1989), p. 9-11 charts.

Aromatherapy: Use essential oils in baths or massage oils, as compresses or body wraps. Use angelica, birch, cardamom, yarrow, caraway, lovage, juniper or fennel.

Flower Essences: Avocado, chaparral, sage, spruce or jasmine are essences for cleansing the physical and nonphysical bodies. Use avocado in particular for blood cleansing.

Gemstones and Gem Essences: Moss agate, calcite, peridot, diamond, herkimer diamond, eilat stone, lapis lazuli or moonstone are all positive as cleansing essence. Hold or wear citrine or bloodstone.

Emotional Healing: There comes a time for the old or negative to be cleansed away so new ideas and patterns can emerge. Use the blood cleansing process in this way, eliminating what doesn't work emotionally and changing to new patterns that do. Decide what you want to banish from your life, and do a ritual on it of banishing and invoking. Decide what you want to institute in its place—the universe allows no vacuums—and bring these into your life now. The New Moon is a good time to start, or the ending moon and continuing into the new moon. Another good time is New Year's Eve.

Boils

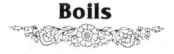

Boils or abscesses, particularly recurrent ones, are a sign that blood or liver cleansing and immune system building are acutely needed. They can come incidentally as infected hair follicle or local irritation, or as staph infections likely to recur, and indications for the serious blood cleansing methods of the previous section. Chronic constipation, which results in a buildup of toxins in the body, may be a factor or cause. Other causes include food or airborne allergies, stress, poor hygiene, bacterial dis-ease, certain drugs, a junk food diet, wound infection, thyroid dis-ease or diabetes. If you are diabetic, boils may be a sign of elevated blood sugar levels. Glandular disturbances also play a part.

The Typical American Diet, high in white sugar, refined flour and saturated fats, is much implicated in boils (as well as in acne, where several conditions are similar). Overconsumption of meat, pork, eggs, milk and dairy products contribute to the toxicity that leads to boil formation, along with a deficiency in the essential fatty acids. A vegetable juice fast, followed by a raw vegetable diet are positive in releasing the toxins and rebalancing the body.

Boils appear suddenly, after itching, mild pain and local swelling. They are round, tender and pus-filled, and last from ten to twenty-five days. Boils usually appear on the face, scalp, buttocks or underarms. Swelling of nearby lymph glands can occur. There are many holistic ways to heal boils quickly.

Vitamins and Minerals: Along with a daily multiple vitamin and mineral supplement, use vitamin A up to 50,000 IU per day for two to four weeks, cutting down to 25,000 IU per day after. Use dry form A if possible. Use a B-complex-50 three times a day, vitamin C (3000-10,000 mg or 3-10 grams), and vitamin E (800 IU per day). Vitamins A or E may also be used directly on the boil. These are all intended for immune system building, and focus on antioxidants for blood and liver cleansing. A highly important mineral to use is zinc (50 mg) three times a day until healed, then 15-50 mg per day after. Coenzyme Q10 or germanium are positive for immune system building and are superior antioxidants. Try evening primrose or black currant oil, as boils may be an EFA deficiency (essential fatty acids).

Herbs: Horsetail grass (silica) or oat straw tea are positive for reducing inflammation, and echinacea tincture is an antibiotic. Use burdock and red clover together in tincture as a blood cleanser, and Oregon grape root or birch tree bark are good cleansers for skin dis-eases. Pau d'arco, goldenseal or chaparral are other herbal antibiotics, but echinacea will usually do the job. When using echinacea, you must stay on it for a minimum of ten days or symptoms will return.

Moist hot compresses or poultices help, including herb poultice choices of: chamomile, plantain, dandelion, burdock, comfrey or calendula, or lobelia and mullein together. A hot black teabag placed on the boil will draw out pus. Use a hot poultice of slippery elm powder made into a paste until the pus is drained, then use it as a cold poultice until the skin is healed.

Naturopathy recommends other poultices, but primary treatment is in cleansing fasts. See the information on Blood Cleansing, and switch to a healthy diet.

Poultices or compress choices are: castor oil, boric acid, tea-tree oil, roast onions, cooked mashed garlic, an oven-heated lemon slice, a fig slice, honey, a slice of pumpkin, finely chopped cabbage or the skin of a hard boiled egg. After the boil breaks, clean the area with two tablespoons of lemon juice in a cup of boiled water, and use twice a day as a compress.

To boost the immune system use Kyolic tablets, about six per day, chlorophyll from alfalfa or wheatgrass to clean the bloodstream, or kelp tablets for balanced minerals. Propolis is an important immune system builder, and glandular extracts may also be important: use raw thymus (500 mg daily) or raw spleen extract. Oil of Bitter Orange is a remedy for staph infections. Take four drops in orange juice three times a day until two or three days after symptoms are gone. This usually works in three to seven days.

Homeopathy and Cell Salts: Use *Belladonna* in the early stages before pus forms; the skin will be painful, red and hot. This will stop the process in many cases. After twenty-four hours or if Belladonna hasn't helped, try *Hepar sulph.* if the forming boil is very painful and tender to the slightest touch, sensitive to cold, and with sharp, sticking or throbbing pains. *Mercurius* is the remedy to use once pus has formed. Use *Arsenicum* at any stage if there is burning pain, relieved by warm applications, or *Lachesis* if the area is bluish or purplish, pus is dark and thin, and the boil is tender—discontinue Lachesis as soon as improvement is noted.

Cell Salts: *Ferrum phos.* is used in the first stages of any dis-ease, including boils. Use *Kali mur.* before pus has formed and *Silica* once the boil bursts to speed discharge and healing. Use *Silica* also for boils that come on slowly without pus development, and for cyst-like lumps that remain under the skin after a boil has mostly healed. *Nat. sulph.* is the cell salt for chronic boil conditions.

Amino Acids: These are important in boosting the immune system, for their sulfur content and antioxidant properties. Use a combination free-form amino acids. Single aminos include cysteine, methionine or arginine.

Acupressure: Do a full foot massage twice weekly, and increase gradually to twice a day. Use a foot massage roller ten minutes a day, if you wish, and pay attention to releasing any points that seem tender or congested. Also pay particular attention to the endocrine gland pressure points (see Immune System Dis-eases), and to the lymphatic gland points (see Blood Cleansing section). Use the Great Eliminator point in the web between thumbs and first fingers.

The illustration shows an applied kinesiology sequence (from *Touch for Health*) that strengthens the kidneys and spleen for toxin elimination. If help is available, hold the calf and wrist points simultaneously, and when they are released, hold the two foot points simultaneously. Work the points, which will be tender, until they stop hurting. If you are working alone, release the calf and wrist points before doing the ones on the foot.

Acupressure for Boils

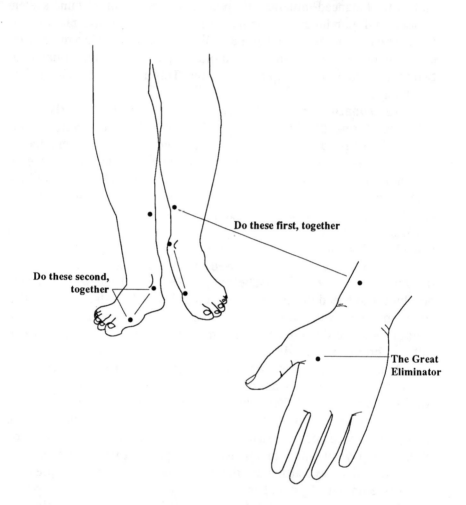

Do these first, together

Do these second, together

The Great Eliminator

These stimulate the blood cleansing and eliminative organs, the kidneys and spleen. Do the points on wrist and calf first.

John Thie, DC, *A Touch for Health, A New Approach to Restoring Our Natural Energies* (Marina del Rey, CA, DeVorss and Co., 1973), p. 64.

Aromatherapy uses essential oils primarily as compresses, but in a diffuser they will aid the immune system. For immune and antiseptic properties use lavender, tea-tree or thyme. Everlasting is an anti-inflammatory, and chamomile is for pain. Thyme or tea-tree make particularly good compresses, and rosemary is for skin rejuvenation and healing.

Flower Essences: Use luffa to regenerate the skin in ulceration or skin dis-eases. Mallow is for the endocrine system and reduces toxemia for skin healing. Amaranthus is used to boost the immune system and repel bacterial inflammations. Jasmine relieves mucus from the digestive system, detoxifies and reduces inflammations.

Gemstones and Gem Essences: Emerald, jade, citrine, ruby, rutilated quartz or amethyst essences help to boost the immune system. Emerald is particularly helpful in removing toxins from the body. Malachite, obsidian, petrified wood or ruby are blood-cleansing essences for infections. Also hold or wear a piece of bloodstone or citrine (natural citrine, not heat-treated amethyst).

Emotional Healing: Boils are anger to the boiling point, boiling over and seething. Find safe ways to release it, instead of bottling it up inside until it boils its way out. The part of the body the boil appears on may also be suggestive. If it's on the buttocks, who or what in your life is a pain in the ass?

Breast Lumps

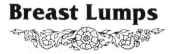

Fifty percent of women will discover a breast lump at some time in their lives, and fifty to seventy percent of women have fibrocystic breasts. With that high a figure, it is difficult to call fibrous breasts a dis-ease. I would consider it, rather, a condition common to women in modern American society and/or an environmental or nutritional pollution symptom. Breast lumps seem to occur under three primary factors: over-estrogen production in the body of a menstruation-age woman, over-ingestion of unsaturated fats in the diet, and use of high amounts of caffeine. Over-production of estrogen and the problem with fats can possibly be traced to the hormones fed to meat and dairy animals, and also to poultry. These pollutant residues remain in the flesh and are concentrated in the fats (including milk fats) that are ingested by meat and dairy eating women.

A vegetarian or organic diet, especially one free of milk products, is sometimes enough to cause breast lumps to disappear by themselves. Stopping coffee, tea, chocolate and colas—all high in caffeine—is enough to change the fibrous breast conditions of many women by itself. Decaffeinated coffee does not seem to cause this condition.

It is normal for women's breasts to feel a little lumpy, particularly around menstruation. Benign breast lumps and cystic breasts may fluctuate with the menstrual cycle but some lumps may also grow quite large. They are fluid-filled and move freely under the skin like an eye under the eyelid; they are tender and may be painful. New cysts rarely form after menopause, and eighty percent of breast lumps are benign. A malignant lump has different symptoms: it does not move freely, is not tender, and does not fluctuate in size or go away. I have had good results in helping women with breast lumps or fibrocystic breasts, using holistic methods and diet change. Begin by stopping caffeine and milk products, eating a diet low in saturated fats, and switching to either vegetarianism or organic meats and poultry. Avoid alcohol and cigarettes.

Vitamins and Minerals: Along with a multiple vitamin and mineral supplement, add a B-complex-50 to the diet to make sure there is enough folic acid and vitamin B-6 nutritionally available. More B-6, up to 200 mg per day, is helpful for hormone balancing, especially if there are menstrual problems along with the breast lumps. Vitamin E is of highest importance in reducing cystic breasts and lumps; use 1000 IU per day in gradual increases for a month, then 600–800 IU per day (use dry form). This alone may correct the condition within a few weeks. Evening Primrose Oil (gamma linolenic acid, essential fatty acids), two capsules three times a day, is a hormone balancer that may also change the condition without other help. Coenzyme Q10 is a powerful antioxidant, along with vitamin E, and may be helpful as well.

Herbs: A tea of one ounce red clover and one ounce blue violet leaf to a pint of water will cleanse the system and dissolve most breast lumps (and uterine or ovarian fibroids). Drink a pint of this daily over several months. These can be used as tinctures also and the herbs can be eaten fresh. Squaw vine or black cohosh herbs are also helpful, as well as mullein, pokeroot or witchhazel as an external poultice. Other suggested herbs are echinacea, goldenseal, blessed thistle, ho shou wu, pau d'arco or pokeroot. Dandelion is listed by some sources as a cancer preventive; use it internally and externally. For ovarian cysts, make a strong tea of raspberry leaf, black currant leaf, witchhazel leaf and powdered myrrh. Strain and mix one cup of this with a cup of cooled boiled water and use as a nightly douche.

Naturopathy: Eat a high fiber, mostly raw foods diet with vegetarian protein to avoid the meat and poultry hormones; avoid saturated fats, dairy, caffeine, smoking and alcohol. Use castor oil packs at least three nights a week; see the Naturopathy methods section for directions. Other poultices to try are Black Ointment, or licorice stick and flaxseed simmered together into a paste. Flaxseed oil taken internally (1–1-1/2 tablespoons per day) is another essential fatty acid. Kelp tablets are an important remedy that can reduce breast lumps and fibroids quickly, as iodine deficiency seems to be a factor in their formation. An alternate way to use this is in the Edgar Cayce remedy Atomidine; follow the directions on the bottle. Bee pollen taken internally is a hormone balancer and may prevent or delay the appearance of malignancies. Coffee enemas, especially with a fast, are helpful, though ingested coffee may be the cause of the lumps.

Homeopathy and Cell Salts: See an experienced homeopath for this one, but here are some possibilities. *Conium* is a remedy for enlarged breasts with hard lumps, painful during and before periods, and with stitching pains. *Calcarea carb.* is for sore, hot swelling in breasts, with many fears and anxieties; it is a remedy for fatty tumors. Use *Belladonna* when breasts are sore, swollen and inflamed, or dry and stony hard and tender. There is heat, redness, throbbing or burning. For uterine fibroids, one remedy is *Calcarea iodata*.

Cell Salts: *Calc. sulph.* is the remedy for cystic tumors or fibroids. Use *Kali mur.* for all dis-eases with swelling. *Silica* is the remedy for cyst-like lumps under the skin, or a swollen, hard, inflamed breast that is sensitive and has burning pain.

Amino Acids: Use a combination free-form amino acids. Single aminos recommended for breast lumps and cystic breasts are methionine, glutathione, and arginine (use with lysine; avoid if you have herpes).

Acupressure: Do full foot acupressure, releasing sore spots—you will find them at the base of the toes. Try the Female Regulating Release from Iona Marssa Teeguarden (*Acupressure Way of Health: Jin Shin Do*, Japan Publications, 1978). See the illustration. The sequence is to balance women's hormones and promote overall good health. Use it also for menstrual imbalances.

Aromatherapy: Scents include melissa, jasmine, rose and rosewood, all for cell regeneration and women's hormones, as well as for women's emotional well-being. Use any of these in baths or massage oils, or slightly diluted as breast compresses. Rose is highly expensive but considered a panacea for all women's dis-eases.

Flower Essences: These include almond and chaparral for the immune and endocrine systems; almond is also for cell regeneration and fear states, and chaparral is for all cysts and tumors. Use hawthorne for cysts and tumors, and pomegranate for all women's issues, both physical and emotional. Pomegranate particularly helps women with nurturing issues.

Acupressure for Breast Lumps

Points Used in Female Regulating Release

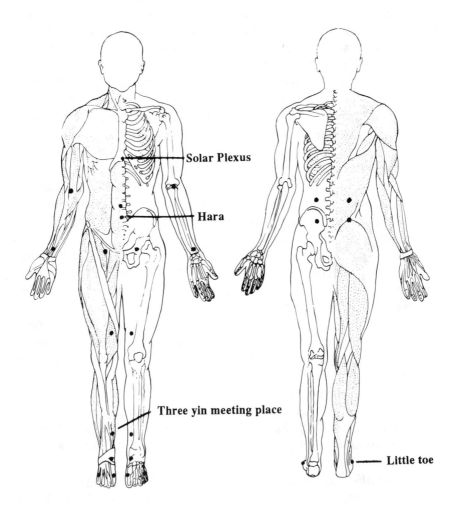

Solar Plexus

Hara

Three yin meeting place

Little toe

Positions are on both sides of the body, and running down the center line on the front. This is a general balancing sequence for women's organs and hormones.

Iona Marsaa Teeguarden, *Acupressure Way of Health: Jin Shin Do* (New York, Japan Publishing Co., 1978), p. 138.

Gemstones and Gem Essences: Use malachite-azurite essence for abnormal cell growth and the metal silver in essence for cysts; beryl, herkimer diamond, kunzite, lapis lazuli, pink tourmaline or moonstone are also positive. These are all women's stones. Try holding an elestial quartz, pink tourmaline or gem rhodochrosite, or wearing one of these on the body.

Emotional Healing: Dis-ease of the breasts is centered in women's need to nurture and be nurtured. Are you in need of receiving (or overneeding to give) mothering, protecting or nourishment? Are you overbearing in your mothering of others, or putting up with someone who is overbearing or overprotective toward you?

Today's attitudes focus on selfishness, telling women who are caring and nurturing that they are codependent and in need of therapy. Nurturing and caring in balance are positive attitudes, whatever the psychology and twelve-step industry say to the contrary. As long as nurturing is not at the expense of one's own needs or manipulative (overbearing) of others, validate its positivity and your right to be who you are. Remember always, and most importantly, to nurture yourself.

Burns

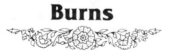

Burns are common kitchen injuries, but can also happen anywhere there is heat, open fires, hot liquid, chemicals or electricity. Sunburn is also a burn and treated as such. There are four classifications of burns, of increasing seriousness. First degree burns involve only the outer layer of the skin; the skin is pink and pressure makes a white spot. With quick treatment, blisters may be prevented. Second degree burns include redness and blisters; the outer two layers of skin are involved, plus hair follicles and skin glands. The blister may scar on healing, should not be broken, and cleanliness is important. Third degree burns involve the entire skin thickness and muscle tissue or a large body area, and medical help is needed. These burns are painless, the nerve endings having been destroyed. There may be oozing, or in extreme cases (fourth degree burns)

white or black charred flesh and dryness. Third and fourth degree burns are serious health threats, with risk of shock, bacterial infection, significant scarring, and loss of muscle function. First and second degree burns respond easily to home healing, and holistic methods help more serious burns significantly.

Immediate essential first aid for all burns is to submerge the burned area in cold water and keep it there for at least ten minutes. This prevents blistering in less serious burns, and lessens tissue damage in more severe ones. Do not put oils or salves on burns, cover or bandage them, or break blisters. If you are burned with hot liquids or chemicals, pull off all wet clothing.

Vitamins and Minerals: After soaking in cold water, pierce a vitamin E capsule with a pin and apply it to the burn every one to four hours. Take vitamin E internally also, (800–1600 IU per day) to prevent scars and speed healing in all burn degrees. Between applications of vitamin E, spray a one to three percent solution of vitamin C and distilled water on the burn, and take vitamin C internally (1000 mg per hour). This reduces pain, swelling and chance of infection, and speeds healing. Vitamin C is used intravenously for severe burns, and in megadoses.[1] Take by mouth, go to bowel tolerance, and decrease slowly after the crisis.

Potassium is important in burn healing take up to 100 mg per day (but not over). Zinc helps tissue repair—use 50–100 mg per day. Vitamin A is helpful for wound healing—use 50,000 IU per day (dry form) for one month, then decrease to 20,000–25,000 IU. Selenium aids tissue regeneration and helps pain, and coenzyme Q10 or germanium is also good for pain relief. Essential fatty acids are recommended, as linseed or evening primrose oil, two to four capsules three times a day. In second or third degree burns, use raw adrenal glandulars, one tablet three times a day. B-complex is good for stress.

Herbs: Aloe vera for burns is many women's first knowledge of herbal healing. Use it alone or mixed with vitamin E, honey or propolis, and use it internally and externally. Use poultices of comfrey alone, or comfrey with wheatgrass, or comfrey with wheat germ oil, vitamin E oil and honey. Honey and calendula also makes a good external burn poultice, as does honey, propolis and zinc, or honey, comfrey and calendula. Vitamin E oil on the gauze keeps the poultice from sticking. Take a half teaspoon of cayenne tincture for shock, or a quarter teaspoon cayenne herb in a glass of water (drink in sips).

Naturopathy: Calendula cerate ointment is a favorite of naturopaths and homeopaths for burn healing, and chlorophyll ointment is also used on

---

[1]Dr. Ross Trattler, *Better Health Through Natural Healing* (New York, McGraw-Hill Publishers, 1985), p. 145.

burns. Make a compress of diluted lemon juice (one part juice to three parts distilled water), or undiluted apple cider vinegar, and apply to burns on a sterile gauze pad. Witchhazel or bicarbonate of soda diluted in water is also used, or castor oil or olive oil. Try a poultice of an onion slice sprinkled with salt or of Redmond clay to draw out inflammation and prevent infection. Many of the poultices described under herbs are also used by naturopaths.

Homeopathy and Cell Salts: Use *Arnica montana* if there is fear or shock, or *Aconite* if the woman thinks she is dying (the injury does not have to be serious for this emotion to occur). Use *Urtica urens* for stinging burns, usually first or second degree, and calendula tincture or ointment externally. Hypericum tincture can be used externally after blisters form for second degree burns; apply it without breaking the blisters, and use *Cantharis* or *Urtica urens* internally. Use calendula tincture after the blisters break, diluted with water, two or three times a day. For third degree burns, use *Cantharis* internally, but only use external calendula after healing has begun. For electrical burns, the remedy is *Phosphorus*, taken two or three times a day for several days. If the burn is a scald accompanied by pain in sinews and tendons, use *Ruta graveolens* internally.

Homeopathic physician Cindy Brown, MD, uses the following protocol for burns:

First Degree:	Calendula tincture or lotion topically, and *Urtica urens* internally every few hours for pain.
Second Degree:	Hypericum tincture or Urtica urens tincture topically, taking care not to break blisters. Calendula tincture topically after blisters break, and *Cantharis*, *Causticum* or *Urtica urens* internally for relief.
Third Degree:	No topical applications, except during the latter part of the healing process to reduce the chance of scarring. *Cantharis* internally for pain.[2]

Cell Salts: Apply *Kali mur.* as a paste (made with water or vitamin E oil) to first or second degree burns.

Amino Acids: Protein is important for burn healing and skin and tissue repair. A combination free-form amino acids capsule is recommended. Cystine is a single amino helpful in burn healing.

[2]Cindy Brown, MD, Personal Communication, August 12, 1991.

Acupressure for Burns

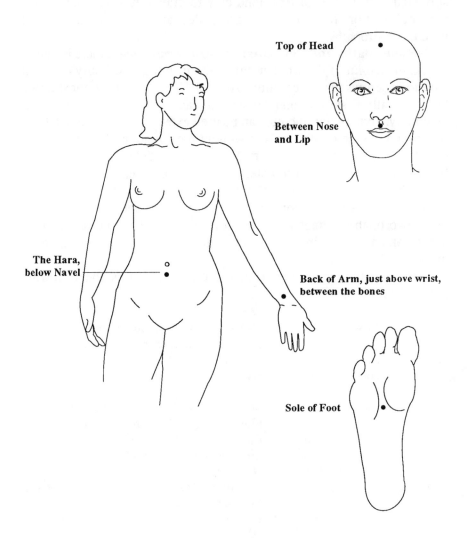

Top of Head

Between Nose
and Lip

The Hara,
below Navel

Back of Arm, just above wrist,
between the bones

Sole of Foot

These points are specifically for treating shock as a result of burns.

Iona Marsaa Teeguarden, *Acupressure Way of Health: Jin Shin Do* (New York, Japan Publishing Co.,
1978), p. 153.

Acupressure: Shock is a complication of more serious burns and can be serious or even fatal. Use pressure points at the top of the forehead (hairline), between the nose and upper lip, below the navel (the hara), and at the bottoms of the feet to prevent shock or bring someone out of it. Help the woman to lie down with feet elevated, and keep her comfortably warm. Give her water (nothing alcoholic) or one teaspoon of apple cider vinegar in water in small, frequent sips. Use *Arnica montana* (homeo-pathic remedy), or Rescue Remedy (flower essence), placed under the tongue.

Aromatherapy: Lavender in a diffuser helps pain and speeds burn healing; it also is an emotional calmative. Diluted with olive oil in a massage oil, it can be applied directly to the skin. Geranium, rosemary or niaouli are also used for cell regeneration and skin healing.

Flower Essences: Rescue Remedy, a Bach Flower Remedy that is a combination of five flowers, is important for any trauma, accident or fear situation. I have used this to bring women as well as pets out of shock and it works immediately. Follow if necessary with homeopathic *Arnica*, but use the flower essence first. A flower essence of aloe vera can be used internally and also rubbed on the skin; it aids cell regeneration and stimulates the central nervous system.

Gemstones and Gem Essences: Botswanna agate, carnelian agate or picture agate essence help to reoxygenate the cells and aid cell regrowth. Botswanna agate is for use in traumatic situations and picture agate helps in the body's ability to use vitamin E. Hold or wear a piece of chrysocolla, chrysoprase, aquamarine or celestite for cooling, balancing of systems, and pain relief.

Emotional Healing: What (or who) is burning you up? Aren't there better ways to deal with anger than to draw fire to you? Go to your altar, light a candle (sic), and tell her/him off, or hit a stack of pillows or phonebooks with your fist or a rubber hose. Release anger in safe ways, say what you need to say or do it physically, but get it out. Fill your aura with blue light.

Cancer

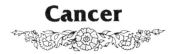

One in three people in the United States will die of cancer, and one in nine women will get breast cancer in her lifetime. The leading cancer cause of death for all women, Black or white, is now smoking-related lung cancer, with breast cancer second. Cancer rates are increasing for women in this country, and estrogen, high fat diets, environmental pollution and smoking are implicating factors. The amount of pollution that we eat, drink, breathe and live with everyday has overloaded everyone's immune systems. Like a cup over-filled, when no more can be dealt with the body reacts. No matter what we do or how healthy we live, there is no escaping the damage to the earth that reflects in our own bodies. Still much can be done. Cigarette smoking is one of the direct causes of cancer, and smoking is deadly for women. It is implicated in the causes of cervical, uterine and ovarian cancers, all other cancers, and in osteoporosis, menopause difficulties and birth defects. If you smoke quit, avoid as many chemicals, food additives and pesticides as possible, and eat a low fat vegetarian diet.

Over-amount of estrogen is considered the leading cause of cancer in women (and of other reproductive system dis-eases). Meat animals and poultry are fed high amounts of this hormone to make them heavier before slaughtering. The residues remain in the fat and meat, putting women who are meat-eaters in danger. The hormone DES, known to cause cervical cancer in the daughters of women prescribed it to prevent miscarriages in the 1950s, is still fed to beef cattle up to ten days before slaughter. Poultry, which is also fed estrogen, contains more fat and stores more of the drugs. The FDA, so quick to harass the vitamin and healthfood industry, does not intervene. A high saturated fat diet (the Typical American Diet), besides being tainted with the estrogens fed to cattle and poultry, is a major source of free radicals in the blood, tissues and cells. Free radicals damage the DNA programming of cell reproduction and protein formation in the body. It is a factor in why a healthy cell will reproduce wildly, becoming a cancer cell. A high fat diet means frequent eating of fried foods, animal fats or oil, and milk products; cooking oils that may be rancid are also a cause of free radical production.

Says MD Cindy Brown:

> For breast cancer, I used to tell my patients that...eating fat
> is like throwing gasoline on a fire. There's evidence from
> extensively studied breast cancer in Japanese women who
> ate the traditional Japanese diet (about 10–12% fat) that not
> only did they have 1/4 the incidence of breast cancer that we
> do, but that on an extremely low fat diet, it seems to behave
> much more benignly, so that their overall cure rates are
> around 75% and ours have remained at 50–55% for the last
> 40 years, in spite of all the so-called advances.[1]

Healing cancer for women means removing as many of the source factors as possible, and protecting women's bodies from pollutants and free radical damage. It includes antioxidant vitamins, herbs that cleanse the system of toxins, and factors that promote healthy cell and protein growth. It means preventing suspicious or precancerous cells from becoming cancerous, and making women who already have cancer as comfortable as possible. There are methods for reducing stress and boosting the immune system, factors in cancer formation and in dealing with the dis-ease itself. There are no easy answers or cures—as long as the planet is choked with poisons, so will her people be—but there is much that women can do in self-healing, even for this most frightening of dis-eases.

Vitamins and Minerals: Along with a multiple vitamin and mineral supplement, vitamins A, E and B-complex are essential in both prevention and treatment. Vitamins A and E are antioxidants, and particularly use a dry form natural E that contains selenium—up to 1600 IU of E and 200 mcg of selenium a day. Use high amounts of vitamin A (50,000–100,000 IU for ten days, decrease to up to 50,000 IU for a month, then use 25,000 IU as a maintenance dose). This is especially good in cervical dysplasia (suspicious Pap smear) for normalizing. Stomach upset and nausea indicate too much, so know when to cut back, and use vitamin A in dry form. Beta-carotene can be added to this, about 10,000 IU per day. Use vitamin C to bowel tolerance, and a B-complex; niacin may be important in preventing precancerous cells from becoming malignant, as may calcium, and calcium is also a pain reliever. Germanium (200 mg) and coenzyme Q10 (60 mg) both help to reduce the side effects of chemotherapy and radiation, and are pain relievers; germanium may be more important. Zinc (50 mg per day) boosts the immune system. For precancerous conditions, vitamins B-6, B-12 and folic acid may be enough to reverse the situation. Do not take supplemental iron if you have cancer.

[1]Cindy Brown, MD, personal communication, August 12, 1991.

Herbs: May Bethel in *The Healing Power of Herbs* offers a cancer healing blend:

1 ounce red clover	2 ounces Oregon grape root
1 ounce burdock seed	1/2 ounce bloodroot

Steep these in a pint of water and a pint of apple cider vinegar for two hours, strain, and take a glassful four times a day for growths or tumors on any part of the body.[2] A tea of red clover and blue violet leaf is also anticarcinogenic, or of red clover, burdock and violet. Pau d'arco, echinacea or chaparral, or a mix of chaparral, burdock, red clover and yellow dock are other herb remedies. For cervical dysplasia, make vaginal suppositories from powdered chaparral and melted cocoa butter. Jason Winters' Tea is a chaparral anticancer formula, and periwinkle tincture is used for leukemia.

Naturopathy: Fasts with daily coffee enemas are important to detoxify the body, and high colonics can also be helpful. Eat a diet of fresh, raw foods as much as possible, a raw vegetable cleansing diet or macrobiotic diet. Castor oil packs can have spectacular results, for either skin or internal cancers, and especially for breast cancer. Shiitake mushrooms, spirulina, wheatgrass juice or aloe vera juice are important immune system builders. For more immune building, use Kyolic tablets (two, three times a day), combination raw glandular complex with extra raw thymus, or kelp tablets (iodine deficiency may be a factor in cancer and fibroid tumors).

Fruit and vegetable juices cleanse and rebuild the body: use beet juice (also prevents chemotherapy side effects), carrot juice (beta-carotene/vitamin A), asparagus juice, raw cabbage and carrot juice together, or grape, black cherry or black currant juice. Eat as much of raw onions and garlic as you can. Raw almonds contain the B-vitamin known as laetrile. A teaspoon of olive oil taken three times daily reduces the side effects of radiation therapy. Black currant oil is effective for precancerous pathologies, for reducing chemotherapy/radiation side effects, and for clearing the cancer itself. Bee pollen prevents or delays the appearance of malignant tumors, and reduces existing tumors in size; it is a preventive for all forms of cancer. Take two tablets to an ounce daily; it also increases appetite.

Homeopathy and Cell Salts: There are a number of homeopathic remedies that have good results with cancer, but they are only available through homeopathic physicians. Some of them include *Carcinosin*, *Schirrhinum* (for breast cancer), *Hydrastis canadenisis* and *Oleum animal* (for nipple pain). More available are *Phosphoricum* for bone cancer, or

[2]May Bethel, *The Healing Power of Herbs* (N. Hollywood, CA, Wilshire Book Co., 1968), p. 136.

Euphorbium for cancer pain (use every two hours).

Cell Salts: *Calc. phos., Silica* and/or *Kali sulph.* are recommended cell salts and use *Kali phos.* for pain and offensive discharges.

Amino Acids: These are listed as highly important both in preventing cancer and in cancer healing. Use a combination free-form or liver amino acids (liver-based aminos also contain B-12, niacin and other B-complex vitamins; see Twin Labs Predigested Liver Amino Acids combination). Single aminos detoxify and protect the liver from free radical formation: L-carnitine, cysteine, methionine, or taurine. For chemotherapy and x-ray side effects, use L-glutathione.

Acupressure: The pressure points shown in the illustration are for pain in any part of the body and from any source. Try also ear acupressure for pain relief, immune stimulation and all-over rebalancing. Massage the whole ear tissue until the ears feel tingly all over. Full foot massage is also helpful and important; work out any sore spots that you find in any of these.

Aromatherapy: Use tea-tree, lemon, lavender or niaoli in massage oils, baths, compresses or diffusers. They boost the immune system, are antiseptic and detoxify. Tiferet-Lifetree has a combination for pain relief and an everyday balancer.

Flower Essences: Aloe vera in essence is indicated for all cancers and tumors and for leukemia, and apricot essence has similar properties to laetrile. Hawthorne reduces cancer spread, but is ineffective for bone cancer or leukemia. Use pomegranate for cancers or tumors of women's reproductive organs or breast cancer. Other essences include: bloodroot, chaparral, sweet corn, hellebore, hyssop, avocado, red clover, mugwort or onion.

Gemstones and Gem Essences: Use azurite-malachite essence for abnormal cell growth and cancer. Other choices are lapis lazuli, moonstone, blue quartz, blue tourmaline or pink tourmaline for cancer and precancerous states. Hold or wear blue tourmaline or gem rhodochrosite; use kunzite for pain.

Emotional Healing: An emotional picture has been defined as the "cancer personality," or someone prone to developing this dis-ease. The typical picture is a woman who has had a deprived childhood, followed by finding something that fulfills her life and is then lost—a lover, job, child, reason for Be-ing. The woman appears to others as a "saint," someone who never gets angry or difficult, but in fact is very angry and has an inability of expressing it. The cancer will appear about a year and a half after the loss, if the anger at the loss is not released. Deep hurt, longtime resentment and secret grief are cancer personality factors.

Acupressure for Cancer
Points to Release Pain

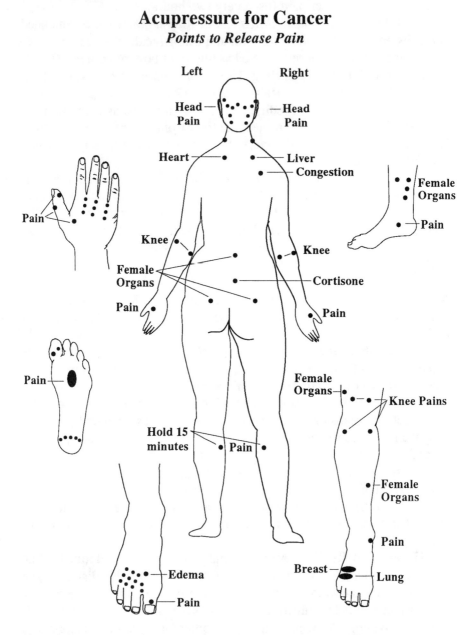

Shown above are several pain control reflex buttons that are stimulated by pressure that causes them to release natural pain-inhibiting chemicals (endorphins) in the brain. Also shown are energy-stimulating reflex buttons and the great eliminator point (autonomic nervous system) in the webs between the thumbs and first fingers.

Mildred Carter, *Body Reflexology* (W. Nyack, NY, Parker Publishing Co., 1983), p. 34.

Meditation is highly valuable and helpful in reducing stress and fear, and in boosting the immune system. Visualize the cancer leaving your body through an imagined release hose, or pac-man type helpers eating the malignant cells. Imagine tumors shrinking until gone. Flood them with blue light. Read Bernie Siegel's *Love, Medicine and Miracles* (Harper and Row, 1986), and join a *holistic* cancer support/emotional therapy group. Releasing the "cancer personality" and emotions of loss and anger are vital to full healing. And know that full healing *is* possible, and happens everyday.

Note: for Skin Cancer, see Skin Dis-eases.

Candida Albicans
Systemic Yeast Infection

Candida can affect many parts of the body and be operant in a number of seemingly unrelated conditions. It can manifest as mouth or foot thrush, skin rashes or dis-eases, as vaginal infections (particularly recurrent ones), chronic fatigue, hypoglycemia, arthritis, sinusitis, digestive upsets or abdominal pain, constipation or diarrhea, joint or muscle pain, cystitis or kidney infections, PMS, depression, hyperactivity, hypothyroidism, adrenal problems, environmental allergies, food sensitivities and even diabetes. Many more women than men are affected, and women who are diabetic or pregnant, have been taking antibiotics or the contraceptive pill, are taking chemotherapy or cortisone (steroids), eat a high sugar and white flour diet, or who are under stress are particularly susceptible. Women who are deficient in the B-complex vitamins or whose immune systems are lowered are also easily prone to developing systemic candida albicans. Longterm system candida has been implicated in mitral valve prolapse, a heart defect.

The cause of candida over-run is intestinal; where the natural balance of bacteria in the gut is disrupted by hormones, antibiotics or refined carbohydrates (white sugar and flour), candida can over-run the system. Once entrenched, it can result in the wide range of symptoms and discomforts listed above and be difficult to diagnose and treat. Medical drugs for candida—Nystatin, Monostat, Nyzoral and Amphotericin B—depress the immune system and develop drug resistant yeast/candida strains. Holistic healing focuses on diet, immune system building, balancing the body's healthy bacteria, and eliminating the yeast by detoxification methods. Systemic candida/yeast is a dis-ease affecting many women, all of whose well-being is much improved by eliminating it. Also see Vaginitis in this book for vaginal yeast/candida remedies.

Vitamins and Minerals: Use a yeast and sugar free (most are) multiple vitamin and mineral complex, and a yeast free B-complex-50. Deficiency in vitamin B-6 is a cause of candida albicans and extra B-12 and biotin are needed. Use zinc for immune building, and vitamin C in high doses, with selenium 100–300 mcg per day. A major candida/yeast treatment is acidophilus, which replaces the beneficial bacteria in the gut. Use nondairy Maxidophilus, Megadophilus or Superdophilus for this. An acidophilus compound from Switzerland called Eugalen Forte, expensive and once very hard to find but becoming easier, is highly positive and worked very well for me. Essential fatty acids (evening primrose oil, salmon oil, linseed oil, Omega-3 or black currant oil) can be extremely effective also. Caprylic acid is one of several things used to eliminate the yeast fungus; follow directions on the bottle. Some of these are not strictly vitamins, but seem to fall most easily into the vitamin category. Digestive enzymes like HCL can make a difference.

Herbs: Pau d'arco, black walnut, white oak bark, buchu, tea-tree tincture or chaparral are all positive in eliminating candida albicans and rebuilding the immune system. Alternate pau d'arco and clove teas or tinctures. There are a number of herbal yeast preparations available in healthfood stores based on these herbs. A plant preparation called stevia can be used as a sweetener to replace sugar in the diet; it is good tasting, nontoxic, nonchemical, and won't feed the yeast. Find it from Sunrider and other companies.

Naturopathy: Eat a diet of vegetables, whole grains and fish, avoiding all sugars (including fruit and fruit sugars), refined carbohydrates, breads, vinegar foods, alcohol and junk foods. Use a diet as free of additives, chemicals and preservatives as possible. If the candida is systemic avoid dairy products, except yoghurt. Once the candida is cleared, many avoided foods can be added back into the diet (not sugar), but watch for allergic reactions and relapses. Many of the foods to stop using in candida albicans are also sensitivities that your body will react to when you use them again. If you have a craving for any food, you are probably allergic to it and/or it is feeding the yeast. Eat cucumber, watermelon (and make the rind into a tea) to help elimination.

A major effective treatment for candida albicans is garlic, usually used as odorfree Kyolic. Take two tablets (or capsules) three times a day. After a few days, you will notice some side effects: flu-like symptoms, depression, a white coating on the tongue, discolored stool, diarrhea or constipation. This is the yeast dying off and leaving the body, and the symptoms will last for around a week. Any yeast-eliminating substance will have this die-off effect. If it gets too uncomfortable, decrease the Kyolic (or other) for a few days but do not stop entirely, then increase it again. This will slow the reaction, but the reaction is positive and means the treatment is working. Once it ends, you will feel a great improvement in well-being. Use this with the above diet, and stay with the diet. Continue taking Kyolic for at least three more months, decreasing gradually after all symptoms are gone to two tablets a day.

Homeopathy and Cell Salts: A nosode of *Candida albicans* is available from homeopathic physicians. See Immune System Dis-eases and Vaginitis for other remedies. Because symptoms can vary so much, general remedies are hard to offer.

Cell Salts: Try *Kali mur*. If there is depression or chronic fatigue with candida, use *Kali phos*. with it; alternate them. Use *Natrum Mur*. when there is a watery discharge from anywhere in the body (sinus, vaginitis, etc.).

Amino Acids: A free-form combination amino acids is important in rebuilding the immune system and detoxifying. Use L-cystine singly.

Acupressure: Use immune building and elimination reflex points, with full foot acupressure twice a week and working gradually up to twice a day. Use a foot roller ten minutes a day as an alternative. Pay particular attention to the endocrine and lymph reflexes (see Immune System and Blood Cleansing sections). The pressure points shown under Boils that work with the kidneys and spleen for eliminating toxins are also positive.

Aromatherapy: Tea-tree oil and thyme are essential oils to use for candida albicans. These are antiseptic, antifungal and build the immune system. Use them in baths and diffusers, and as compresses for external infections (skin); they must be diluted. Also try lavender or myrrh; they are antifungal.

Flower Essences: Amaranthus or sweet corn (zea mays) stimulate the immune system. Pomegranate eliminates toxins and is positive for women in any dis-ease.

Gemstone and Gem Essences: Try cinnabar as an essence, and hold or wear bloodstone. Citrine in essence or worn in the aura will help in eliminating toxins while using treatments.

Emotional Healing: Holistic physician Christiane Northrup notes that:

> Approximately 70 percent of my patients with chronic candidiasis come from alcoholic homes, so it is also important to change negative, immune suppressive thought.[1]

Louise Hay verifies that by describing an emotional state of frustration and anger, demanding and mistrust in relationships, and feeling very scattered. Try giving more and trusting more, and working through the old hurts. Where symptoms are vaginal and chronic, I would suspect that many women are incest survivors. Love and appreciate yourself and others, be less demanding, and work on a positive life outlook.

Cataracts

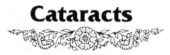

Cataracts are almost considered a given for women over sixty, but the evidence is that they are preventable, even reversible in early stages, and that poor nutrition and toxicities are the major cause. Malnutrition in elders is a pervasive poverty problem in affluent America, and the high sugar, high fat, white flour American diet is as much to blame for malnutrition as it is for cataract formation. A collection of toxicities and elimination problems are also implicated; primary are sorbitol, a sugar substitute used by diabetics that crystallizes in the eyes, and galactose (milk sugar) intolerance. Other toxicities and food intolerances, fatty acid intolerance, high cholesterol, improper calcium assimilation, hormone imbalance, liver dis-ease, chronic constipation, heavy metal toxicities, low-level radiation exposure or x-rays, many medical drugs, adrenal exhaustion, trauma, poor circulation and spinal alignment, and free radical damage are all contributing factors.

Replace free radical-causing substances (saturated fats, sugar, sorbitol, milk products, food toxicities) with a balanced high nutrition diet and

---

[1]Francine Rota, "50 Ways to Better Women's Health," in East/West Journal, November 1990, p. 48.

proper elimination, to detoxify the body. A chiropractor or osteopath can help normalize circulation and the spine, as well as aid stress and adrenal exhaustion, elimination, and many other factors. In as wealthy a society as the United States, nutritional deficiency dis-cases have no need to happen, but they are pervasive—particularly among the poor, elders, women and children and the nonwhite. What the media promotes as a good diet is determined by food industry interests, not real human needs. Information is becoming more available and more real on nutrition, but poverty and the Typical American Diet are still with us, and women on foodstamps or Social Security just don't have enough to eat.

Vitamins and Minerals: These go along with, but are not a substitute for, a good diet. Use a high quality multiple vitamin and mineral supplement; if you are an elder and have difficulty digesting pills and tablets, look for vitamins in soft gel or capsule form or even liquids. Major vitamin deficiencies in cataracts include vitamin C and B-2. Use at least 3000 mg per day of vitamin C with bioflavinoids, a B-complex-50 three times a day, and additional B-2 (15–50 mg), B-6 (50–100 mg) and B-1 (50 mg). Use 25,000–50,000 IU of vitamin A daily in dry form, and vitamin E (increase gradually to 400–800 IU per day) with selenium (200 mcg per day). Minerals are highly important; use a calcium/magnesium tablet, 50 mg of zinc daily, and 3 mg of copper. Manganese is also helpful, and so is lecithin. Vitamin A eyedrops, called Conjunctisan A, are important.

Herbs: Use cineraria eyedrops for several months. Bilberry herb can help in removing chemicals from the eye. Other herbs include gingko biloba, eyebright, rosemary, or chaparral, all used as tinctures internally. Eyebright tea can be used as an external eye compress. Greater celandine is an ancient cataract remedy and still effective: collect the fresh leaves, press them, and use the resulting juice as an eyedrop two or three times a day. Rosehip tea, high in bioflavinoids and vitamin C, also helps to clear cataracts. Aloe vera juice used as an eyedrop and also taken internally has had good results. There is a Chinese herb called Hachimijiogan, also.

Naturopathy: Start with a seven day cleansing fast using vegetable juice or organic fruit juices. A fast this long should be under supervision. If you are diabetic or debilitated only fast with expert help. Use warm water enemas every other day. Follow the fast with a raw foods diet for at least two weeks, and with emphasis on raw vegetables, nuts, fresh fruits, broiled fish and seaweeds after. This is to aid in elimination of toxin buildup and to establish a high nutrition maintenance diet. Avoid coffee, tea, sugar, alcohol and smoking, as well as sugar substitutes (use stevia, a healthy herbal sweetener instead), fats and milk products. Do not take antihistamines.

There are several naturopathic eyedrop methods. Use warm castor oil packs and castor oil dropped into the eyes nightly; wash eyes nightly with coconut milk, then put warm cloths over them for fifteen minutes; or use a drop of raw honey or a poultice of grated potato in the eyes twice a day. Another choice is to use this recipe from naturopaths Mildred Jackson and Terri Teague:

> Place the yellow side of a piece of organic orange peel over the eye and leave overnight. On the second night, use the white side of a fresh piece of organic orange peel. If the peel over the eye creates a great deal of heat, remove it and try again the next night. Continue each night alternating the side of the peel until condition is cleared. Use fresh peel each night and use only organic oranges as commercial oranges have been sprayed with chemicals.[1]

Edgar Cayce's Atomidine, kelp or chlorophyll are also positive.

Homeopathy and Cell Salts: Use the following combination of cell salts, powdered, in just enough distilled water to dissolve. Take ten drops three times a day internally (not in the eyes) for at least a month.[2]

Ferrum phos. 30X	*Kali phos.* 12X
Natrum phos. 12X	*Mag. phos.* 6X
Natrum mur. 12X	*Silica* 12X

Amino Acids: Protein deficiency is a nutritional factor in cataract formation, and a liver-based combination amino acids is highly important. Single aminos for cataract healing include: methionine, cystine, lysine, and glutathione.

Acupressure: Use reflex massage on the toes and fingers, and their bases in the feet and palms. Massage the points for about three minutes, several times a day for the first two weeks, then continue three times a day for the next several months. Also work the webs between the fingers. Some of these points will feel very sore.

Aromatherapy: Use fragrances to stimulate the pituitary (third eye). These include frankincense, sandalwood and myrrh. Breathe them or use a diffuser. Never use essential oils in the eyes themselves.

---

[1]Mildred Jackson, ND and Terri Teague, ND, DC, *The Handbook of Alternatives to Chemical Medicine* (Berkeley, CA, Bookpeople, 1975), p. 65.

[2]Moshe Olshevsky, CA, PhD. *et al., The Manual of Natural Therapy* (New York, Citadel Press, 1990), p. 282–263.

Acupressure for Cataracts

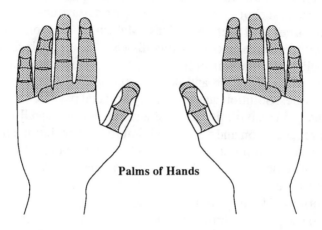

Palms of Hands

Fingers, thumb and base of fingers on palms and the webs between fingers. Pay particular attention to finger tips.

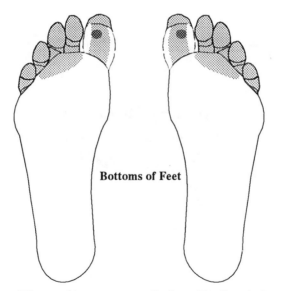

Bottoms of Feet

Toes and base of toes; pay particular attention to toe-tips.

Mildred Carter, *Body Reflexology* (W. Nyack, NY, Parker Publishing Co., 1983), p. 34.

Flower Essences: Use harvest brodiaea essence internally and dropped into the eyes with eyebright herb or comfrey poultices. This also works on the emotional level of the dis-ease. Use lemon essence to detoxify and dissolve scar tissue, or Queen Anne's lace or nasturtium.

Gemstones and Gem Essences: Malachite, turquoise or solution quartz are the gem essences for this dis-ease. Make malachite essence using a polished stone left in the water for no more than half an hour. Malachite expels radiation and heavy metal toxins and regenerates the cells and tissues. Solution quartz aids physical and psychic vision, detoxifies, and helps in assimilation of minerals. Turquoise is an all-healer, used for tissue regeneration and nutrition; it improves circulation and protects from environmental pollutants and background radiation. Stones of amethyst, moonstone, lapis or malachite worn on the body or held in the aura are also positive.

Emotional Healing: Emotional indications for cataracts include an inability to see positive things for one's future, and a pessimistic outlook on life. There is confusion as to one's purpose and an inability to see future joy. Experience the joys of each day and tomorrow will take care of itself. Know that you are protected and loved by the Goddess, live in the here and now, and believe that the future holds many good things to come.

Cervical Dysplasia
See the sections on Cancer, Menopause, and Warts

Chronic Fatigue Syndrome

Chronic fatigue, usually identified with the Epstein Barr Virus, affects tens of thousands of people, three times more women than men. It can also be a result of a number of other things besides Epstein Barr, including adrenal exhaustion, anemia, systemic candida albicans, heavy metal poisoning, hypoglycemia, hypothyroidism, environmental allergies and food sensitivities, and nutritional deficiency or assimilation problems. A few—but very few—cases of chronic fatigue syndrome are mental and nervous disorders; this is a physical dis-ease. Symptoms include extreme exhaustion, flu symptoms with swollen glands, recurrent colds, intestinal problems, anxiety, depression, irritability and mood swings, aching muscles or joints, headaches, memory and concentration loss. The prolonged symptoms result in immune system burn-out and endocrine and adrenal exhaustion. The constellation of symptoms persisting for longer than six months and an elevated antibody count are the basis for labeling this dis-ease. Some women recover eventually, others do not, and while chronic fatigue is not life threatening, it is *quality* of life threatening.

There is more than a virus (EBV) operating here. The past ten to twenty years have seen the appearance of a number of immune deficiency and autoimmune dis-eases that were previously unknown or rare. AIDS is the most publicized example, but lupus, multiple sclerosis, candida, the increase in cancer and arthritis (especially in children), hypoglycemia, environmental and food allergies, and diabetes can be no coincidence. All of these dis-eases point to the pollution and toxification of the planet. The human immune system can only handle so much poisoning and malnutrition before it breaks down. This breakdown is exactly what we're seeing, and chronic fatigue syndrome has become a classic example. Since there is no way to escape the poisoning until we clean up the planet, holistic methods are the best that can be offered for healing these dis-eases.

Vitamins and Minerals: Along with a high quality diet, use a good multiple vitamin and mineral supplement. With it use vitamin C with bioflavinoids to bowel tolerance (5-10 g daily). Use a B-complex-50 to - 100 three times daily, with pantothenic acid B-5. Use vitamins A, E and coenzyme Q10 as antioxidants—50,000 IU of dry form vitamin A for a month, then decrease to 25,000 IU, use 800 IU of vitamin E and 75 mg of CO Q10. Potassium is highly important, and so are zinc, calcium and magnesium. Make sure your multiple vitamin includes the trace minerals.

Because sixty percent of chronic fatigue can be traced to candida albicans, use acidophilus to return the bacterial balance to the intestines. (See the section on Candida Albicans; all of the remedies there are also applicable.) Digestive enzymes are positive for many women with this dis-ease, and essential fatty acids (black currant oil). Egg lecithin, used by some AIDS patients, can be helpful. [1]

Herbs: Make a decoction of dried cayenne flowers, a teaspoon to a gallon of water; boil for a minute or two, then cool. Strain out the herb and place in the refrigerator. Build up your tolerance for this very hot drink slowly, starting with a teaspoonful a day in the morning. Your face will get red and you'll feel hot all over. Increase amounts until you can drink a juice-glassful a day. Cayenne is a potent antiviral and antibacterial; it protects against secondary infections, builds the immune system, and will gradually inactivate the EBV virus. It may irritate the stomach.

Other herbs to try in tincture include: pau d'arco, tea-tree, chaparral, burdock root, echinacea, goldenseal (not if you are hypoglycemic) dandelion or poke root (for the liver and iron deficiency). Drink aloe vera juice; read the directions on the bottle and make sure it contains no additives. Blood-cleansing herbs, particularly red clover and burdock, or red clover and blue violet leaf are helpful. See the herbs for Candida Albicans and Blood Cleansing, and for Immune System Dis-eases.

Naturopathy always starts with diet and does so here. Eat a diet of primarily raw foods, whole grains and fish, and if you eat meat or poultry eat organics. Use fresh whole foods without additives or preservatives and avoid junkfoods totally. Avoid fried foods, refined sugar and flour, alcohol, aspirin, soft drinks, caffeine, fats and shellfish. Take supplemental iodine in the form of kelp tablets (six to eight a day), Atomidine or Lugol's Solution (one drop in water or juice taken twice a week with meals). If your mouth starts to taste metallic, use it less. Chlorophyll in the form of spirulina, wheatgrass, Kyo-green or Green Magma is important.

Kyolic is also important, for candida control and to build the immune system. It is an antiviral, antibacterial and antifungal. Take two tablets three times a day with meals. Another suggestion is apple cider vinegar, one teaspoon taken in water three times a day or apple cider vinegar baths using a half pint of vinegar to a tubful of water. Two teaspoons of honey with meals (or in the vinegar water) are antibiotic and antiviral. Use raw glandular complex, or raw thymus and raw spleen.

Do an elimination diet to test for food allergies and see the Liver Detoxification section for reducing heavy metal pollutants.

Homeopathy and Cell Salts: Careful constitutional treatment by an

---

[1]James Balch, MD and Phyllis Balch, CNC, *Prescription for Nutritional Healing* (Garden City Park, NY, Avery Publishing Group, Inc.., 1990), p. 135–136. I owe much of this book's vitamin information to this excellent source.

experienced homeopath is recommended; treating symptoms, even with a nosode, is less desirable. Some symptomatic remedies, however, follow. If your symptoms include sore throat, swollen glands, chilliness with fever, thirst, restlessness and fatigue, try *Arsenicum*. *Aconite* is for swollen glands, sore throat and fever with thirst after exposure to cold drafts; the woman has fear of dying. If there are weakness and fatigue, swollen glands, red and swollen throat with pus, and sensitivity to both heat and cold, try *Mercurius*. Use *Sulfur* when symptoms linger, the throat burns and feels dry, there is reduced appetite and increased thirst. The woman has discomfort for warmth and is generally lethargic.

Cell Salts: Use three of each of the these twice a day: *Kali phos.*, *Natrum mur.*, *Ferrum phos.*, *Kali sulph.*, and *Natrum sulph.* For acute symptoms that are flu-like, use *Ferrum phos. Silica* is a blood cleanser for poor assimilation and weak memory.

Amino Acids: Take a free-form amino acids combination, and consider the following singly: asparagine and aspartic acid together, or isoleucine with leucine and valine.

Acupressure: Do full foot acupressure working up to twice a day and pay particular attention to the endocrine glands reflex points (see Immune System section). Work the thymus, spleen and adrenal points in particular. Use the *Touch for Health* fatigue sequence illustrated, pressing the upper points on both hand and foot first, then the lower points at the base of the small toe and little finger. You will need help to do these simultaneously.

Aromatherapy: Take baths with tea-tree oil, lemon thyme, clove, lavender, basil or yarrow. Geranium and rosemary together are also positive. Make a massage oil of the following in an olive oil base: 4% bryony, 3% eucalyptus, 3% lavender and 3% rosemary. There is a combination for invigorating available from Tiferet-Lifetree.

Flower Essences: Try any of the following: amaranthus, cotton plant, date palm, pansy, sweet corn (zea mays), sugar beet, bo tree, McCartney rose or peach.

Gemstones and Gem Essences: Blue tourmaline, soapstone or sulfur are essences for the endocrine system, and emerald, jade, picture jasper, blue quartz or citrine are for immune building. Also see the stones for Candida Albicans. Hold or wear rhodochrosite.

Emotional Healing: A lack of enthusiasm and profound boredom for life are emotional coordinates for chronic fatigue. There is resistance and a lack of love for one's life or what one does in it. Perhaps some changes in environment—in more ways than one—are in order? Do what you love and the money and wellness will follow. Energy and enthusiasm go together.

Acupressure for Chronic Fatigue

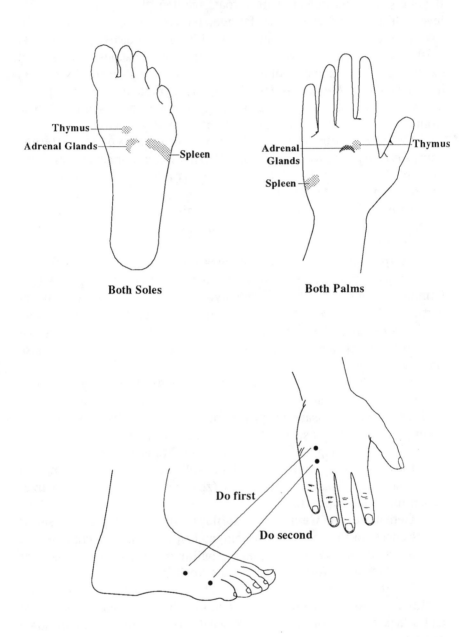

Thymus

Adrenal Glands

Spleen

Both Soles

Adrenal
Glands

Thymus

Spleen

Both Palms

Do first

Do second

John Thie, DC, *A Touch for Health, A New Approach to Restoring Our Natural Energies* (Marina del Rey, CA, DeVorss and Co., 1973), p. 80.

Colds and Sore Throats

A cold is the body's way of releasing toxins and should be supported, rather than suppressed. Naturopaths see it as the *cure* of dis-ease, rather than dis-ease itself. In a healthy woman, a cold a couple of times a year lasts for a week and is a total housecleaning of the body. The release of mucus is a mechanism for detoxifying. Cold viruses surround us all the time; there are hundreds of different forms. We get sick when the body needs elimination or rebalancing. A high carbohydrate or high dairy diet on top of fatigue, stress, constipation or the need for a cry or a rest will start a cold. A cold that affects the chest or lungs, a fever above 102°F for more than three days, or a strep throat are conditions indicating intervention. For other colds, use healing conservatively, rest, speed elimination by fasts or enemas, and just wait it out.

If you have colds frequently, consider allergy analysis, immune building methods and looking at your diet and lifestyle—do you get enough sleep, are you eating quality food, do you smoke, are you too often constipated? Children who get recurrent colds may have thyroid imbalances. Aspirin should not be used for cold treatment in young children; it can cause Reye's Syndrome, a much more serious dis-ease. Avoid anti-histamines that suppress colds and may result in illness deeper in the body. There are dozens of holistic remedies for colds and sore throats. Choose from among those that follow.

Vitamins and Minerals: A 1000 mg (1 gram) vitamin C and bioflavinoids tablet taken hourly with *lots* of water or calcium/magnesium can stop a cold if used early enough, at the very first symptoms. During a cold, go to bowel tolerance but decrease slowly. Some women report the same cold-stopping effect with vitamin A, using a 25,000 IU capsule hourly (for no more than three days), then decreasing to 25,000 IU per day. The two vitamins may be used together, and most women will respond to one or the other. Again the trick is to start very early, at the first signs and symptoms. This will also work for sore throats and strep throats, and for these add zinc gluconate lozenges. Dissolve one under the tongue every three hours for three days, then every four hours for a week. Vitamin B-5, pantothenic acid, is a natural antihistamine.

Herbs: There are any number of herbs and herbal cold combinations. To stop a cold or sore throat at the very beginning, make capsules of two parts goldenseal and one part ground cayenne and take two every three hours. Ginseng with vitamin C will also stop a cold. Use ginger root tea or hot compresses, peppermint, elder blossom or yarrow. For fever, take a catnip tea enema and 1/4–1/2 teaspoon of lobelia tincture every three or four hours—don't overdo the lobelia or it will cause vomiting. Use boneset for achy flu symptoms, or sage or yarrow. White willow is an herbal aspirin and decongestant, horehound and wintergreen open the sinuses (use sparingly), and slippery elm lozenges are great for sore throats. Make a tea of cinnamon, sage and bay and add a tablespoon of lemon juice to it, or sage, garlic and lemon tea, for cough, congestion, flu and to sweat out fevers.

For strep throats use goldenseal and echinacea together, preferably in tincture, suck zinc gluconate lozenges, and massage the throat with Tiger Balm or Sunbreeze. Gargle with goldenseal and myrrh tincture, diluted with water. Sage tea also makes a good gargle; also use internally. Hyssop and white horehound together are good for chest colds; use hyssop, white willow and echinacea together for tonsillitis, sore throats, strep or chest congestion. Use ephedra for chest colds, sinus congestion and sinus headache; if too much a stimulant, use it with catnip. Mullein is used for coughs, diarrhea, runny nose and sore throats.

Here is Joy Gardner's recipe for Lung Tea in *The New Healing Yourself* (The Crossing Press, 1989, p. 69): bring six cups of water to a boil and add a tablespoon each of mullein, coltsfoot and comfrey leaves. Simmer for ten minutes, then add a tablespoon each of cornsilk and lobelia and two tablespoons of peppermint. Brew for five minutes more, strain, and add as much honey as you want. This tea is good for any cold, and particularly for chest colds.

Naturopathy: Use a three day liquid fast with grapefruit juice, potassium broth, herb teas, hot water, lemon and honey, or hot water, apple cider vinegar and honey. After three days go to a *cooked* vegetable diet to slow eliminations. Another cold fast is a mucus cleansing fast: use grapefruit in the morning, a plate of steamed onions for lunch and supper, fresh carrot juice at midmorning, and potassium broth at midafternoon and evening.[1]

Garlic is important both in preventing colds and reducing their severity. Take Kyolic, two tablets with each meal, or eat two cloves of raw garlic two or three times a day until the symptoms have been gone for a few days. Place a cup of chopped garlic over olive oil on your feet and bind in place as a night poultice, or hold a peeled garlic clove in your mouth between tongue and cheek, nicking it with your teeth occasionally, and

[1]Dr. Ross Trattler, *Better Health Through Natural Healing* (New York, McGraw-Hill Book Co., 1985), p. 589.

replacing it every few hours. Another very powerful raw garlic remedy is to combine a crushed garlic clove, 1/2 teaspoon of ground cayenne, the juice of one lemon, a gram of powdered vitamin C, and a teaspoonful of honey. Take three times a day with meals.

Chew honeycomb or use propolis as an antihistamine and immune system booster. Used early enough it can stop a cold from developing and is also good for sore throats. A teaspoon of honey in the juice of one lemon, or honey with a teaspoon of apple cider vinegar in a glass of water can be used every two hours for colds and strep throats; gargle with it every half hour for strep. Another good sore throat gargle is a half teaspoon of sea salt and a half teaspoon of peroxide in a half glass of warm/hot water. Dip a slice of raw onion in hot water and remove the onion; sip all day for "streaming colds."

With all of these choices, there still are more. Use castor oil packs, apple cider vinegar compresses, baths or body rubs, or a lobelia and hops throat compress for sore or strep throats and colds. Take a hot bath containing a cup of sea salt and a cup of baking soda, stay in the tub for twenty to twenty-five minutes, then go to bed and sweat out the cold. A coffee enema can also stop an early cold or speed the healing of a developed one.

Homeopathy and Cell Salts: *Allium cepa* is the most common remedy for cold symptoms; use it for burning discharge from the nose with sneezing and teary eyes. Use *Aconite* in the first stages, for fever, cough, sore throat and stuffed nose, especially after exposure to dry, cold winds. *Bryonia is* for chest colds, with excessive thirst for cold drinks and a dry, painful cough. Use *Gelsemium* for flu-like colds, with sneezing, profuse runny nose, rough throat, chills and fever, headache and aches al over. The woman feels dull and dopey. *Phosphorus* is for colds with cough and respiratory inflammation, laryngitis and hoarseness. Try *Nux vomica* when the nose pours like a faucet and you are very irritable, or *Arsenicum* when you are restless, chilly and weak with burning eye and nose discharges, worsening at night.

Cell Salts: *Ferrum phos.* is for early onset, and for all colds, congestions, coughs, flu and fevers. Alternate it with *Kali mur. Natrum mur.* is for runny colds with loss of sense of smell. Use *Natrum sulph.* alternated with *Kali sulph.* at the end of a cold with profuse discharge.

Amino Acids: Use a free-form amino acid combination to detoxify and rebuild the immune system.

Acupressure: Avoid full foot or hand massage with colds, but let the body detoxify at its own speed. For sore throats including strep throat use a tongue depressor or spoon handle on the back of the tongue and press out the tender spots. Look for tender reflexes for lungs and bronchial tubes in the area just below the collarbone on the front of the body, and on both sides of the back of neck and between the shoulder blades for cold congestion, flu symptoms, the throat and voice. Use the autonomic nervous system reflex deep in the webs between thumbs and first fingers for sinus congestion, and points on the face in a straight line down from the eyes between nose and mouth. (See illustration.)

Aromatherapy: Try essential oils in a vaporizer or diffuser, particularly eucalyptus, lavender, pine, spruce, ginger or rosemary. Use basil essence when the cold is accompanied by depression, insomnia or mental fatigue, and eucalyptus for colds with cough, flu, sinusitis, throat infections or other respiratory symptoms. If the cold has diarrhea, constipation, nausea, vomiting or lack of appetite, use black pepper essence in a massage oil. For sore or strep throats, the oils are geranium, ginger, eucalyptus, myrrh, pine or spruce; these can also be used as compresses, diluted slightly.

Flower Essences: Jasmine is the primary essence, to regulate mucus in the system and for cold symptoms, sore throats, sinus and lung congestion. Use this in daytime; it's a stimulant. Pansy overcomes the cold virus.

Gemstones and Gem Essences: Essences of beryl, jet, meteorite or sulfur are for colds and flu; for sore throats use aquamarine, beryl, coral, lapis lazuli or moonstone essence. Hold or wear lapis or moonstone to help sinus congestion, and sodalite drains the lymphatic system.

Emotional Healing: A cold can be the need for a good rest, and taking time to go to bed at first onset may be enough to stop it. It is also mental confusion and disorder in one's life, a feeling of too much at once or beyond one's control. A combination of suppressed anger and helplessness causes congestion and inflammation, as well as sore throats. Throat dis-ease is a need to cry, express oneself, or say something that's being held inside; it can be blocked creativity or blocked anger.

Acupressure for Colds

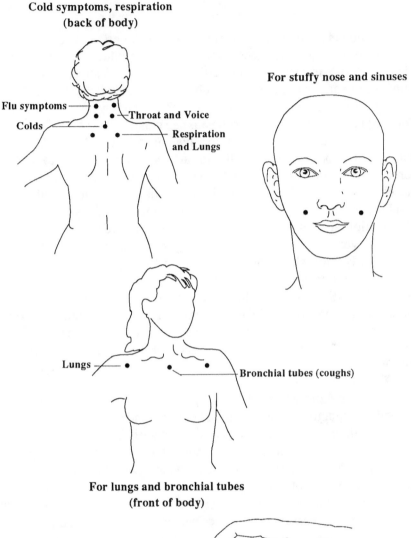

Cold symptoms, respiration
(back of body)

For stuffy nose and sinuses

Flu symptoms

Colds

Throat and Voice

Respiration
and Lungs

Lungs

Bronchial tubes (coughs)

For lungs and bronchial tubes
(front of body)

Web of hand between thumbs and first fingers

Iona Marsaa Teeguarden, *Acupressure Way of Health: Jin Shin Do* (New York, Japan Publishing Co., 1978), p. 67; Mildred Carter, *Body Reflexology* (W. Nyack, NY, Parker Publishing Co., 1983), p. 191; Pedro Chan, *Finger Acupressure* (New York, Ballantine Books, 1974), p. 33-35.

Constipation

Constipation is another dis-ease of the Typical American Diet, a result of refined flour and sugar, excess meat and milk products and not enough fiber. Lack of exercise, liver or gallbladder dis-ease, stress and anxiety, spinal subluxations or defects, hypothyroidism, anemia, lack of digestive enzymes, food allergies, pregnancy and not enough water are all causes. Too frequent use of laxatives or enemas can make bowel action "lazy" and result in chronic constipation or laxative dependency. When waste does not leave the body quickly, the liquids are reabsorbed and the toxins they contain are reabsorbed with them. The straining of constipation results in more serious dis-eases—diverticulitis, appendicitis, hemorrhoids, hiatal hernia, and varicose veins. Bowel cancer may be a result of chronic constipation and low fiber diets. Other dis-eases due to too infrequent bowel movements include headaches, gas, insomnia, indigestion, bad breath, body odor, skin problems, and sinusitis.

Acupressure, acupuncture, deep muscle massage and chiropractic or osteopathic adjustments are highly effective in aiding constipation. Colonic therapy removes old waste matter and helps to reshape the bowel. Eating a high fiber diet of raw whole foods is often the answer to even chronic bowel problems, and exercise and consuming enough water (eight cups a day) are also important. There are a number of other holistic helps for this discomfort and dis-ease.

Vitamins and Minerals: Avoid mineral oil laxatives as they strip the body of vitamins; take fiber bulk laxatives and cleansers at a different time than vitamin tablets, which are washed away by them. Along with a multiple vitamin and mineral supplement, take a vitamin B-complex-50 with extra B-5 (500 mg) and B-12 before meals. Lecithin or brewer's yeast can resolve many women's constipation, and high amounts of vitamin C are laxative. Vitamin E (400–800 IU), calcium and magnesium (1500 mg calcium/750 magnesium) prevent colon cancer. To these add 50 mg of zinc per day. Iron supplements may cause constipation; use only organic iron (hydrolized protein chelate), or a commercial preparation called Floradix. Digestive enzymes often solve the problem, but avoid HCL (hydrochloric acid) if you have ulcers. Some constipation is an imbalance of intestinal bacteria, and can also be caused by systemic candida: take acidophilus as Megadophilus, Maxidophilus or Superdophilus. There may be some initial diarrhea before balance is reached.

Herbs: Aloe vera juice, two ounces of the pure juice three times a day, is a laxative and cleans out the bowels. Do not use this if pregnant or nursing. Other laxative herbs include: senna, fennel, licorice, cascara sagrada, rhubarb, buckthorn, psyllium seed, ginger, barberry, elderberry or dandelion. Cascara sagrada and rhubarb are the most often used. Vervain helps to remove colon obstructions (and blackstrap molasses enemas). Comfrey and pepsin, often sold as a combination, is helpful for indigestion and a laxative, and alfalfa is a cleanser and detoxifier for all organs.

Naturopathy: Many of the most effective remedies come under this category. Begin with a three-day fruit juice cleansing fast and use nightly enemas of blackstrap molasses or warm water with it. Follow with a three-day apple and apple juice mono diet, and take two tablespoons of olive oil on the evening of the third day. Starting in the mono diet, take 25 drops of cascara sagrada tincture in water four times per day. Continue this for two or three weeks, then go to three times a day for two weeks. Reduce again if movements are regular, and decrease again in two weeks; after two more weeks stop.[1] Institute a diet high in raw vegetables, fruits and whole grains, and drink eight glasses of water, fruit juice or herb teas daily (black teas, coffee and alcohol don't count).

Other remedies include: a teaspoon of olive oil daily before breakfast for chronic constipation, and one to two ounces as a laxative. Blackstrap molasses can be used in the same way, as well as in water for enemas. Two glasses of cold water before breakfast, or warm water with lemon juice, will stimulate the bowels. Dried apricots, raw sauerkraut, raw spinach, dried figs, papaya, spanish onion, garlic, two or three fresh tomatoes eaten before breakfast, half a cup of bamboo shoots per day, okra and persimmons all have laxative action. Drink a cup of prune juice or eat half a cup of stewed prunes on an empty stomach.

Many of the bulk/fiber laxatives are naturopathic or herbal preparations. Try glucomannan, Aerobic Bulk Cleanse, Reneu's Inner Cleanse, psyllium seed, flaxseed, agar agar or bran with water before breakfast. Do not take vitamins at the same meal. The principle of these is that they swell in the intestine and cause the muscles to empty the bowel. Cod liver oil in liquid or capsules also empties the bowel, and also try an abdominal castor oil pack followed by an enema or colonics the next day. Green magma, wheatgrass or Kyo-green are chlorophyll supplements and also are laxative, as are kelp or other seaweed preparations.

Homeopathy and Cell Salts: Constitutional homeopathic treatment is recommended here, but some symptomatic remedies follow. *Bryonia* is

---

[1]Dr. Ross Trattler, *Better Health Through Natural Healing* (New York, McGraw-Hill Book Co., 1985), p. 190.

used when stools are large, hard and dry; the woman is insecure and holds back. *Lycopodium* is for ineffectual urging with small hard, incomplete stools and constipation in pregnancy. Use *Nux vomica* for ineffectual desire and urging, with incomplete and unsatisfying movements. *Calcarea carbonia (Calc. carb.)* is the remedy for stool that is hard at first, then pasty, then liquid. Use *Alumina* for dry stools with total lack of intestinal activity.

Cell Salts: *Kali sulph.* is for chronic constipation, and *Ferrum phos.* is for inertia of intestinal muscles. *Natrum mur.* is the remedy if the tongue is white, there are hard dry stools, and for constipation alternating with diarrhea. The indication for *Kali phos.* is offensive odor to stools. For elders use *Calc. phos.* and for children *Natrum phos.* When constipation always occurs before and during menstruation, the remedy is *Silica*; partially expelled stool recedes again.

Amino Acids: Use a liver-extract amino combination for the B-complex vitamins and its detoxifying and nutritive properties.

Acupressure: Do full foot reflexology, paying particular attention to the small and large intestinal points, the liver, rectum and ileocecal valve. Do pressure massage working up to twice a day and working out sore reflex points. There are body reflexes on both sides of the navel and about four inches below it on the front, and on the back find the reflex meridian between the coccyx (tailbone) and the anus. Use the Great Eliminator point in the webs between thumbs and first fingers, and also do pressure massage on the hands, using the body map to locate the eliminative organs.

Aromatherapy: Make a massage oil of twenty drops of marjoram and five drops of rose in two ounces of vegetable oil. Single aromas, for massage oils, baths or diffusers, include fennel, marjoram, angelica, aniseed or carrot seed.

Flower Essences: Pomegranate is indicated for constipation, as the primary essence. Cedar, sage or aloe vera are also positive.

Gemstones and Gem Essences: Coral, emerald, green jasper, picture jasper and sulfur are laxative, and the metals copper or platinum in essence. Hold or wear yellow or yellow-green gemstones to stimulate the digestive system and aid in elimination.

Emotional Healing: Constipation can be stinginess, hoarding or a fear of poverty; it can be a refusal to let go of the past or of old ideas. Know that there is always enough and the past is over. Do an uncording ritual (see *Casting the Circle: A Women's Book of Rituals*) for letting go of what (or who) is gone, and create affirmations about affluence and free flow. There is always enough, and letting go of the past makes way for the future.

Acupressure for Constipation

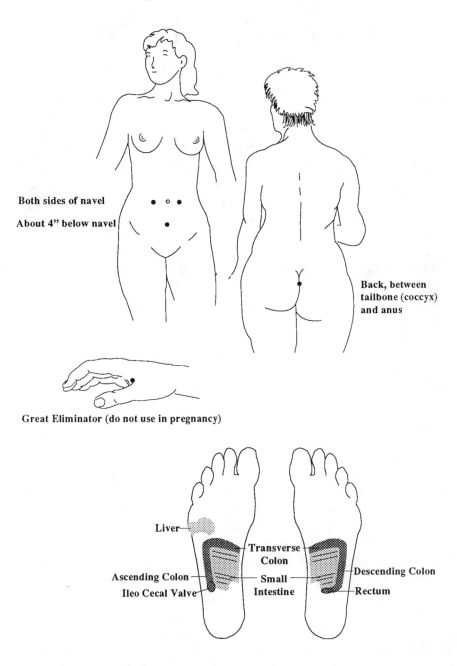

Both sides of navel

About 4" below navel

Back, between
tailbone (coccyx)
and anus

Great Eliminator (do not use in pregnancy)

Liver

Transverse
Colon

Ascending Colon

Descending Colon

Ileo Cecal Valve

Small
Intestine

Rectum

Cathryn Bauer, *Acupressure for Women* (Freedom, CA, The Crossing Press, 1987), p.135; Pedro Chan, *Finger Acupressure* (New York, Ballantine Books, 1974), p. 40-41.

Coughs and Flu

Coughs and flu usually go together, but coughing can have a number of causes. It is the body's way of removing dust or mucus from the bronchi and airways, and can be a sign of irritation in the lungs, throat or bronchial tubes. Coughs can be a sign of asthma or lung dis-ease, but more often are symptoms of allergies or chest colds. Influenza (flu) is a viral dis-ease of the respiratory tract, involving headache, weakness, achiness, fever and chills. There is a dry throat and cough, sinus and chest congestion, tiredness, and sometimes nausea or vomiting. Like the common cold, which also may include coughing, the flu is brought on by a variety of changing viruses that make successful vaccination difficult. Many women who take flu vaccines end up with the flu, and homeopaths have a horror of the whole vaccination practice. Coughs and flu are usually self-limiting dis-eases, lasting under two weeks, but occasionally can become more serious. Where there is blood in the sputum, coughs lasting longer than two weeks, flu or cough in debilitated women or elders, or persistent coughing in children, expert help is needed. Otherwise, like the common cold, rest and healing will suffice. A number of holistic remedies for cough and flu are given here, and also see the section on Colds.

Vitamins and Minerals: The vitamin program is similar to that of colds and sore throats. Along with a multiple vitamin and mineral supplement, use vitamin C (1000 mg hourly) at the start to try to stop it completely. Drink a lot of water with this and decrease it slowly. Use C to bowel tolerance during the dis-ease. Vitamin C helps to lower fever, boost the immune system, and flush toxins from the body; it is also antiviral. Vitamin A is another immune booster and antioxidant; take 25,000 IU daily and add more with beta-carotene. Zinc gluconate lozenges are used with sore throats and coughs and are highly important in flu healing. Dissolve one lozenge under the tongue every two hours. The B-complex vitamin B-5 is an antihistamine, and B-6 is also important; use them with a full B-complex-50. Gamma linolenic acid (black currant oil) is recommended.

Herbs: Ginger root tea or tincture taken frequently at the start of a cough or flu can sometimes stop it, as can the cayenne and goldenseal capsules described under Colds. Five drops of cinnamon oil in a teaspoon of water taken several times a day at the early start can also sometimes stop the flu. For coughs, use coltsfoot, slippery elm bark (in tea or lozenges), ginger root, gum plant, licorice (not for women with high blood pressure), ephedra (for bronchodilation), mullein, squill, or wild clover. Wild cherry is a sedative and expectorant; use coltsfoot for the lungs. St. John's wort controls coughing and stimulates sweating for fevers. Use herbal cough syrups of licorice, wild cherry or coltsfoot, and capsules of cayenne to break up the worst coughs and congestions.

For flu symptoms, make a tea of an ounce elecampane root in a pint of water; boil for fifteen minutes. Strain and add a teaspoon of honey and two teaspoons of lemon juice. Drink a cup warm three times a day. Boneset is good for all flu symptoms and achiness and is recommended, as well as elder flower, and the two may be used together. Echinacea or goldenseal, ginger tea or yarrow are positive, and peppermint tea will cause sweating and aid nausea. To reduce fever, take catnip tea enemas with 1/4–1/2 teaspoon of lobelia tincture every three or four hours. Use yarrow, peppermint and elderberry together from the first signs of flu on, and clover or alfalfa tonics help in recovery. For lung congestion use fenugreek, comfrey and slippery elm together. Or use sage, garlic and lemon tea for flu and coughs; pour six cups of boiling water over two heaping tablespoons of sage leaves, two chopped garlic cloves and the juice and pulp of half a lemon. Add honey to taste and steep for five minutes. Drink a cup per hour hot and stay in bed to sweat.

Naturopathy: For coughs, boil a lemon for ten minutes, then juice it, put the juice in a glass and add one ounce of vegetable glycerin or fill the rest of the glass with honey. Take a teaspoonful several times a day. For a similar recipe, cook the juice of a lemon, a cup of honey and half a cup of olive oil until blended, and take a teaspoonful every two hours. Or: peel and chop six onions and place them with half a cup of honey in a double boiler top. Cover and simmer for two hours, strain and pour into a covered jar. Take a tablespoonful warm every two or three hours.

Garlic is an important remedy for colds, coughs and flu—it is antiviral, antibacterial and an immune builder. Use two Kyolic tablets three times a day with meals and see the raw garlic remedies listed under colds.

In early flu stages, take a hot bath with epsom salts, or a cup of sea salt and a cup of baking soda. Stay in the tub for twenty to twenty-five minutes and then go to bed to sweat out the toxins. Withhold food but drink lots of herb teas and fluids. Once respiratory symptoms have developed, apply castor oil packs to chest and throat (apple cider vinegar compresses may also be used). Again stay on a liquid (no milk) diet until symptoms are relieved, then reintroduce foods slowly.

Homeopathy and Cell Salts: *Oscillococcinum* is a homeopathic remedy that can stop the flu if taken early enough. Nosodes of *Bacillinum* or *Influenzium* are available from homeopathic physicians. Use *Baptisia* for headache, aching limbs and fever, or *Arsenicum* for chills, restlessness, anxiety or stomach upset. *Aconite* is for early stages of both flu and coughs, or use *Nux vomica* in early stages where there is irritability. *Bryonia alba* is for chest colds with dry painful cough and thirst for cold drinks. *Eupatorium* is the remedy for flu with aching bones and muscles, runny nose, and fever with chills; use *Gelsemium* for sneezing, runny nose, rough throat, chills and fever, aches, headaches and flu symptoms. *Ipecac* is for moist, rattling coughs with choking and nausea. Use *Kali bichromium* when cough is worst first thing in the morning and produces a stringy, thick, gluey sputum. *Drosera* is for violent coughs, barking coughs, and whooping cough.

Cell Salts: *Natrum mur.* is the primary cell salt for flu; take it every hour at onset until improvement, then three times a day for two more weeks. If there is no improvement, alternate *Natrum mur.* with *Calc. phos.* and *Kali phos.* until there is, then go back again to *Natrum mur.* only.

For coughs, use *Ferrum phos.* if feverish and sore, *Kali mur.* if there is a white, stringy expectoration, or *Natrum sulph.* with green or yellow-green expectoration. Use *Mag. phos.* for dry spasmodic cough or whooping cough, *Natrum mur.* for watery expectoration with a salty taste, or *Silica* for a smothering cough at night.

Amino Acids: A free-form amino acids combination is important for its B-complex vitamins, immune building factors, ability to control fevers, and ability to detoxify the body.

Acupressure: For flu and coughs look for tender pressure points above the breast bone and on the back just above the shoulder blades. A reflex point in the opening of the collar bone will stop coughing. Use the points on the wrist and behind the big toe together (you will need help for this) and then the points at base of thumb and base of ring finger together. (See illustrations.) Also see the pressure points illustrated for Colds and Sore Throats.

Aromatherapy: Use eucalyptus in a vaporizer or diffuser twice a day. Lavender is also important. Other oils include bergamot, rosemary, cypress or myrrh. Tiferet-Lifetree has a respiratory combination.

Flower Essences: Jasmine regulates mucus in the system, and manzanita is for the lungs.

Gemstones and Gem Essences: Use beryl, jet, meteorite or sulfur in essence, or the metals copper or gold. Hold or wear a piece of azurite to clear and decongest the sinuses, chest, throat and lymphatic system. Aquamarine will help sore throats or coughs.

Acupressure for Coughs

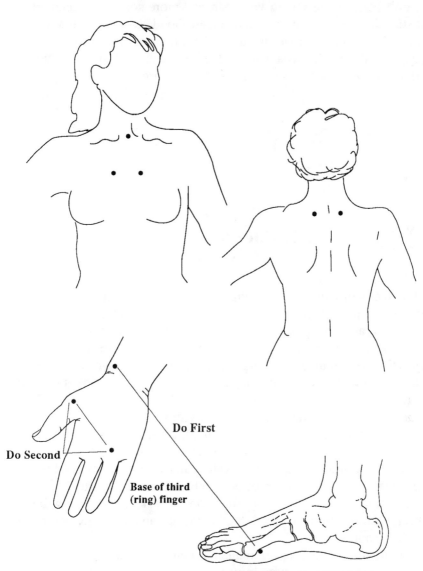

Do foot and wrist points together, first, then do thumb and base of ring finger together

John Thie, DC, *A Touch for Health, A New Approach to Restoring Our Natural Energies* (Marina del Rey, CA, DeVorss and Co., 1973), p. 36; Pedro Chan, *Finger Acupressure* (New York, Ballantine Books, 1974), p. 36.

Emotional Healing: Flu is running with the herd and accepting mass negativity and beliefs: if the radio says the flu is going 'round, you will get it. Don't believe everything you hear, and more so, don't accept every statistic. You are an individual and you are Goddess—not the mass mind. Coughs can come from words unsaid, held back or choked on, anger or blocked creativity. Say what you need to say and make time to do your real work in the world. (Also see Colds and Sore Throats.)

Cystitis
Bladder Infections

Thirty times more women than men experience cystitis or bladder infections (urinary tract infections), and forty percent of women will suffer it chronically at some point in their lives. Many bladder infections are caused by an imbalance in intestinal flora, the after-effect of taking antibiotics or other medical drugs. A majority of women who have chronic bladder infections seem also to have systemic candida albicans (see that section in this book) and/or food allergies. Birth control pills can be a factor, poor-fitting diaphragms or allergy to spermicides, liver congestion, caffeine or alcohol (they are irritants), constipation, need for spinal adjustments, stress, or frequent sexual activity (lesbian or heterosexual). A simple lack of drinking enough water can cause or aggravate this disease, and nylon underpants or pantyhose that restrict airflow to the vaginal area also make it worse. Wiping from front to back on the toilet will help to keep bacteria out of the urethra and bladder, and urinating before and after intercourse.

Symptoms of cystitis are frequent urination, usually with burning or pain. You may have the urge to urinate again as soon as the bladder is voided, or feel an urge but nothing comes. There may be pain or cramping in the urethra, above the pubis, and/or in a line running along the pelvic bones. The urine may have a strong smell, look cloudy, or contain blood or fragments. There may be no other symptoms than frequency, and the abdomen may feel or appear to be bloated. An untreated bladder infection can spread to the kidneys, a more serious infection. If pains run along the back at about waist level, the tubes leading from bladder to kidneys are involved, or the kidneys themselves.

Vitamins and Minerals: Along with a multiple vitamin and mineral supplement, vitamin C is the big one here. At first sign of a bladder infection, take 1000 mg per hour and *lots* of water, and this may be enough by itself to stop it. For prevention, take at least 1000 mg of C per day. Along with the vitamin C, particularly in megadoses, also use a B-complex-50 or -100, and 600 IU of vitamin E. The target B-vitamins are choline, folic acid, B-2, B-5 and B-6. Use zinc (50 mg) for immune building and calcium/magnesium (1000–1500 mg calcium with half the amount of magnesium); for chronic inflammations use 25,000 IU of beta-carotene daily. Acidophilus in the form of Megadophilus or Maxidophilus is recommended, taken internally, and can be used as a douche. If you are taking antibiotics, this is essential. After the infection, stay on these for immune building and prevention.

Herbs: Juniper berries, buchu, cornsilk, marshmallow root, nettles, parsley, dandelion or uva ursi are used for bladder infections, as well as the herbal antibiotics goldenseal, echinacea or pau d'arco. Use bearberry, couchgrass and yarrow together, or bearberry, sage and horsetail. Use a comfrey poultice over the bladder area externally, and if there is blood in the urine use shepherd's purse.

Naturopathy: Eat a whole foods diet of vegetables, vegetarian protein, whole grains, unsaturated oils and some fresh fruit. Drink water, fruit or vegetable juices, or herbal teas. Avoid constipation. To acidify the urine and stop a bladder infection, cranberry juice is primary. Use the unsweetened stuff from healthfood stores and drink a sixteen ounce glass hourly from the first sign of an infection. It will usually stop it within a couple of hours. Once stopped, continue the juice for prevention at least twice a day. Cherry juice, lemon juice and water, buttermilk (acidophilus), or two teaspoons of apple cider vinegar in a glass of water will do the same things. If you have nothing else available, drink a sixteen ounce glass of plain water hourly, and make sure you are drinking at least eight glasses of water or liquids per day. Avoid caffeine, alcohol, citrus and soft drinks; they are kidney and bladder irritants.

Kyolic is important in ridding the body of candida albicans and the infection bacteria (E. coli): it is an antibacterial and immune system builder. Use two tablets three times a day with meals. Watermelon, and watermelon seed or rind in tea, or watermelon pills are diuretic and cleanse the urinary tract. Eat a lot of onions and use an onion poultice for the kidneys. Castor oil packs are also effective. Drink carrot juice, beet juice or cucumber juice; avoid dairy products, hot spicy foods and sugar. Take a hot bath with two cups of baking soda in it, soak for half an hour, then shower off.

Homeopathy and Cell Salts: Use *Cantharis* for cystitis with frequent, painful urination, or *Causticum* for cystitis that is chronic with involuntary discharge of urine. *Aconite* may be used at first onset. *Sarsaparilla is* the remedy when pain is worst at the end of urinating, or *Staphysagria* for "honeymoon cystitis." *Mercurius* symptoms are worse at night and include burning, uncontrollable urges, dark urine, passage in small amounts, and pain worse when not urinating or at the beginning or end of urination. *Nux vomica* cystitis has burning or pressing pain during urination, needle-like pain, and the attacks occur after taking alcohol, coffee or medication. The woman requiring Nux is always irritable. *Apis* is used in severe pain, strong urging with little urine flow, and the abdomen is sensitive to the touch.

Cell Salts: *Ferrum phos.* is for tender kidneys and first onset. *Kali sulph.* is the remedy for difficult urination and *Natrum sulph.* for kidney stones. Or use the following combination: *Kali mur.*, *Ferrum phos.*, *Kali phos.*, and *Mag. phos.*

Amino Acids: A full combination amino acids builds the immune system, detoxifies, repairs tissue, and contains the B-complex vitamins and sulfur. Single aminos include methionine and cystine.

Acupressure: Look for tender areas on the feet and hands and pay particular attention to the liver, bladder, kidneys and urinary tract on the body map. Massage the reflexes in the wrists, and use the Great Eliminator/ autonomic nervous system point between the thumbs and first fingers. Also look for tender points between the third and fourth toes. See the illustration for other reflexes.

Aromatherapy: Use eucalyptus, juniper and thyme together in a bath, or take a bath with lavender essence or sandalwood (make sure it's the pure essential oil). Others include birch, cajeput, cedarwood, tea-tree or lovage.

Flower Essences: Chamomile strengthens the kidneys, and eucalyptus is for kidney and urinary tract inflammation.

Gemstones and Gem Essences: Lodestone and magnetite are the gem essences, in addition to the metal silver. Hold or wear bloodstone, jade, citrine, topaz or amber calcite.

Emotional Healing: What (or who) is pissing you off? Withheld anger is an invitation to cystitis, usually anger at a lover. Release the need to blame others and express the anger and hurt. Many women with chronic cystitis have herstories of sexual abuse.

Acupressure for Cystitis

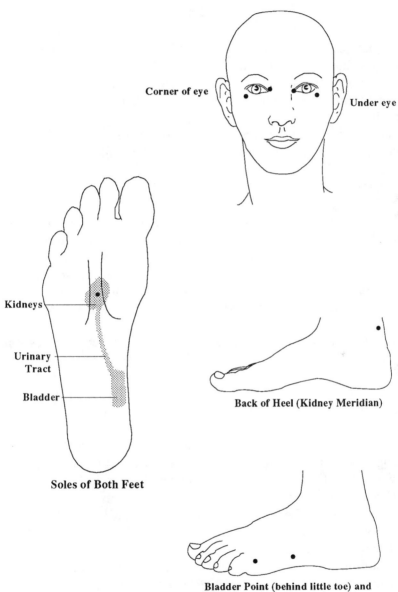

Corner of eye

Under eye

Kidneys

Urinary Tract

Bladder

Soles of Both Feet

Back of Heel (Kidney Meridian)

Bladder Point (behind little toe) and
Bladder (behind ball of foot on side)

Cathryn Bauer, *Acupressure for Women* (Freedom, CA, The Crossing Press, 1987), p. 51 and 120.

Depression

Depression is considered a mental and nervous dis-ease, a reaction to not admitting sadness or guilt to oneself or others. The experts, however, seldom use a political analysis to explain its incidence in women, or consider the number of physiological factors that add to or cause it. Women in this high stress society are in a position of working twice as hard to earn half as much—monetarily, socially, politically and in civil rights. We have a society where women do most of the work—and all of the disagreeable and low-paying work—and are the lowest paid and most often unemployed. We fight daily for reproductive and sexual freedom, and for the everyday perks that men take for granted or don't even notice. On top of all this, we hold most of the responsibility for making a home for ourselves and our families, for bringing peace to the world (the men certainly won't do it), and for bearing and raising new lives. The majority of poor in affluent America are single or lesbian women, women with children, and elder women, Black and white. Is it any wonder that the majority of those who seek psychological help are women and that twice as many women as men are on tranquilizers and antidepressants?

There are a number of physical reasons for women's depression, also. Some of them include endocrine imbalances, chronic fatigue syndrome, heredity, heavy metal toxicity, high sugar diets, chronic headaches or migraines, endometriosis, hypoglycemia or diabetes, candida albicans or food sensitivities, mononucleosis, any physical dis-ease, and winter in cold climates. Stress and nutritional deficiencies are major causes. Yet, in a world where there could be peace, freedom for all, an end to homelessness and hunger, sexual and reproductive rights, racial equality and job parity, there would be a lot less depression in women.

The remedies below are for mild to moderate depression and can also be used with psychotherapy. Depression that is severe can be a life-threatening dis-ease, requiring expert help to heal. Use conventional and holistic methods together for best results.

Vitamins and Minerals: The B-complex vitamins are essential in healing depression; use a B-complex-100 three times a day. Specific B-vitamins include B-1, B-3 (niacin), B-6, B-9 (folic acid) and B-12. Women with menstrual problems or on the pill need B-6 (250–500 mg total per day) and folic acid (400 mcg total daily). Lecithin is important for brain and nerve function but is not for use by manic depressives; niacin is a calmative and necessary for women with migraines (use 100 mg per day total). A B-complex-100 will do the job without others added for most women. Use vitamin C for stress (1000–3000 mg per day or go to bowel tolerance). A complete calcium/magnesium supplement can make a great difference for many women and is recommended, in addition to a multiple vitamin-mineral supplement.

Herbs: Calming tension can also relieve depression; for stress try passion flower, scullcap, catnip, or chamomile. Herbs for lethargy include a mix of gotu kola, damiana, lavender and rosemary, or poplar bark with gentian root, or agrimony with centaury. Single herbs include borage, vervain, lavender, lime blossom, black cohosh (for hormone balancing, particularly for women over forty), cloves, balm or peppermint. Burn myrrh as an incense and also drink it as a tea. See the section on Stress, as well.

Naturopathy: Eat a high protein, grain and raw vegetable diet, without additives, salt, unsaturated fats, chemicals, refined flour or sugar, alcohol or caffeine. Do an elimination diet to check for food allergies, and a candida cleanse if indicated.

In addition, spirulina, essential fatty acids (black currant oil or primrose oil), and/or bee pollen or propolis will all be helpful. Since poor assimilation can be the source of nutritional deficiency, try a glass of water with a teaspoon of apple cider vinegar and a teaspoon of honey with meals. Make a vegetable juice of watercress, spinach and carrots in a juicer, or eat bananas to stimulate the antidepression hormones of the brain. Cloves added to other herb teas also aid depression, and foods with oregano.

Homeopathy and Cell Salts: The following remedies are for mild to moderate depression. Remember that there may be an aggravation, a worsening before there is relief. Depression responds very positively to expert homeopathic treatment and this expert help is recommended. Use *Arsenicum* for anxiety and depression, exhaustion and restlessness, especially with chills or when worse between midnight and 2 AM. *Ignatia* is for depression following a grief or end of love affair; there is disappointment, anger, anxiety or headaches. *Passiflora* is a mild sedative, and *Pulsatilla* is for depression with weeping, especially in women of light coloring. Use *Aurum metallicum* for suicidal feelings, or *Calcarea carbonica* for sadness, melancholy, heavy feeling in limbs and weepiness. If your symptoms are silent, melancholy and peevish, and distant music causes sadness, the remedy if *Lycopodium*.

Cell Salts: *Natrum mur.* is for recurring unpleasant memories, and consolation causes weeping. *Calc. phos.* is for great depression with difficulty in performing daily life. *Kali phos.* is for stress and depression. Also try Combination Cell Salts (Bioplasma), or Calmes Forte.

Amino Acids: These are highly important for depression, stress reduction, nutrition and brain function. Use 750 mg of GABA (Gamma-aminobutyric acid) with niacinamide and inositol as a tranquilizer. This can take the place of many medical drugs. For personality disorders, use glutamic acid, and tyrosine for brain function. Avoid phenylalanine, as many depressed women are allergic to it; if you are manic depressive avoid choline (vitamin), ornathine and arginine (aminos). Try a combination amino acids otherwise, and monitor your response.

Acupressure: Do full foot or hand acupressure and pay particular attention to the reflexes for the sinus, pituitary, cerebrum, cranial nerves, thyroid, adrenals, liver and thymus. For releasing grief, try acupressure points below the collar bone on both sides near the shoulders (you will know them by the soreness), and on the back beside each shoulder blade (see illustrations). Work the points for the entire endocrine system on hands, feet and body.

Aromatherapy: Take one drop each of the following essences on a brown sugar cube: chamomile, jasmine and bergamot. Use any of the following in baths, diffusers, or a drop near the body to inhale: lavender (recommended), clary sage (recommended), jasmine, basil, bergamot, rose, melissa, chamomile, orange or neroli. Tiferet-Lifetree has a relaxing combination that treats depression.

Flower Essences: Blackberry is for depression from grief; borage opens the heart and drives away sorrow; dill is for stress and manic depression; and hellebore is for depression from aging or a broken romance. Use peach for mood swings and to bring a sense of joy. Scullcap in essence tones the nervous system, and sugar beet is for depression due to blood sugar disorders. In the Bach Flower Remedies, try Star of Bethlehem for grief, trauma or loss, or Sweet Chestnut for despair and anguish.

Gemstones and Gem Essences: A number of gem essences are used including: botswanna agate, moss agate, azurite, chrysoprase, coral, eilat stone, garnet, herkimer diamond, labradorite, lapis, onyx (for grief), peridot, rose quartz, rutile quartz, sapphire or topaz. Hold a piece of apophyllite or chrysocolla and/or wear turquoise.

Emotional Healing: Standard definition is not acknowledging one's sadness, grief or guilt. Add to these emotions women's anger and rage, and the inability (or fear of repercussions) at expressing these powerful emotions. Release grief by a good cry or a ritual letting go, and guilt by working on self-love. Release anger by speaking it out, and doing safe actions (hitting a punching bag or pillow) to express it. Another way of ending depression is to do some activism; get involved in changing the things you are depressed about. First understand what it is that you are angry or sad about, then do work on releasing the depression and pain.

Acupressure for Depression

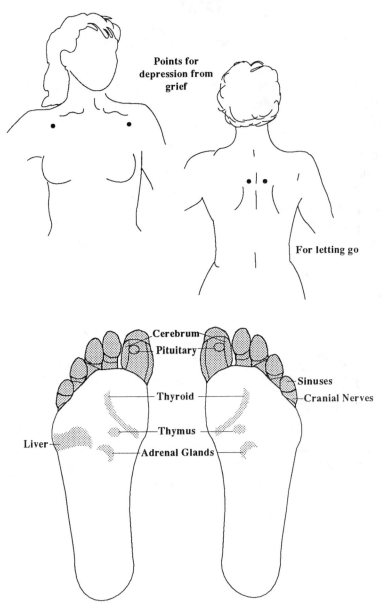

Points for depression from grief

For letting go

Cerebrum
Pituitary
Sinuses
Cranial Nerves
Thyroid
Thymus
Liver
Adrenal Glands

Foot Reflexes for Depression

Iona Marsaa Teeguarden, *Acupressure Way of Health: Jin Shin Do* (New York, Japan Publishing Co., 1978), p. 150; Moshe Olshevsky, CA, PhD., *et. al.*, *The Manual of Natural Therapy* (New York, Citadel Press, 1989), p. 298.

Diabetes
Adult Onset

About five percent of people in the United States are diabetic, another five percent may have adult onset diabetes that is undiagnosed, and twenty million more may have impaired glucose tolerance ability. Eighty percent of diabetics are fat, a metabolic condition that goes with the dis-ease. Most women who develop adult onset diabetes have experienced a severe emotional shock in the preceding year, and reduction of fear and stress is important for their healing. Diabetes results when the pancreas produces insufficient amounts of insulin, preventing the body from utilizing glucose. There are two types of diabetes, juvenile and adult onset. Juvenile diabetes occurs usually in children or young adults, and may be linked to viral infection or chemical toxicity; as adults they will be insulin dependent. Once beginning the use of injected insulin, it is almost always lifelong. Adult onset diabetes occurs later in life, usually in women with a family heredity of the dis-ease. Diet and healing methods can often control blood sugar levels so that insulin is not required. The information here is for both types of diabetes, but primarily for adult onset.

Diabetes is a dis-ease of civilization with adrenal exhaustion, liver congestion or toxicity, endocrine depletion, and poor diet leading to pancreatic insufficiency. Stress is a major cause, along with refined carbohydrates, caffeine, alcohol, street drugs, and nicotine. Food allergies and environmental sensitivities can be factors. Early holistic care of mild adult onset diabetes can often result in total cures; in prolonged cases or where there is insulin dependency, degenerative factors can be reduced along with the amounts of insulin required. Diabetes is a serious dis-ease requiring expert supervision. *Holistic therapies may lower insulin need and change blood sugar values. Monitor carefully and frequently.*

Vitamins and Minerals: Along with a multiple vitamin and mineral supplement, the following are important. Chromium (Glucose Tolerance Factor) is a mineral that helps to stabilize blood sugar and is essential for diabetics; take 200 mcg daily. Use 15–30 mg of zinc daily, 1500 mg calcium/750 mg magnesium, and essential fatty acids (evening primrose oil or black currant oil)—two capsules three times a day. Of the minerals, manganese and potassium are also important. Use vitamin A (25,000 IU per day) but not beta-carotene; diabetics cannot convert it to A. Also take a B-complex-50 two or three times a day, plus lecithin. B-complex lowers the need for insulin, detoxifies stress, and helps diabetic neuropathy. B-6 (250–500 mg total daily) helps to prevent arteriosclerosis. Vitamin C with bioflavinoids reduces insulin need, and helps stop diabetic cataracts use 3000-12,000 mg daily or go to bowel tolerance. Vitamin E (800 IU daily, particularly E with selenium) also lowers insulin need and promotes organ healing. Germanium in addition is positive, and digestive enzymes may also help. Avoid PABA, fish oil capsules, and large amounts of niacin.

Herbs: Dandelion stimulates pancreatic activity, as does buchu, and both are good in early stages. Use fenugreek and cornsilk together, goats rue or mullein, goldenseal (antibiotic), alfalfa, parsley, periwinkle, huckleberry leaves, ginseng, juniper, cedar berries or uva ursi. Yarrow contains some of the same active ingredients as insulin; drink four cups of yarrow tea per day and eat three Jerusalem artichokes with it.

Naturopathy: Eat a diet high in unrefined carbohydrates, with most of the protein from vegetable (grain and bean) sources. Use whole grains, yoghurt, nuts, tofu, fish, organic fowl or meat, raw or lightly steamed vegetables, and fiber. Frequently eat foods that are insulin producing: Jerusalem artichokes, brussels sprouts, cucumbers, green beans, garlic (lots of it), oatmeal or oat flour products, soybeans, or avocado. Avoid fruits and fruit juices, all refined sugar and white flour products, white rice, alcohol, street drugs, smoking, and saturated fats. Eat several small meals a day, with as much as three-quarters of the diet in raw foods.[1] Also use spirulina, berries, brewer's yeast, bananas, cheese, sauerkraut, watercress, parsley, and organic juices.

Use iodine in the form of kelp tablets or Atomidine. To replace sugar as a sweetener, try stevia, an herbal that helps to balance glucose; avoid sorbitol chemical sugar substitutes; they cause cataracts. Try raw pancreas glandular extract and/or pancreatic enzymes for digestion. Stop smoking.

Homeopathy and Cell Salts: See an experienced homeopath for diabetes, but some remedies include: *Syzygium* as a general remedy, and *Codeinum* for depression and skin irritation in diabetes.

Cell Salts: Use ten tablets of each twice a day: *Kali phos.*, *Natrum Mur.* and *Ferrum phos.* Use *Natrum Sulph.* for over-urination and to help the liver.

Amino Acids: Try 500 mg of carnitine and glutamine twice a day on an empty stomach. Avoid L-cystine. Try a combination free-form amino acids and monitor the results.

Acupressure: When using acupressure for diabetes, monitor insulin

---

[1]Dr. Ross Trattler, *Better Health Through Natural Healing* (New York, McGraw-Hill Book Co., 1985), p. 209–211.

and blood sugar levels carefully. Insulin need may decrease. If you use this form of healing, you must use it consistently. Look for sore spots starting on the left side of the front of the body below the ribs. After releasing these, move an inch toward the center of the body and press again, then move across the body to a little above the navel. Press each sore spot to release it. There are kidney-adrenal points just below the eyes, points for the internal organs on top of the head, and a point for the spleen and pancreas just above the lip in the center. See the illustration for these, and bladder meridian points on the back. Do full foot or hand reflexology, starting with twice a week and working up to twice a day.

Aromatherapy: Massage the whole body daily with an oil containing the following essences: eucalyptus, geranium and juniper, 4% of each in olive oil. This can also be used in baths.

Flower Essences: Apricot strengthens the pancreas and balances blood sugar; banana is for sugar assimilation and skin reactions; ginseng regenerates the pancreas and associated organs; sugar beet essence produces insulin in the body. Others include marigold for pancreatic inflammation, pomegranate for insulin production and absorption, and Queen Anne's lace for emotional understanding of the diabetic process.

Gemstones and Gem Essences: Moss agate, amethyst or rhodochrosite are the gem essences. Hold or wear rhodochrosite, malachite, citrine or amber.

Emotional Healing: Most adult onset diabetes occurs after a major emotional shock, such as the loss of a mate. There is deep sorrow and longing for what might have been, a yearning for the sweet ideal in life now lost. The woman is starving for affection (sweetness) and has a perception that no more is left. Find joy in little things. There is sweetness everywhere. Remember to love yourself.

Acupressure for Diabetes

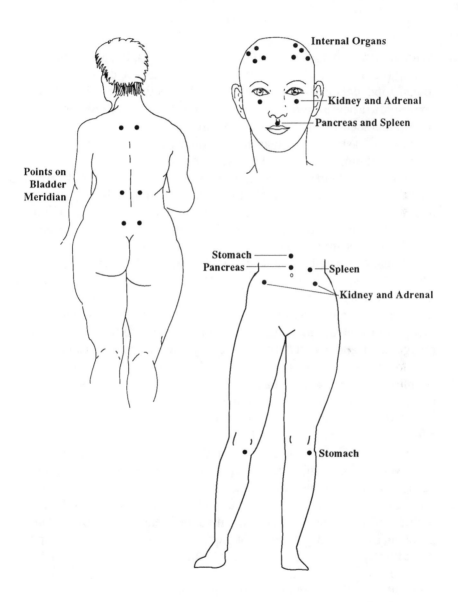

Internal Organs

Kidney and Adrenal

Pancreas and Spleen

Points on
Bladder
Meridian

Stomach
Pancreas

Spleen

Kidney and Adrenal

Stomach

Mildred Carter, *Body Reflexology* (W. Nyack, NY, Parker Publishing Co., 1983), p. 156-160; Moshe Olshevsky, CA, PhD., *et. al.*, *The Manual of Natural Therapy* (New York, Citadel Press, 1989), p. 255.

Diarrhea

Acute diarrhea in adults, lasting two or three days, is the body's way of getting rid of toxins or unwanted substances. It can be caused by laxative foods, food poisoning, bacterial or viral infection, "change of water" (exposure to a new bacteria, for which the body hasn't developed antibodies), food intolerance usually from wheat or milk, antibiotics, intestinal parasites, overeating, gastritis, pancreas/adrenal/digestive malfunction, excess vitamin C or zinc, or emotional causes. If diarrhea becomes chronic, there is severe pain, blood in the stool, fever above 101°F, stools look tarry and black, if you are not urinating, or if there is obvious dehydration, expert help is needed. Otherwise, it is best to withhold foods, drink lots of liquids, and let the body purge itself for the first day or two before treating.

In children, diarrhea lasting longer than twenty-four hours is serious, and should be treated immediately in infants, who can dehydrate rapidly. The high cause of infant mortality in third world countries is primarily due to diarrhea dehydration, which can usually be remedied with the following emergency formula. Dissolve a teaspoon of salt and a tablespoon of sugar in a pint of boiled water. Allow to cool in a covered bottle (store in the refrigerator), and give it to the child every few minutes in teaspoonfuls. If a child or infant does not respond to this or holistic methods within a couple of hours, seek expert advice. If a nursing infant has diarrhea, check the mother's diet for possible source.

Vitamins and Minerals: Persistent diarrhea causes a deficiency in every nutrient, particularly minerals. This same diarrhea may also be caused by deficiencies, particularly of the B-complex vitamins folic acid, B-1, B-6 or niacin, magnesium (from taking an imbalance of too much calcium without enough matching magnesium), iron, and/or potassium. Take a full B-complex-50 and up to 100 mg of potassium per day, along with a multiple vitamin and mineral supplement. If malabsorption is a problem, use a liquid B-complex and/or a liquid multiple. Take acidophilus in the form of Maxidophilus or Megadophilus to replace friendly intestinal bacteria, and charcoal tablets—every four hours with water but not at the same time as other supplements or medications—until the diarrhea stops. If acidophilus aggravates the diarrhea, the cause of the diarrhea is dairy intolerance.

Herbs: Carob powder in water is a good diarrhea remedy, as is blackberry tea or slippery elm tea or capsules. Other teas or tinctures include cinnamon (1/4 teaspoon to sweeten other teas), catnip, peppermint, raspberry, strawberry leaf, chamomile, oak bark, tormentil, ginger, or black elder bark. Make a cayenne and cinnamon tea: boil two cups of water and add 1/2 teaspoon cinnamon and a dash of cayenne. Simmer for twenty minutes, cool and strain, and take two tablespoons every hour. To make slippery elm tea, use an ounce of the powdered herb in a quart of water and simmer it down to a pint. Take a teaspoon every half hour. Slippery elm can also be used as a food for infants and debilitated women. For dysentery, use juniper berries or whole Canadian thistles boiled in milk or slippery elm.

Naturopathy: Help the body to eliminate what it is trying to purge by going on a fast, and even use enemas to speed the process. (Do not use enemas if colitis is suspected.) It is highly important to drink plenty of fluids; use bottled water and a teaspoon of apple juice every fifteen minutes. After the fast there are a number of foods that will help: apples (remove the skin), applesauce, bananas, carob or amaranth powder, barley water, carrot and cabbage juice, yoghurt, sauerkraut and tomato juice (a tablespoon of each every hour), rice water, kefir milk, blueberries or huckleberries. Try blackberry juice or blackberry wine, also, for diarrhea after radiation.

Eat a teaspoon of chopped garlic and a teaspoonful of honey three times a day between meals. Garlic (or odorless Kyolic) tablets are antibacterial. Eating a clove of raw garlic a day while traveling will help prevent dysentery, as will acidophilus or vitamin C. A glass of water with two tablespoons of epsom salts in it is effective also for dysentery. For simple diarrhea, food poisoning or dysentery, put a teaspoon of apple cider vinegar in a glass of water and take a sip every five minutes. It will remineralize the body and balance electrolytes and fluids. Kelp tablets are also important for replacing lost minerals.

Homeopathy and Cell Salts: Some of the many remedies for diarrhea include *Arsenicum* for violent and frequent diarrhea with nausea and vomiting, nighttime diarrhea recurring after food or drink, or for food poisoning. Use *Cinchona officinalis* for slimy watery diarrhea after eating fruit, or *Colocynthis* for violent fluid stools after every food or drink. For slimy stools, abdominal pain, and painful spasms in the anus, the remedy is *Mercurius*. Use *Podophyllum* for watery, profuse offensive stools in the morning or for teething children. Try *Veratrum album* for profuse rice water stools with exhaustion and/or vomiting; the woman needs to be very cold. *Sulfur* is for frequent diarrhea at night or early morning, driving the woman from bed, with back pain, abdominal pain and/or anal spasms.

Acupressure for Diarrhea

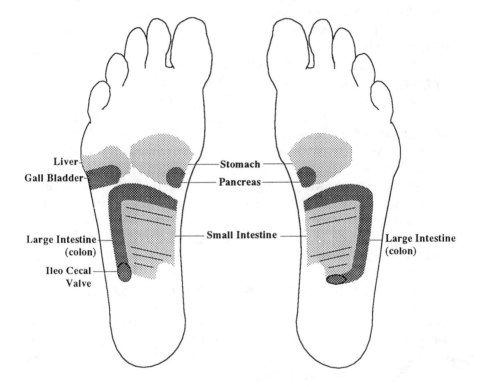

Liver
Gall Bladder
Stomach
Pancreas
Large Intestine (colon)
Small Intestine
Large Intestine (colon)
Ileo Cecal Valve

See the same body map on the hands

Moshe Olshevsky, CA, PhD., *et. al.*, *The Manual of Natural Therapy* (New York, Citadel Press, 1989), p. 34.

Cell Salts: Take *Ferrum phos.* at the start, *Natrum phos.* if there is acidity, and *Natrum sulph.* with biliousness.

Amino Acids: Use a combination liver-based amino acids for B-complex vitamins, tissue repair and rebuilding. They are powerful as antioxidants and nutrients.

Acupressure: The pressure points are similar to those for constipation, as they bring the organs into balance. Do full foot or hand massage, paying particular attention to the small and large intestines, stomach, liver, gall bladder, pancreas and ileocecal valve.

Aromatherapy: Cardamom, chamomile or ginger root are used in baths, massage oils or diffusers. Inhale at separate times rosemary and black pepper fragrances.

Flower Essences: For emotionally caused diarrhea, try the Bach remedies: for diarrhea caused by stress use Vervain. For diarrhea brought on by uncertainty, indecisiveness or hesitancy, use Scleranthus. In other than Bach essence flowers, try green rose, dill, nasturtium or bloodroot.

Gemstones and Gem Essences: Take beryl in essence for diarrhea, and the metal copper for dysentery. Hold or wear black tourmaline, tourmaline quartz, or smoky quartz.

Emotional Healing: What (or who) do you want to get rid of or get over with in a hurry? What can't you hold onto? What are you running away from? There is fear and rejection here. Eliminate the cause to eliminate the diarrhea.

Fever

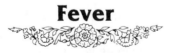

Fever is a symptom of the body's attempt to fight off an infection or toxin. Without the fever, the immune system has less way to combat the dis-ease, and fever itself is not the dis-ease but the method of curing it. Normal body temperature varies slightly with the individual in a range from 98–99°F. A temperature under 102°F in adults or 103°F in children is not serious, but prolonged fever (one to four days is normal) that does not sweat out or a fever beyond 103°F requires intervention. The process runs in stages. First the woman feels chilly and seeks a warm bed and rest. Weakness and body aches encourage inactivity, the mind is sluggish, and she has no appetite. There may be headache, nausea or vomiting. In the next stage the fever has peaked and sweating begins, followed by greater comfort; the chills and aching stop, and the temperature returns to normal.

Aspirin to bring down a fever stops the natural immune process and results in a longer illness. Holistic methods reduce fevers and encourage sweating to speed the process but do not halt or abort it. The reason for the internal heat is to kill the infectious bacteria or virus, and the sweating eliminates toxins. Fevers in infants and children need to be watched carefully; they can go high quickly and result in convulsions. Above 106°F, there can be brain damage in children or adults. In all fevers, withhold food but drink lots of fluids to prevent dehydration and support the body in the immune process.

Vitamins and Minerals: During a fever, withhold multiple vitamin and mineral supplements, iron and zinc. Use vitamin C to bowel tolerance and drink plenty of bottled water, herb teas or juices with it. Use vitamin A, up to 50,000 IU per day for as long as a week, then decreasing to 25,000 IU daily in dry form. Both of these are immune system builders and infection fighters. Use a B-complex, and 400–800 IU of vitamin E per day.

Herbs: There are a number of herbs that will support the body in the fever process, causing the temperature rise to peak and the sweating stage to begin. Choose one of the following: Elderflower and peppermint, catnip and peppermint, or elderflower and lime blossom are frequently used fever combinations that are highly effective. Other herbs as tinctures or teas include boneset, yarrow, raspberry, catnip, feverfew, yellow dock, echinacea, ginger, pleurisy root, lemonbalm or vervain. Use sage, garlic and lemon tea, or sage, lavender and rosemary. Drink any of these teas hot and frequently, and stay in bed to sweat. Lobelia tincture (1/4–1/2 teaspoonful every four hours) will cause sweating and break a fever. Use half doses of any of these for children.

To make elderflower and peppermint tea, use four tablespoons of peppermint leaf and four tablespoons of elderflower to two cups of water. This is a very strong tea. To make sage, garlic and lemon tea, pour six cups of boiling water over two heaping tablespoons of sage leaves, two finely chopped garlic cloves, and the juice and pulp of half a lemon. Sweeten with honey to taste, and steep for five minutes.[1]

Naturopathy: Do a liquid fast for the duration of the fever, withholding solid food but drinking lots of pure liquids. Do not use milk, coffee, black tea or alcohol. Hot water and lemon juice, pure unsweetened grape juice at room temperature, apple juice diluted with water, or a teaspoon of apple cider vinegar and a teaspoon of honey in a glass of tepid

---

[1]Joy Gardner, *The New Healing Yourself* (Freedom, CA, The Crossing Press, 1989), p. 105–106.

water all will support the fever process and speed it. Vinegar-honey water works especially well. Catnip tea enemas will also break a fever and speed the release of toxins from the body.

Take odorless garlic (Kyolic) or raw garlic in any of many forms (see Colds and Sore Throats for recipes). Use a garlic or onion poultice to the soles of the feet. Garlic is antibacterial and antiviral, as is onion. Use bee propolis or royal jelly, amazing immune system boosters highly effective for fevers and infections.

Take a tepid (body temperature, 98.6°F) epsom salts bath for half an hour, then go to bed to sweat out the fever under blankets. Use tepid plain water compresses to face and body, or lie in a tepid tub of water. Get out if you feel chilled and wrap up in bed. Use a brisk towel rub to dry.

Homeopathy and Cell Salts: *Aconite* is for sudden onset of any disease after exposure to dry cold winds; there is anxiety, restlessness and fear with a dry cough or dry mouth. Use *Belladonna* for fever with flushed face, red-hot-dry skin and dilated pupils. There is agitation, restlessness and mental dullness; there may be muscle twitching. *Nux vomica* is for chills greatly worsened by moving the blankets; there may be digestive symptoms, over-indulgence before onset, and irritability. If the woman or child is irritable and whiny, craving affection, her remedy may be *Pulsatilla*. Use *Bryonia* if the woman has fever, headache, sore throat, upset stomach or rheumatic inflammation; she is thirsty, irritable and wants to be left alone, and feels worse with the slightest motion.

Cell Salts: *Ferrum phos.* is for fevers with slower onset than the suddenness of *Aconite* or *Belladonna*. Try *Natrum sulph.* for chills and fever, flu, fever with upset stomach, and for intermittent fevers.

Amino Acids: Take a combination free-form amino acids on an empty stomach three times a day.

Acupressure: Use pressure only on the pituitary points of the hands, feet and face. These are located in the pads of the thumbs and big toes, in the slight depression under the nose, and in the (third eye) center of the forehead. Press these points without massaging them every few minutes until the fever breaks. The webs between thumbs and first fingers are also fever points, as are the outside of the elbows, and just above the shoulder blades on the back. (See illustration.)

Aromatherapy: Essential oils to reduce fevers are used in baths, as massage oils for body rubs, and as compresses, as well as to smell in the air. If in bed, place a drop on the pillow. Use bergamot, chamomile, ginger, eucalyptus, cypress, peppermint or tea-tree.

Flower Essences: Dandelion causes deep relaxation and reduces fevers, and ginseng regenerates the endocrine system, also with fever reduction.

Acupressure for Fever

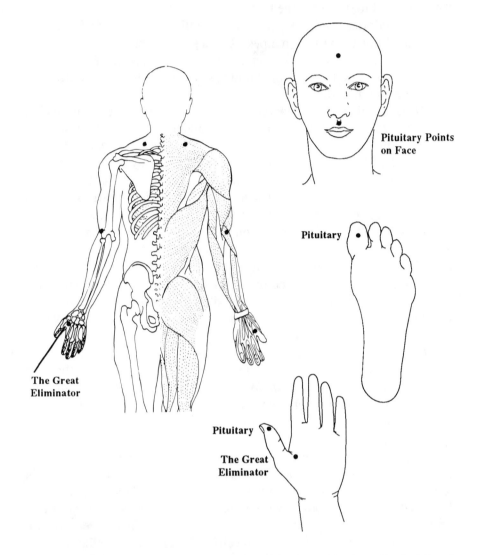

Pituitary Points on Face

Pituitary

The Great Eliminator

Pituitary

The Great Eliminator

The Great Eliminator: Located on the outside of the hand between the thumb and index fingers, just below the junction of the first and second metacarpals. It is an important general tonic point that helps to regulate the autonomic nervous system, and has been used traditionally for fever and colds. It should not be used on pregnant women.

Iona Marsaa Teeguarden, *Acupressure Way of Health: Jin Shin Do* (New York, Japan Publishing Co., 1978), p.134-135; Mildred Carter, *Hand Reflexology: Key to Perfect Health* (W. Nyack, NY, Parker Publishing Co., 1983), p. 169.

Gemstone and Gem Essences: In gem essence, use chalcedony, coral, red jasper, lapis lazuli, jet or ruby, as well as the metals copper, silver or gold. Hold or wear lapis, chrysocolla, aquamarine, sapphire, sodalite or blue tourmaline. Moonstone also balances the endocrine system, and is a stone for the pituitary.

Emotional Healing: What (or who?) is burning you up? Fevers are anger and frustration, and infections are anger, irritation and annoyance. Release anger in safer ways than turning it inward; end the frustration by changing what can be changed and walking away from the rest. Maybe it's time to have that upfront fight with your mother or lover. Get it over with and clear the air.

Fibroid Tumors
Uterine, Ovarian & Fallopian tube cysts
See the sections on Breast Lumps, Cancer, Menstruation and Menopause

Hair Loss
Alopecia

Hair loss is not only male heredity and vanity, but a dis-ease that affects many women. There are several cases where hair loss is expected. It is normal to lose significant amounts of hair in the last few months of pregnancy or for three or four months after childbirth. The hair usually regrows by the time the baby is six months old, and hormonal changes are the cause. It is also normal for women after menopause to experience thinning hair, particularly to the front, and greying hair with age. This is also hormone-related, and much can be done to prevent and often reverse it. Radiation to the head or chemotherapy for cancer will cause hair loss, often total, which regrows after the therapy is stopped. Beyond these things, sudden falling out of women's hair in large quantities or in patches is called alopecia and can be caused by a number of factors. With holistic methods the loss can usually be stopped and very often the hair will regrow, though usually less fully than before.

Glandular imbalances are a major cause of hair loss in women, with the adrenals, thyroid (low thyroid) or pituitary glands involved. Stress, which depletes these glands, and emotional or physical trauma or shock are other causes. Hypoglycemia is another important factor. Nutritional deficiencies can cause both hair loss and greying in women. Other factors include poor scalp circulation (cranial-sacral massage work is wonderful), illness or surgery, diabetes, too harsh shampoos, hair dyes and hot dryers, fevers, heavy metal poisoning, anemia, alcohol and smoking. I have experienced hair loss due to adrenal exhaustion and stress, and the hair has regrown with vitamins, diet and herbs.

Vitamins and Minerals: A multiple vitamin and mineral supplement is important here, as are additional B-complex vitamins. Deficiency in the B-complex is the major nutritional reason for women's hair loss. Use a B-complex-50 to -100 two or three times a day. Use additional pantothenic acid (B-5, 500 mg three times a day) for stress and hypoglycemia. You can go as high as 2000 mg daily, and this can also return the color to greying hair. Use additional B-6 (50 mg three times a day); draining of B-6 in women on the pill can cause hair loss. Use B-3 (niacin) in the same amounts. Niacin is a relaxant and the niacin flush brings blood to the scalp. Biotin, inositol, PABA and folic acid are also essential: use 1/2 teaspoon of inositol, 5 mg folic acid, 50 mcg biotin, and 300 mg of PABA two or three times a day. Vitamin E, (400–800 IU daily) is helpful, as is vitamin A in dry form (25,000 IU per day). Minerals that are important include a calcium/magnesium supplement (magnesium deficiency can cause hair loss), zinc and iron. For greying hair the target vitamins are also B-complex-50, with folic acid, B-5, PABA and trace amounts of copper. Essential fatty acids in the form of evening primrose oil, fish oils or wheat germ oil are helpful for both hair loss and greying. Use a biotin shampoo and conditioner and avoid chemical shampoos, dyes, hot dryers and harsh brushing. Coenzyme Q10 will oxygenate the scalp.

Herbs: Make the following herbal preparation. Take a heaping tablespoon each of dried nettles, yarrow and rosemary (for light hair) or black walnut (for dark) and put it into two cups of water in a nonaluminum pot on the stove. Bring to a boil, then shut off the flame and let it cool. Strain out the herbs and place the liquid in a pint plastic container, adding water to fill it. Use as a hair rinse after every shampoo; don't rinse it off. It will stimulate growth, make the hair shine and stop dandruff. Over a period of a few months it regrew my hair.

Other herbs include horsetail grass for calcium, silicon taken internally, cleavers internally, and use herbs for reducing stress (see Stress section). Use sage tea as a rinse for dark hair or chamomile for light hair, use comfrey rinse for dry hair, or lavender rinse for oily. Rub aloe vera gel, castor oil or wheatgerm oil into the scalp the night before shampooing, and shampoo the next morning. Another scalp rinse infusion is rosemary, raspberry and red sage.

Naturopathy: Emphasis is on a diet of whole foods, organic meats and fowl for protein if you are a meat-eater, and particularly fish. Some beneficial foods include onions, garlic, egg yolks, mustard greens, alfalfa, raw greens, carrots, seafoods and sea vegetables, seeds, whole grains and wheatgerm. Brewer's yeast or lecithin is helpful. Kelp tablets (6–8 per day, or more) or Edgar Cayce's Atomidine or 636 are iodine and mineral supplements particularly recommended for the thyroid. Use a glass of water with a teaspoon of apple cider vinegar and a teaspoon of honey with meals; it remineralizes and aids assimilation of vitamins, minerals and other nutrients. Use apple cider vinegar as a hair rinse.

When washing hair, alternate hot and cold head sprays in the shower, starting with hot and always ending with cold, three or four times. Massage the scalp daily with the fingers or a vibrator to increase circulation. Drink barley water, soy milk or a green drink (spirulina, Kyo-green, wheatgrass juice) three times a day. Raw glandular extracts can be very helpful; try for ninety days: thyroid (where there is deficiency), adrenal or pituitary. Take a teaspoonful of olive oil, wheatgerm oil or fish liver oil daily. A quarter cup of onion juice with a tablespoon of honey can be used as a daily scrub massage.

Homeopathy and Cell Salts: Try *Kali carb.* for dry, falling hair or *Bryonia* for falling hair that is oily. *Phosphorum acidum* is the remedy for hair loss following stress or the death of someone close. *Sepia* is when hair loss is associated with PMS, and there are chills, crying or irritability. Take these in 6X potency (*Phosphorum acidum* and *Bryonia* can even be used in 1X) two or three times a day until there is improvement. Use along with herbs and vitamins.

Cell Salts: *Silica* is for the hair and *Kali phos.* is for stress. These can be alternated. *Calc. phos.* is a general tonic and stimulant.

Amino Acids: Use a combination free-form or liver-based amino acids for protein and nutrition; this is highly important in stimulating hair growth and recoloring grey hair. Single aminos are: methionine, cysteine or tryptophan (it will be on the market again eventually).

Acupressure: Take handfuls of hair and pull gently over the whole head. The full body organ map is located in the scalp as it is in the hands, ears and feet, and this exercise stimulates the whole body while bringing blood to the scalp. Use a wire brush or your loose-fisted hands in a tapping motion over the scalp to do more of the same. Next, place the fingernails of one hand against the fingernails of the other and buff them together rapidly for a few minutes, then relax. Do this a couple of times a day.[1] Do foot, hand or body acupressure paying particular attention to the endocrine glands (see Immune System section). Work the pituitary points in the pads

Acupressure for Hair Loss

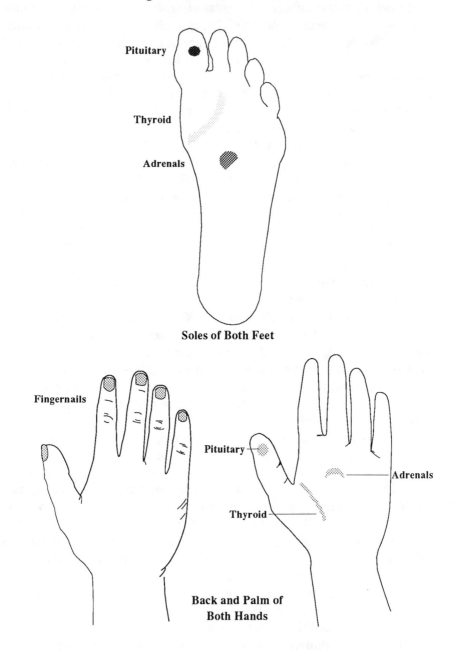

Pituitary

Thyroid

Adrenals

Soles of Both Feet

Fingernails

Pituitary

Adrenals

Thyroid

**Back and Palm of
Both Hands**

Mildred Carter, *Body Reflexology* (W. Nyack, NY, Parker Publishing Co., 1983), p. 215-216.

of the big toes and thumbs, plus the adrenal and thyroid points.

Aromatherapy: Put three to four drops of cedarwood or rosemary, bay, clary sage or ylang ylang in a tablespoon of olive oil. Rub into the hair the night before shampooing.

Flower Essences: Take cedar in essence internally or on the scalp to balance hormones and stimulate hair growth. Cotton flower is for protein content, balances hormones, and brings more lifeforce to the hair; use internally and externally. Lemon is for nutrient assimilation, and star tulip nourishes hair growth (but use with other methods). Try henna essence for greying hair.

Gemstones and Gem Essences: The metal brass, or gemstones jet or onyx are used in essence for hair loss; use pearl for the adrenals. Hold or wear black tourmaline or amethyst.

Emotional Healing: Fear and anxiety are a major cause of hair loss in women, as well as of greying hair. There is a belief that strain and pressure are necessary in daily living. Can you learn to relax and trust life? Can you make things easy?

Headaches

Simple headache is a pain in the head, sinuses, around the eyes, or from muscular constriction of the neck. It may occur with indigestion and often is caused by digestive disturbances or constipation. Other causes of headache include stress and tension (a major cause, particularly in women), poor posture, jaw, neck or spinal misalignment or injury, eyestrain, sinusitis, insomnia, food sensitivities or allergies to food/s or additives, hypoglycemia, or menstrual disorders. Overuse of vitamin A (it takes a lot of it longterm to result in symptoms) and some medical drugs can result in headache as a side effect. Chocolate, caffeine, red wine, fluorescent lighting, computer screens, chemical fumes, hangovers and MSG (monosodium glutamate) used in Chinese restaurants are common headache causes. Environmental allergies, pollution, liver toxicity, anemia, mold allergies and high blood pressure are other causes. More women than men are subject to both headaches and migraines, perhaps because of women's internalization of stress and anger. (See Migraines.) Along with the

---

[1]Mildred Carter, *Body Reflexology* (W. Nyack, NY, Parker Publishing Co., 1985), p. 215–216.

holistic methods described below, prevent constipation and see a chiropractor, osteopath or acupuncturist if headaches are frequent. Neuromuscular massage or sacral-cranial work is also very helpful. Learn to meditate and do it nightly to reduce stress. Avoid aspirin and use herbs instead.

Vitamins and Minerals: Use a quality multiple vitamin and mineral supplement. I like Schiff's Single Day for its inclusion of 75 mg of B-complex, important in headache, migraine and stress control. Add a B-complex-50 to -100 and this alone may be enough to stop many women's headaches. B-complex is the anti-stress vitamin. Take additional niacin (500–200 mg per day) when headaches are acute, and a sublingual vitamin B-12. B-6 can also be a factor, particularly when headaches are menstrual-cycle related or you are on the pill. Use vitamin C daily (1000 mg or more) and a complete calcium/magnesium supplement. Take a calcium/magnesium hourly (even better with vitamin C) during a headache; it may stop it. Coenzyme-Q10 or germanium oxygenates the blood, and is a pain and stress reducer. Vitamin E, gradually increasing up to 800 IU per day, improves circulation, reduces high blood pressure, and is an antioxidant. Potassium (under 100 mg daily) may be helpful. The multiple, B-complex and calcium/magnesium are the essentials.

Herbs: Two categories of herbs are helpful, as well as a series of headache relievers. The categories are stress reducers and liver cleansers. Stress reducers are used for most headaches; they ease pain and muscle tension and are emotional calmatives. They include: scullcap, passion flower, valerian, hops, catnip, feverfew, limeblossom, melilot, chamomile or lavender. Some good headache combinations include: scullcap, hops and catnip together; scullcap, catnip and valerian; limeblossom, rosemary and lavender; scullcap and feverfew; or scullcap and passion flower. Liver cleansing headache herbs include: peppermint, celandine, chamomile, culvers root, fringe tree, goldenseal, pulsatilla (pasque flower), senna (for constipation), burdock, or lobelia.

Take passion flower or rue for headaches with eyestrain (do not use rue in pregnancy), betony for headaches with dizziness, black cohosh for menstrual-related headaches particularly in women over forty, lady's slipper for headaches in menopause, or mistletoe for headaches from high blood pressure or too much blood to the brain. Valerian is for pain, and white willow is an herbal aspirin. My favorite of all of these is scullcap alone, or with passion flower or feverfew. Feverfew dilates the blood vessels to the brain, willow contracts them; use feverfew at onset, and willow after the headache settles in.

Naturopathy: Eat a whole foods diet high in protein and raw vegetables, avoiding sugar, refined flour products, alcohol, caffeine, cheese, processed foods or foods with preservatives, overuse of salt, citrus, nitrite food additives, MSG and artificial sweeteners. Do a fruit juice (noncitrus) cleansing fast for three days with coffee or warm water enemas, and reintroduce solid foods slowly, watching for allergic reactions. Many headaches and migraines are food allergy related; avoid reacting foods.

Where digestion is a factor in headaches, drink a glass of water with a teaspoon of apple cider vinegar and a teaspoon of honey in it daily with meals. During a headache, use apple cider vinegar as a compress to the forehead, and/or inhale the fumes from boiling half water and half apple cider vinegar in a nonaluminum pot. (Inhale for seventy-five breaths; the headache is gone within half an hour.) Another way to relieve a digestive-caused headache is to place a half teaspoon of lemon juice and a teaspoon of baking soda in a glass of tolerably hot water. Drink it bubbling, and repeat every fifteen minutes until the headache is gone. Use hot and cold water compresses alternating to the neck and shoulders to relieve muscle tension, and cold compresses to the head. An ice cold foot soak for five minutes followed by a warm bed will usually stop a headache, too. To stop a severe headache or abort a migraine, induce vomiting with lobelia or ipecac.

Homeopathy and Cell Salts: *Arnica* is for headache after an injury or that feels bruise-like. *Pulsatilla* is for headache with watery eyes and indigestion, worse in stuffy rooms and lying down. Use *Belladonna* for bursting headaches, aggravated by light, noise and jarring; the woman has a red, flushed face. *Ignatia* is for bandlike pressure across the forehead with dizziness and nausea. Take *Aconite* at onset, or with the emotion that the woman thinks she is dying. *Nux vomica* is for splitting headache after eating, with nausea and vomiting; there is constipation and irritability. *Bryonia* is for sharp, severe headaches, aggravated by the slightest movement, even turning the eyes; the woman is thirsty.

Cell Salts: Take every half hour: *Ferrum phos.* and *Kali phos.* until pain is gone. Use *Natrum sulph.* for bilious headaches with a tendency to vomit, or *Kali mur.* for sick headaches. *Kali phos.* is for nervous tension headaches.

Amino Acids: Tryptophan will be back on the market eventually; vitamin B-3 is its closest substitute for now. GABA is a stress reducer and antidepressant. Avoid tyrosine and phenylalanine.

Acupressure: Massage the neck and shoulders at first sign of a headache and work out the tender reflexes you will find along the muscles on both sides of the spine. Massage the second joint of each thumb, alternating right and left for two minutes each and five times on each hand. Work the webs between thumbs and first fingers (not in pregnancy). Press

Acupressure for Headaches

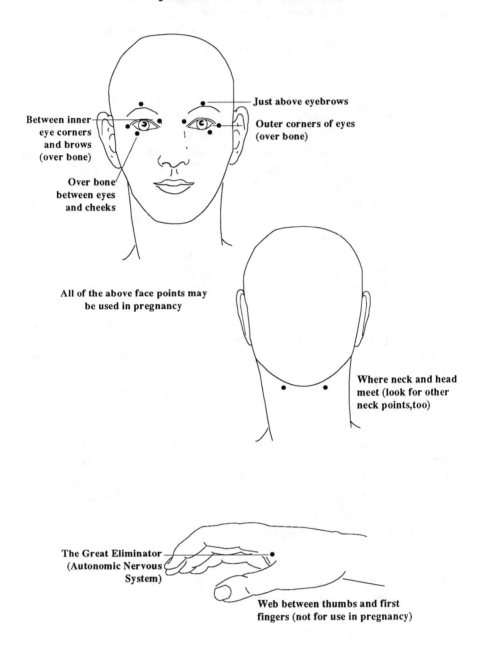

Just above eyebrows

Between inner eye corners and brows (over bone)

Outer corners of eyes (over bone)

Over bone between eyes and cheeks

All of the above face points may be used in pregnancy

Where neck and head meet (look for other neck points, too)

The Great Eliminator (Autonomic Nervous System)

Web between thumbs and first fingers (not for use in pregnancy)

Cathryn Bauer, *Acupressure for Women* (Freedom, CA, The Crossing Press, 1987), p. 87; Pedro Chan, *Finger Acupressure* (New York, Ballantine Books, 1974), p. 54-57.

your thumb against the roof of your mouth for four or five minutes, moving to other spots on the roof occasionally; this releases nerve pressure to the head. Look for tender pressure points on the bony structures around the eyes and along the eyebrows; these are good for all headaches, and particularly for sinus and eyestrain headaches. (See illustration.)

Aromatherapy: Rub a few drops of peppermint oil, chamomile essential oil or lavender oil on your temples and use them in a diffuser. Other scents include rosemary, cardamom, rosewood or melissa. These can be used in baths or massage oils as well, or as compresses. A headache combination is available from Tiferet-Lifetree, containing lavender, marjoram, aniseed, niaouli, basil and peppermint.

Flower Essences: Grapefruit blossom essence is for tension headaches.

Gemstones and Gem Essences: Gem essences of hematite, kunzite, or amethyst are helpful for headaches. Hold or wear turquoise, chrysocolla, kunzite, rose quartz, aquamarine, or blue or pink tourmaline.

Emotional Healing: Your abilities and ideas are being denied and you feel invalidated and manipulated, or you are invalidating yourself. You are a perfectionist too critical or self-critical, or you are ego-sore from being criticized. There is fear and anger here, at yourself and others. Know you are Goddess, you are perfect, walk away from others' games, love yourself and just relax. Surround yourself with blue light before going to work and feel protected all day. Do the Self-Blessing every night and meditate before bed. Let life's stresses roll off you like water off a duck's back. Be compassionate with yourself and with others.

Heart Dis-Ease

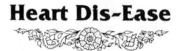

One in three people in America dies of heart dis-ease, one in three of cancer, and one in three of anything else. Formerly a men's dis-ease, heart disorder is increasing in women as a cause of death and particularly in Black women. Like cancer, it is a dis-ease of civilized countries where the diet is high in white sugar, saturated fats and refined flour. Before 1910, the year that industrial flour refining was first implemented, incidence of heart dis-ease, cancer and immune disorder dis-eases was very low. Many of the dis-eases that are major killers today were rare or nonexistent before 1910. The refining process strips essential nutrients from grain, particularly B-complex vitamins and vitamin E, that are required for healthy heart function. The growing of grain on demineralized soils that are loaded with chemicals and pesticides results in further deficiencies and toxicities. In addition, the feeding of hormones and antibiotics to meat and dairy animals to fatten them faster or increase milk production results in the saturated fats problem. An enzyme in homogenized milk, xanthine oxidase, can clog the arteries and cause heart damage. While saturated fat consumption in the United States has increased only ten percent in the last hundred years, consumption of refined carbohydrates and sugar in the American diet has increased seven hundred percent.[1] The implication here is that the Typical American Diet is the cause of so many American deaths. We are an affluent society dying of malnutrition and nutritional deficiency dis-eases. There is a definite link between sugar consumption and high triglycerides in heart dis-ease.

The holistic remedies listed in this section are for women who have had heart attacks, and are also heart attack preventives. Heart dis-ease is a serious condition requiring expert supervision.

Vitamins and Minerals: Along with a multiple vitamin and mineral supplement, B-complex is essential. Use 25–50 mg with each meal and extra B-1, B-6, B-3 and folic acid. Vitamin B-3 (niacin) reduces incidence of angina; work slowly up to 400–500 mg a day, but only if you do not have rheumatic heart dis-ease. B-6 lowers cholesterol and prevents blood clots, and folic acid (B-9) is a vasodilator (use 75 mg per day total). Pangamic acid (B-15, 150 mg per day) helps heart healing, lowers cholesterol and oxygenates the blood. It also lowers the side effects of medical heart drugs. Lecithin, comprised of two B-complex vitamins inositol and choline, is a fat emulsifier; take two capsules or a tablespoonful with meals. Use vitamin C with bioflavinoids (1000 mg three times a day); it lowers triglycerides, strengthens capillaries, and keeps plaque from forming on arterial walls. Take a natural vitamin E with selenium, increasing gradually from 100 IU per day, adding 100 IU weekly, to a total of 800–1000 IU daily (with 200 mcg of selenium). These are the essentials.

Beta-carotene (vitamin A, 10,000–25,000 IU per day) reduces heart attacks in high-risk patients with angina, chest pain or obstructive artery dis-ease. Use essential fatty acids (Omega-3, EPA, black currant oil, primrose oil, olive oil). Calcium chelate with magnesium chelate or orotate regulates heart rhythm and decreases blood cholesterol. Most heart patients are chromium deficient (use 200 mg per day), potassium deficient

---

[1]Dr. Ross Trattler, *Better Health Through Natural Healing* (New York, McGraw-Hill Book Co., 1985), p. 321

(90 mg) and may be copper deficient (3 mg).Coenzyme Q10 and germanium oxygenate the blood and help to prevent additional heart damage after a heart attack, and Kyolic (odorless garlic) reduces cholesterol and lowers blood pressure.

Herbs: Hawthorn berries strengthen the heart, lower cholesterol and high blood pressure and regulate the heart rate. It can be used daily longterm in tincture, capsule or decoction two or three times a day and is the most primary of heart-healing herbs. Lily of the valley regulates heart action and is similar to digoxin (use this under expert advice only). A combination of scullcap, cayenne and goldenseal strengthens the heart, as does motherwort. Peppermint tea calms palpitations and tension about the heart and prevents heart attacks. Rosemary and elder are for edema. Use black cohosh with yellow jasmine for angina, and cactus grandiflorus for angina with irregular heartbeat; alfalfa decreases blood cholesterol and adds minerals. Alfalfa added to other herbs helps in their assimilation. Angelica relaxes the heart and builds infection resistance, and mandrake root lowers high blood pressure and strengthens the heart. Parsley tea is a heart toner.

Naturopathy: Eat a whole foods diet, at least fifty percent of which is raw vegetables. The diet should be high in fiber, and the protein mostly vegetable protein. Foods that lower cholesterol and triglycerides include: tofu, beans and soybeans, peas, cold water fish, brewer's yeast, nuts except peanuts, bran, onions, garlic, wheat germ, sprouts and lecithin. Avoid sugar, refined grains, hydrogenated fats, fried foods, salt, alcohol, caffeine, red meat and dairy products (except yoghurt, kefir or buttermilk). Take occasional vegetable juice fasts. Use spirulina, wheatgrass juice or other green drinks, iodine in the form of kelp or Atomidine (with angina take 1 drop twice a day for five days, stop five days and repeat five times). Grape juice, citrus juice or pectin are helpful, as are essential fatty acids and EPA. Women with heart dis-ease should *never* smoke.

Drink two ounces of the following before each meal to strengthen the heart and circulatory system: half cup each of tomato juice and lemon (or orange) juice, a tablespoon brewer's yeast, and six tablespoons of wheat germ oil.

Homeopathy and Cell Salts: For acute situations of angina or heart attack, especially the first time, use *Aconite*: symptoms are stitching pain in chest, anxiety, fear of dying, restlessness, and fever. *Latrodectus mactans* is for violent chest pain radiating down the left arm to the fingers, with numbness, extreme anxiety, nausea, and rapid, weak pulse. *Arsenicum* is for chest constriction with a burning sensation; the woman is cold, anxious and restless. Use *Lilium tigrinum* for the feeling that the heart is in a vise, full to bursting, and a cold feeling around the heart; the woman has a herstory of gynecological problems. Try *Cactus grandiflorus* for acute and chronic functional heart disorders, with constriction like iron bands, palpitations and sometimes asthmatic breathing. *Crataegus* (hawthorn) is a strengthener for the heart muscle.

Cell Salts: *Mag. phos.* is for spasmodic darting pains, *Natrum phos.* for rheumatic heart pain, and *Calc. fluor.* is for impaired circulation and heart muscle weakness. For arteriosclerosis use *Silica*.

Amino Acids: Take a free-form amino acids combination. Of single aminos, taurine corrects heart arrhythmia, carnitine (1500–3000 mg daily) decreases blood cholesterol and triglycerides and is useful in angina; take with vitamin C. Histidine and proline are also positive, as is methionine.

Acupressure: In acute situations of heart attack or angina, massage the heart pressure points on the left hand at the base of the third and fourth (little) fingers. (This is also on the left foot.) Then go to the pituitary reflex in the pads of both thumbs (and big toes). If someone can help, have her hit the flat of her hand on the back where the head joins the neck; this point can stimulate a failing heartbeat. There is another spot on the back, left side, just above the shoulder blade. These are emergency measures, to use before the paramedics come. To slow a too rapid heartbeat, make a fist with the thumb on the outside, and press the wrist of the left hand. See these emergency points, and points to tonify the heart daily, in the illustrations.

Aromatherapy: Melissa, ylang ylang or rose are the essential oils for use in diffuser or massage oils. Jasmine, lemon or marjoram are also positive, and lily of the valley is a heart stimulant.

Flower Essences: Try centaury agave, hawthorn, angelica, bleeding heart, mallow, peach blossom, bloodroot, dill or sunflower. Bach Flower Remedies help the emotions; use Rock Rose for panicky people, or Heather with Rock Water for overanxiousness. Olive is for physical exhaustion, and Rescue Remedy is for acute situations.

Gemstones and Gem Essences: Gem essences of emerald, sapphire, malachite, green or black tourmaline, ruby or garnet are positive. Hold or wear rose quartz, pink tourmaline, kunzite or emerald.

Emotional Healing: The heart is the center of love both given and received, self-love, love for others and universal love. Heart dis-ease is a lack of joy or hardening of the heart; the woman does not give of her heart or receive into it, or has lost her heart's love. There is stress, strain, emotional pain or blockage of emotions, loss or grief. Learn to relax, to go through the process of feeling and of letting go and grieving. Learn to love yourself, others, the Goddess, and your life; learn to love living in the world. The best way to have a healthy heart or to heal a broken one is to love.

Acupressure for the Heart

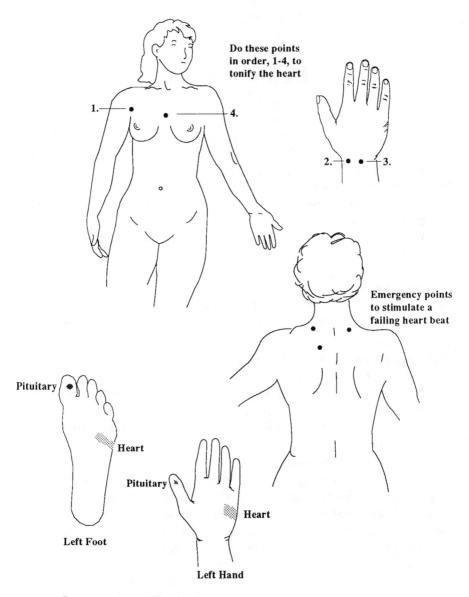

Do these points in order, 1-4, to tonify the heart

Emergency points to stimulate a failing heart beat

Pituitary

Heart

Pituitary

Heart

Left Foot

Left Hand

Do acupressure on these hand or foot points in an emergency

Mildred Carter, *Body Reflexology* (W. Nyack, NY, Parker Publishing Co., 1983), p. 132-133; Cathryn Bauer, *Acupressure for Women* (Freedom, CA, The Crossing Press, 1987), p.126.

Hemorrhoids

Hemorrhoids are varicose veins of the rectum—swollen veins that may protrude beyond the anus. They are painful, and burn or itch, sometimes bleeding with bowel movements. The primary causes are poor diet, leading to constipation and straining, which in turn lead to laxative dependency. Constipation weakens the rectal and intestinal muscles, and laxatives stretch them so that more laxatives are needed for bowel evacuation. Lack of exercise, pregnancy, improper lifting, weak abdominal muscles, or stress, fatigue and tension that cause the muscles to constrict are other causes. Like so many modern ills, hemorrhoids are another dis-ease of industrialized civilization, with its refined flour, low fiber diet and sedentary lifestyle. Prevention of hemorrhoids is easier than curing them and usually means a high fiber diet and avoiding constipation. Surgical removal of hemorrhoids only gets rid of the current immediate problem, not the cause—they often come back and the surgery creates more scarring. Some women who experienced incest have rectal and intestinal dis-eases as adults, due to damage of too young tissues and emotional backlash to the childhood pain. Awareness, therapy and holistic healing methods can help tremendously. Also see the section on Constipation in this book.

Vitamins and Minerals: Along with a complete vitamin and mineral supplement, use a complete B-complex-25 to -50 up to three times a day, plus additional B-6, up to 50 mg three times a day with meals. Use a vitamin C with bioflavinoids (1000–3000 mg per day). A 100 mg rutin tablet three times a day may be enough to cure hemorrhoids—rutin is a bioflavinoid. All women should be on a calcium/magnesium supplement; it helps constipation, and is a preventive for colon cancer. Vitamin E promotes normal healing; use 400-800 IU per day. Vitamins A and D heal the mucous membrane; use 25,000 IU per day of A in dry form or beta-carotene, and 600 IU (total) of D. Liquid lecithin applied daily is an external healer for hemorrhoids and may totally eliminate them. It is also helpful used internally.

Herbs: Plantain, witchhazel, white oak bark, calendula, comfrey, pilewort, elderberry, goldenseal and black walnut are all external choices. Make an infusion, strain and cool it, then dab it on or use the not-too-hot herbal tea dregs as a poultice. Make a strong infusion of elder and honeysuckle flowers together, combine pilewort and witchhazel externally, or aloe vera and goldenseal together. Calendula comes in salve form, and once you have used the comfrey dregs externally, drink the tea. An herbal salve of comfrey and goldenseal, or comfrey, goldenseal and plantain (a number of these are available) is soothing and pain relieving. Goldenseal constricts the swollen veins.

Naturopathy: Eat a high fiber diet primarily of raw vegetables and whole grains. Avoid constipation at all costs, and if using laxatives use the bulk fiber ones rather than other types. Drink six to eight glasses of water, fruit or vegetable juices, or herb teas daily. Use a teaspoon of olive oil, castor oil or linseed oil daily to prevent constipation and lubricate the bowels. Try alternating hot and cold sitz baths or compresses to cause the hemorrhoids to shrink or recede. Cayenne and garlic enemas, or lemon juice and water enemas are recommended. See the fasts and enemas listed under Constipation.

A peeled clove of garlic held in the rectum will reduce hemorrhoids; change two or three times a day. Use papaya juice, lemon juice, castor oil or witchhazel externally, or cut a piece of raw potato into a bullet shape and use it as a suppository. Use cottage cheese or raw chopped cranberries as a poultice, or a compress of roasted onions to draw out inflammation. Place a quarter cup of liquid witchhazel in warm water and use as a sitz bath for fifteen minutes twice a day. This is described as curing hemorrhoids completely in a few days. Or use Batherapy, a mineral bath powder, as a sitz bath.

Homeopathy and Cell Salts: Try Hyland Pile Ointment, a homeopathic preparation from Standard Homeopathic, or Hamamelis ointment. Paeonia is an external ointment to use when there is severe pain and extreme sensitivity to touch.

Internally, use *Sulfur* where there is constipation and itching but no bleeding. For protruding hemorrhoids with bleeding and diarrhea use *Hamamelis* or *Aloe* three times a day until there is improvement. For nonprotruding piles in women of sedentary habits, try *Nux vomica*, and if hemorrhoids appear after childbirth use *Pulsatilla.*

Cell Salts: Use *Calc. Fluor.* for nonbleeding hemorrhoids, and if bleeding use *Ferrum phos.* Both can be used together, alternating.

Amino Acids: No specific amino acid is recommended here, but a combination contains the B-complex vitamins and is important for tissue healing.

Acupressure for Hemorrhoids

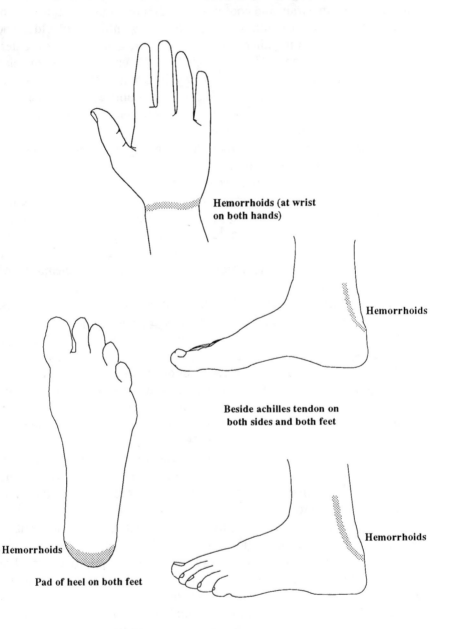

Hemorrhoids (at wrist on both hands)

Hemorrhoids

Beside achilles tendon on both sides and both feet

Hemorrhoids

Pad of heel on both feet

Hemorrhoids

Also see section on Constipation

Mildred Carter, *Body Reflexology* (W. Nyack, NY, Parker Publishing Co., 1983), p. 179-180; Moshe Olshevsky, CA, PhD., *et. al.*, *The Manual of Natural Therapy* (New York, Citadel Press, 1989), p. 43.

Acupressure: See the section on Constipation and use the illustrations as a guide to working the reflexes of the entire eliminative system. Full foot or hand acupressure is recommended. For hemorrhoids specifically, find the areas at the bend of both wrists, or on the bottoms of the feet at the heels. It may take digging with a crystal or other hard object to place enough pressure to find and release these points under the callouses. On the upper parts of the feet, on both sides of both feet along the Achilles tendons will be other tender areas. Again, use pressure to work the points until they release. Do this a couple of times a day.

Aromatherapy: Take baths or sitz baths containing cypress, frankincense and juniper essential oils together, or cypress or juniper individually.

Flower Essences: Use redwood internally, and mallow both internally and externally.

Gemstones and Gem Essences: Coral in essence or the metal copper is used for hemorrhoids and varicose veins. Hold or wear hematite, black tourmaline, tourmaline quartz, onyx or bloodstone.

Emotional Healing: The cause of hemorrhoids may be anger from the past, feeling burdened and fearing to let go. There may be physical or emotional damage from childhood incest. The traumas of the past are over, and you have survived them and are whole. Learn to trust again and to let go. Understand that you were not to blame. Forgive yourself.

Herpes

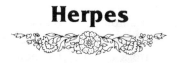

There are three main types of herpes: cold sores on the lips, genital herpes that is usually sexually transmitted, and herpes zoster which is shingles. The same virus causes chicken pox, and once it enters the cells it becomes permanently incorporated with cell DNA and cannot be cured. After the infection is established, acute flare-ups of cold sores can be triggered by a fever, cold or sore throat, or stress. Cold sores may be sexually transmitted. Genital herpes is transmitted by sexual contact (sometimes by oral sex with someone with cold sores). Shingles is reactivation of the chicken pox virus. The dis-ease settles in the nerves. The emphasis in this section is on genital herpes—though valid for the other forms—and on controlling and limiting the recurring flare-ups. Despite the "permanent" prognosis, much healing can be done with optimistic results.

Genital herpes affects over thirty-five percent of the American population, and half a million new cases are diagnosed yearly. Most new cases occur in white women between twenty and forty years old. The first attack is the worst, occurring within three weeks of exposure, but the virus can lie dormant for years before it surfaces. There is fever, swollen glands, and weakness and sickness for as long as two weeks, though some women may not experience this. Subsequent attacks tend to be less severe and usually recur when the immune system is low or the woman is tired and under stress. Frequency varies from several times a month to once in years, and outbreaks usually stop after menopause. Some women never have a second attack. The infection is contagious during outbreaks, and a few women (eleven percent) can be "asymptomatic shedders"—they can transmit the dis-ease when they do not have blisters or lesions. If you are pregnant and have herpes, you will probably have a cesarean birth to protect the infant (justified if sores are active at delivery).

Symptoms of a herpes attack are blisters on the genitals, vagina, buttocks, thighs, anus and navel. Burning sensations can be felt before the blisters erupt, and there may be extensive pain in the nerves of the groin. Lesions dry and crust over in ten to fourteen days. Stress, exhaustion, overwork, fever, citrus fruits, sunburn, menstruation, acid diet, vitamin deficiencies (B-complex), excess l-arginine, friction from clothing, and sexual contact can trigger an attack. Of as much concern as the physical is the woman's emotional state, and depression and low self-image go along with the dis-ease. Women who are depressed tend to also have more outbreaks that are more severe.

Vitamins and Minerals: Along with a multiple vitamin and mineral supplement, the following are indicated. Vitamin A (25,000–50,000 IU daily) in dry form or as beta-carotene prevents the infection from spreading, and A can also be used topically. Use a B-complex-50 to -100 three times a day; it reduces stress and the frequency of outbreaks and is essential in depression. Additional B-1 (200–300 mg per day total), B-6, B-12 (up to 2000 mcg) and folic acid are helpful. Use vitamin C with bioflavinoids (1000–5000 mg per day or to bowel tolerance during attacks); zinc up to 100 mg per day during attacks and 50 mg otherwise (use zinc lozenges for mouth sores); and vitamin E (400–800 IU per day) with selenium (200 mcg). Vitamin E can also be used directly on the sores. These are for cold sores, genital herpes and herpes zoster, and are important.

Acidophilus is recommended, four capsules four to six times daily during outbreaks and two capsules three times a day otherwise. This needs to be fresh and kept refrigerated. Egg lecithin, and essential fatty acids (evening primrose oil, black currant oil or fish oils) are cell protectors. Use a daily calcium/magnesium tablet.

Herbs: Several herbs are used topically including licorice root gel, echinacea tincture (unless its stinging is too painful), butternut, comfrey, goldenseal made into a paste with water, black walnut or slippery elm. Aloe vera gel (make sure it's pure), or tinctures of calendula, hypericum, wild indigo or myrrh are also used topically; use witchhazel and myrrh together. Internally, use burdock root tea, red clover, sassafras, chaparral, white oak, pau d'arco, echinacea or Oregon grape root in teas or tinctures or goldenseal in capsules. These are blood cleansing herbs and herbal antibiotics. Use one of each.

Naturopathy: The most important news for herpes is Kyolic (odorless garlic), which holistic physician Christiane Northrup says can cure it totally:

> At the onset of any tingling, I have patients take twelve Kyolic capsules by mouth, then three every four hours (while awake) for three days. Almost all my patients who have used this remedy have no further outbreaks.[1]

She believes that Kyolic is the most effective longterm treatment, though it will not stop an attack already in progress. I would also recommend a maintenance dose of four to six tablets/capsules per day after the initial treatment.

Eat a whole foods diet low on dairy products, sweets and sugars, refined flour, alcohol and citrus fruits. Use a lot of yoghurt, kefir or acidophilus milk. Avoid chocolate, coffee, nuts, red meat, chicken, tomatoes, seeds and peas. During the primary infection do a vegetable juice fast (beet and carrot juice are good) and a daily coffee or herbal enema. Drink lots of burdock tea as a cleanser.

Raw thymus tablets (500 mg twice day) boost the immune system, and kelp or Atomidine add minerals and iodine to the diet. Lemon juice (or echinacea or tea-tree oil) applied to tingling will reduce the blister formation and duration. Warm salt, soda or epsom salt baths reduce discomfort while blisters are active.

Homeopathy and Cell Salts: An experienced homeopath can find the precise remedy here, as so often outbreaks are connected to emotional states, and these states are reflected in specific remedies. *Rhus. tox.* is the primary remedy for small, inflamed blisters in clusters, filled with a

---

[1]Francine Rota, "50 Ways to Better Women's Health," in *East/West Journal*, November, 1990, p. 51.

yellowish fluid; there is achiness, and discomfort is improved by moving around. Try *Arsenicum album* if the sores burn intensely but feel better for applying warmth. If sores are painful to cold and touch and pus forms rapidly, try *Hepar sulph.* Use *Graphites* if eruptions ooze a honey-colored sticky fluid, and individual ulcers are large (pea-sized) and itch. *Petroleum* is a genital herpes remedy for moist sores that ooze and itch, worse in the open air and better for warmth. *Dulcamara* is useful when the outbreak seems to have been triggered by a sudden change from warm and dry to cold wet weather. Try *Sepia* if no other remedy seems to fit.

Cell Salts: *Natrum mur.* is indicated in herpes accompanied by a feeling of rejection. *Silica* is for sores with pus formation, and use *Ferrum phos.* at the onset. The three may be alternated.

Amino Acids: The arginine-lysine balance is a major factor in the treatment of herpes. When the amount of lysine in the body is greater than that of arginine, the herpes virus is suppressed. It is therefore highly important to supplement with 500–1000 mg of lysine per day, taken with vitamins C and A, and to eat the diet indicated above. The foods listed to avoid are primarily arginine producing foods (nuts, grains, meat, chicken, dairy, corn, chocolate and seeds). Another important amino acid with herpes is GABA (gamma-aminobutyric acid); it helps tremendously with depression, stress and the emotional factors of the dis-ease and can also reduce attacks by doing so. There are amino acid combinations available without arginine, and these are recommended.

Acupressure: The liver, spleen and lung meridians are affected in herpes and these are what an acupuncturist would focus on. Use full foot reflexology for ten minutes twice a day, paying attention to these organs on the body map, as well as to the endocrine glands and lymphatics. Also see the points used for depression as well as the points for pain (in the section on Cancer). Work on building the immune system. Anywhere you find a tender spot, massage it out.

Aromatherapy: Use bergamot, eucalyptus and geranium together in baths, as well as to inhale in a room diffuser. Lemon and tea-tree are also positive—both are antiseptics, and diluted may be used on the lesions as a compress.

Flower Essences: Pansy overcomes viruses and mobilizes the immune system; squash or papaya are for sexual dis-eases and ease crises concerning identity and sexuality. In any time of stress, trauma or despair, consider Bach's Rescue Remedy.

Gemstone and Gem Essences: Atacamite or spessartine garnet are gem essences for herpes. Also hold or wear emerald, watermelon tourmaline or black tourmaline.

Acupressure for Herpes

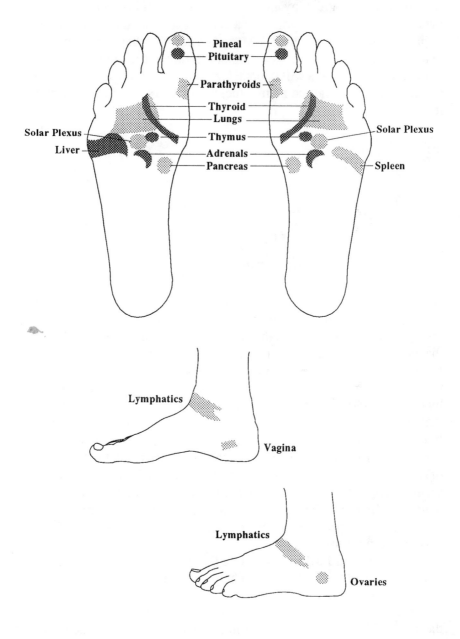

Emotional Healing: Herpes is a rejection of the genitals or sexuality, a buying into mass shame and public guilt about sex. Women are indeed sexual Be-ings, and this is not something to be ashamed of but something to take great joy and pride in. All acts of love and pleasure are the Goddess' rituals. Do you need a dis-ease to proclaim your shame? Or to justify a wish to be celibate? Many women who develop herpes do so in a relationship where sex is a problem. Heal your feelings about sexual guilt and the outbreaks will happen less and less. Herpes is not a punishment; it's a virus, and too many others share it for you to be ashamed of it.

Hiccoughs

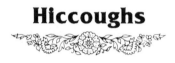

Hiccoughs are caused by spasms of the diaphragm, the big muscle between the abdomen and the lungs. As the diaphragm contracts, air breathes in involuntarily and the vocal cords snap shut, causing the sound that goes with the spasm. There is also irritation to corresponding nerves. Hiccoughs are common in children who take in a lot of air through their mouths, and in adults may be caused by indigestion and stomach gas, or by carbonated drinks in excess. Overeating or overdrinking will distend the diaphragm causing hiccoughs, and the condition is usually self-limiting. Prolonged, longterm cases happen occasionally and can be caused by serious disorders, but most hiccoughs respond to any of dozens of self-help methods. These can be lots of fun to read about and all of them seem to work. A high carbon dioxide level in the blood stops hiccoughs, which is why breath holding and breathing into a paper bag are popular. If hiccoughs happen frequently, consider better eating habits and see the section on Indigestion.

Vitamins and Minerals: While this isn't a vitamin deficiency disease, a couple of things here might help, particularly if hiccoughs happen often. Calcium/magnesium tablets, recommended for all women daily as osteoporosis prevention, have antispasmodic action on all the muscles of the body. This little bit of help may be enough to prevent recurrent hiccoughs, and is also an aid to indigestion. It is best not to try taking pills during a hiccoughs attack, for fear of choking on the tablet going down.

Proteolytic enzymes (digestive enzymes) help to prevent formation of gas and therefore to prevent hiccoughs, and the B-complex vitamins are important for every aspect of digestion. Niacin (B-3) is a muscle and nervous system relaxant. Acidophilus is important for women subject to indigestion and gas; it balances the healthy flora of the intestinal tract. Use the usual multiple vitamin and mineral supplement, with a daily B-complex-50 and calcium/magnesium to stop hiccoughs, and add digestive enzymes and/or acidophilus if gas and indigestion are recurrent.

Herbs: Dill leaf tea, a teaspoon to a cup of boiling water, sipped slowly will equalize the blood carbon dioxide and stop most hiccoughs; it is also good for indigestion and gas. Chew dill seeds, caraway seeds or mint leaves. Other teas include peppermint, catnip or fennel. Inhale a few grains of ground black pepper; the resulting sneeze will usually stop the hiccoughs.

Naturopathy: Here's where the remedies get interesting. The selections given here are ones that work and are not too outrageous. Put a teaspoon of apple cider vinegar in a glass of warm water and sip slowly, or a teaspoon of sugar in half a glass of warm water. Lie on the floor without a pillow and drink a half glass of water, lifting only your head to swallow; by the time the water is gone, the hiccoughs should be. Chew and swallow ice for ten or fifteen minutes, or lie on your left side for that amount of time (or do both?). Take a hot bath. Swallow a teaspoon of fresh onion juice, or a teaspoon of dry sugar. Drink a glass of water that has a tablespoon sticking out of it, with the spoon handle pressing against your left temple. Drink a glass of orange juice.

Homeopathy and Cell Salts: For hiccoughs after overindulgence try *Nux vomica*; the woman is irritable and there is indigestion, gas or muscle spasms. *Pulsatilla* is the remedy for women of usually light coloring who have digestive disturbances after eating rich or fatty foods. If adult, she is of a mild nature, craving affection; if a child, she is whiny and fussy. Her symptoms may change to different parts of the body. *Ignatia* is used for loud and noisy hiccoughs; use *Rathnia* for violent ones. Use homeopathic Ginseng tincture for all cases; see the dosage on the bottle.

Cell Salts: *Mag. phos.* is used every fifteen minutes in acute attacks.

Amino Acids: A free-form amino acids combination will help the digestive system, and every other body system, overall. It provides a high level of protein and B-vitamins.

Acupressure: There are a number of acupressure points that will stop hiccoughs, and this is a remedy of choice. Look for sore meridian points above and below the breastbone, halfway between the bottom of the breastbone and the navel, and on the back between the shoulder blades

Acupressure for Hiccoughs

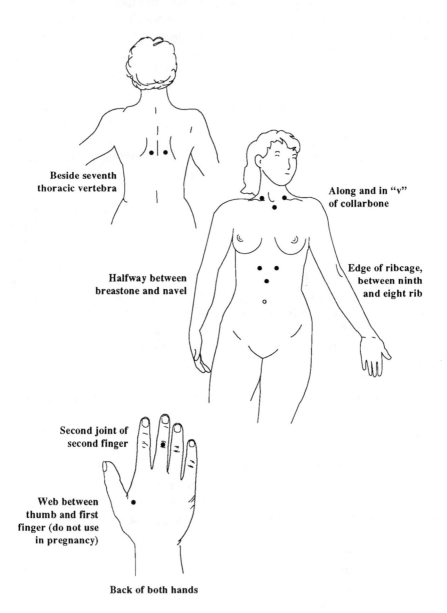

Beside seventh thoracic vertebra

Along and in "v" of collarbone

Halfway between breastone and navel

Edge of ribcage, between ninth and eight rib

Second joint of second finger

Web between thumb and first finger (do not use in pregnancy)

Back of both hands

Iona Marsaa Teeguarden, *Acupressure Way of Health: Jin Shin Do* (New York, Japan Publishing Co., 1978), p. 68; Pedro Chan, *Finger Acupressure* (New York, Ballantine Books, 1974), p. 62-64; Mildred Carter, *Body Reflexology* (W. Nyack, NY, Parker Publishing Co., 1983), p. 139; Joy Gardner, *The New Healing Yourself* (Freedom, CA, The Crossing Press, 1989), p. 226.

(three-quarters of the way down the line of the blades). Or work the second joint of the second finger of both hands, the index finger, and the webs between thumbs and first fingers. Massage the center of the soles of the feet (the diaphragm), or press between the nose and upper lip. Another reflex is reached by grasping the tongue with a clean cloth and pulling out as far as possible. Work a point for thirty seconds, then stop and go to another point (or the other hand or foot) for thirty seconds, then repeat. It may take a few repetitions but any of these points will work.

Aromatherapy: Sniff basil, sandalwood or tarragon essential oils; basil and sandalwood may be used together.

Flower Essences: Daisy relieves hiccoughs and deepens shallow breathing.

Gemstones and Gem Essences: Use beryl in essence.

Emotional Healing: The breath has the ability to take in life. Are you trying to take in too much at once? Take it slow and easy—but take it.

High Blood Pressure
Hypertension

High blood pressure usually goes along with atherosclerosis, the narrowing of the arteries with cholesterol plaque. Unreduced high cholesterol leads to heart attacks, and unreduced high blood pressure leads to heart dis-ease, kidney failure and strokes. Sixty-one million Americans have high blood pressure, more and more of them women, and Black women are particularly at risk. Besides high cholesterol, other factors include smoking, overuse of stimulants, alcohol and caffeine, drug abuse, the contraceptive pill, steroids, high unsaturated fat diets, high salt intake, fiber deficiency, excess weight, and lack of exercise. A deficiency in the essential fatty acids may be a significant cause of hypertension; this deficiency is partly caused by the losses in refining flour. Processed foods are loaded with salt, which overused becomes a poison, and there may be a genetic factor with salt consumption the trigger. High fat diets—meat and dairy products, unsaturated fats—are a precipitating factor in cholesterol formation which narrows the arteries and results in high blood pressure. Stress overall is a significant cause, and women live with it always.

Normal blood pressure in women reads slightly under 120/80, a reading of 140/90 is considered suspicious, and anything above is high. There are often no symptoms to hypertension at the beginning. Later symptoms include headache, dizziness, nervousness, irritability, ringing ears, energy loss, fatigue, insomnia and intermittent pressure rises that later become persistent. How many women have been dosed with tranquilizers who have high blood pressure instead? And there is more:

> The most revealing and upsetting fact of all is that in my experience over 85 percent of all cases of high blood pressure are both treatable and preventable without drugs and most physicians know it. The problem is that both the prevention and treatment of hypertension require lifestyle changes which are both difficult and time-consuming to accomplish.[1]

These changes are doable. They include a vegetarian or near-vegetarian diet with increase of dietary fiber and exercise, reduction of stress and excess weight where it is a health factor, and eliminating excess salt, smoking, alcohol, sugar, saturated fats, refined carbohydrates and caffeine. The Typical American Diet is killing one in three of us with high blood pressure and heart dis-ease when wellness without drugs is within reach.

Vitamins and Minerals: Begin with a high quality daily multiple vitamin and mineral supplement, one with a high level of B-vitamins (Schiff's Single Day lists 75 mg of each). Use an additional B-complex-50 to -100 and lecithin up to 15 g per day (it reduces cholesterol). Additional niacin is recommended (100–400 mg twice a day total) and also reduces cholesterol. Calcium, magnesium and vitamin D remove salt from the body, and deficiencies in these have been linked to high blood pressure. Use up to 3000 mg of calcium with half the amount of magnesium and 600 IU of vitamin D (these may all be available in one complete calcium tablet). Use potassium up to 100 mg per day and 50 mg daily of zinc. Take a vitamin C with bioflavinoids (3000–6000 mg per day; stop at bowel tolerance or sooner) to repair the capillaries and reduce blood clotting.

Vitamin E with selenium is highly important: start with 100 IU twice a day and work up slowly to 800–1200 IU, adding 100 IU per week. A gradual increase is essential, as doing it rapidly will raise some blood pressures temporarily. Vitamin E is the most significant item for lowering hypertension. Choose a quality E, though it may be more expensive, as rancid E (a problem with some cheap ones) causes more damage than

---

[1]Dr. Ross Trattler, *Better Health Through Natural Healing* (New York, McGraw-Hill Book Co., 1985), p. 365.

good. Selenium (200 mcg daily) reduces heart dis-ease and increases the pressure-lowering ability of E; some better E's will come with it. Coenzyme Q10 (100 mg daily) or germanium (90 mg daily) are antioxidants and oxygenators, and recommended. Essential fatty acids, as primrose oil, black currant oil, flaxseed oil or even olive oil are also highly important in reducing blood pressure. If you also have high cholesterol, add chromium (200 mcg per day), and the Coenzyme Q10 is essential.

Herbs: Dong quai, a Chinese herb known as the women's ginseng, is important for many women in reducing high blood pressure, and also in reducing menopause symptoms without estrogen drugs. It is an estrogen precursor, a balancer but not an estrogen itself. Try it in tablets or tinctures, and the tablets can be made into a tea (which tastes wonderful, like celery). Some women cannot tolerate it, however. If you feel increasingly tense, irritable, jumpy and insomniac with it, stop and switch to black cohosh. Black cohosh is a progesterone precursor, the opposite of estrogen and again a balancer rather than the hormone itself. This will reduce high blood pressure and treat menopause symptoms in the women who react well with it—usually the women who cannot take dong quai. Do not use it in licorice root combinations, however, as licorice raises blood pressure. These are the two primary herbs to try.

Another antihypertensive herb is hawthorn berries, which helps heart dis-ease, reduces cholesterol deposits in the arteries and lowers blood pressure. Lime blossom, watercress, suma, rosemary, raspberry leaf, passion flower, mistletoe, and nettles are other choices. Celery, dandelion and parsley are diuretics; scullcap, chamomile and passion flower are calmatives; and lime blossom, hawthorn and yarrow may be used together. Sassafras and prickly ash together also reduce blood pressure. Drink alfalfa tea or take three or four alfalfa tablets daily to control both high and low blood pressure and to strengthen the arteries. Alfalfa also increases the assimilation of other herbs, is high in minerals and vitamins, and it tastes good. Rosemary after a stroke will help to return motion, speech and memory.

Naturopathy: If you are taking blood pressure drugs and beginning alternative therapies, you will need to monitor your blood pressure frequently and carefully. Brief fasts are helpful at the beginning of holistic therapies, and will decrease pressure rapidly; they are also used when going off the drugs eventually, when the blood pressure is controlled. Do these under expert supervision, with gradual decreases of the medical drugs. The beginning three day fast is usually of grapefruit or apple juice. After ending the fast, return to solid foods slowly and begin a whole foods diet. Also learn to meditate or do yoga daily; they are major anti-stress factors and blood pressure reducers.

Kyolic (odorless garlic) is highly important in reducing blood pressure and cholesterol; take two capsules three times a day. You can also use raw garlic (about three cloves a day), or garlic and parsley perles; they are not odorfree, however. A woman I worked with took dong quai and Kyolic only, and moderated her diet—she was off blood pressure medications within four months and has stayed off them.

Cucumbers and cucumber juice—a whole raw cucumber or half a cup of juice daily—will help to lower blood pressure. Drink a cup of potato water (the cooled water from boiling scrubbed unpeeled potatoes) daily, or eat two apples a day. Drink a glass of water containing two teaspoons of apple cider vinegar and a teaspoon of honey four times a day. It is high in potassium and minerals, blood cleansing, a digestive and will lower blood pressure. Kelp tablets, five to eight a day, or chlorophyll (Kyogreen, spirulina, wheatgrass, barley grass juice) are also helpful. Pick from any of these choices.

Homeopathy and Cell Salts: *Thyroidinum*, homeopathically made from thyroid gland, is listed as primary for many women with hypertension. *Nux vomica* is used for intermittent high blood pressure, particularly after overindulgence, and *Crataegus* is a cardiac restorative. Where the pulse is full, strong, or hard and there is anxiety and restlessness try *Aconite*. A French preparation of mistletoe called *Guipsine* may be used at two pills four times a day for a few days, then decrease. Expert help is recommended.

Cell Salts: Use *Kali phos.* and *Calc. phos.* alternating twice daily. *Kali mur.* dissolves blood clots and is also used for stroke recovery.

Amino Acids: Take taurine (50–100 mg per kilogram of body weight) in three divided doses per day. L-carnitine, glutamine and glutamic acid (500 mg of each daily) aid in preventing heart attacks and detoxify the body (this comes as a combination), and methionine is also positive. A combination free-form or liver extract amino acids is highly recommended, but if you are taking MAO inhibitor drugs avoid tyrosine.

Acupressure: This method can have major effects in reducing high blood pressure, but avoid it totally if your rate exceeds 200/100. There are a number of points on the back of the body that will lower blood pressure. You may need another woman's help with some of them. The points are located just above the shoulder blades, at the back of the shoulders just below the arm-shoulder joints, in the crease of the elbows, at the outside top of calves below the knees, and just below the outer ankle bones on the feet. There is a spot on the back of both hands where the bones or the thumbs connect to the lower hands that balances the autonomic nervous system. Work any of these points or work them in series, or work what you can reach. You will know them by their tenderness.

Acupressure for High Blood Pressure

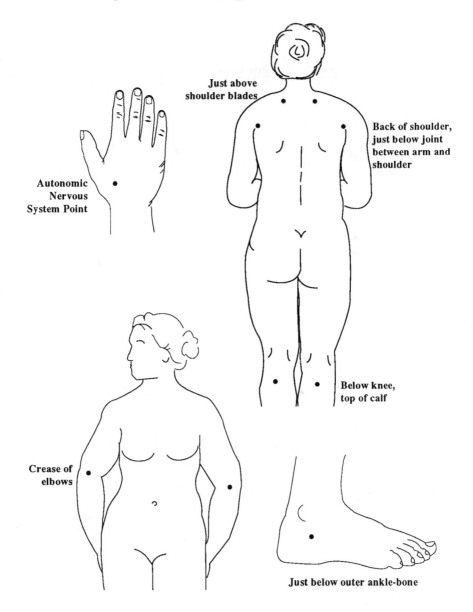

Just above
shoulder blades

Back of shoulder,
just below joint
between arm and
shoulder

Autonomic
Nervous
System Point

Below knee,
top of calf

Crease of
elbows

Just below outer ankle-bone

Note: If blood pressure exceeds 200/100, do not do acupressure

Iona Marsaa Teeguarden, *Acupressure Way of Health: Jin Shin Do* (New York, Japan Publishing Co., 1978), p. 70-76; Moshe Olshevsky, CA, PhD., *et. al.*, *The Manual of Natural Therapy* (New York, Citadel Press, 1989), p. 117.

Acupressure for High Blood Pressure

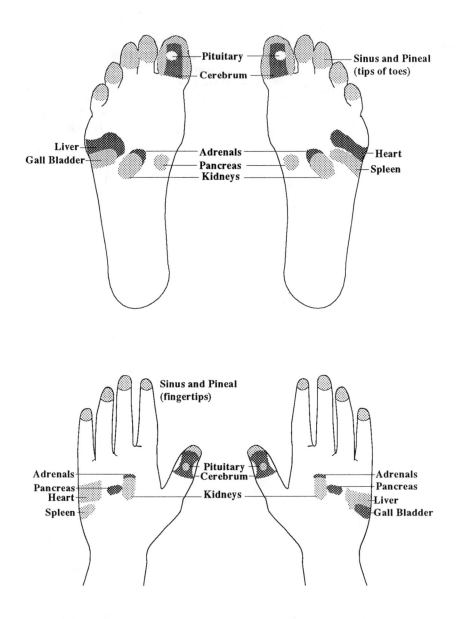

Moshe Olshevsky, CA, PhD., *et. al.*, *The Manual of Natural Therapy* (New York, Citadel Press, 1989), p. 117.

Also do full foot or hand reflexology paying particular attention to the pineal, pituitary, cerebrum, heart, spleen, adrenals, kidneys, pancreas, liver and gall bladder reflexes. Press each point for two minutes, then use a reflex roller for five minutes twice a day on each foot. The point for the autonomic nervous system is only on the hands. On the ears, along the curved vertical groove on the back at almost the center, is another acupressure point for lowering blood pressure. All of the hand, foot and body reflex points are also located on the ears.

Aromatherapy: Use two drops each of hyssop, lavender, marjoram and melissa in baths or to inhale. Use each separately in a massage oil. Ylang ylang also lowers blood pressure, as does lemon.

Flower Essences: Bleeding heart or centaury agave are the primary essences. Both regulate blood pressure, aid in vitamin and mineral absorption, and regenerate; bleeding heart heals the heart physically and emotionally. Spiderwort or lemon lower cholesterol, hops strengthens the blood vessels, daffodil lowers blood pressure and eases stress, and angelica heals the autonomic nervous system and is positive for all cardiovascular diseases.

Gemstones and Gem Essences: Amber, moss agate, beryl, coral or rose quartz strengthen the blood vessels, and coral lowers cholesterol. For arteriosclerosis use picture agate, beryl, chalcedony, or petrified wood in essence. Hold or wear aquamarine, beryl, rose quartz or kunzite.

Emotional Healing: There is suppressed anger, hostility, resentment or rage at someone who is running your life; you can't tell her off without hurting her, and you love her. It's time to take your life back, re-empower yourself, and trust in the Goddess to shoulder the burdens with you. Release anger in positive ways without turning it inward or onto others, and trust in yourself and in the love of the universe. Do it gently but firmly and the one you love will go along.

Hypoglycemia

Hypoglycemia is a factor in such dis-eases as chronic fatigue syndrome and migraines, and may be the real reason behind a number of other dis-eases from emotional instability and depression to alcoholism, allergies, asthma attacks and seizures. Chronic stress, either a cause or a result, goes along with it. Symptoms appear when blood sugar levels drop, from missing a meal or between meals, or from foods that cause an over-production of insulin (sugars, chocolate, refined carbohydrates). In normal physiology, the body's blood glucose level remains even, with insulin secretion and a complicated hormone balance controlling the process. In hypoglycemia, the pancreas produces too much insulin, an over-reaction to what is needed at the time, and too much glycogen (sugar) is removed from the blood. The results are very similar to what happens when a diabetic receives too much insulin or takes insulin without food to balance it. In the hypoglycemic, the blood sugar levels are on a rollercoaster of highs and lows, and the woman experiences a variety of unpleasant symptoms that make normal life impossible. The opposite of diabetes, most doctors consider it either a non-dis-ease or a pre-diabetic state, neither of which is correct.

Many women who are hypoglycemic think they are suffering from other dis-eases that the low blood sugar imitates. They may think they are "losing their minds" or need mental help, and may end up on tranquilizers that make everything worse (I have been there). They may suffer from migraines, headaches or seizures, asthma attacks or anxiety attacks, insomnia, ulcers, sweet or alcohol craving and food binging, and most have food sensitivities that are part of the problem. They crave the foods that trigger the reactions in a physically addictive way. Symptoms of low blood sugar include: dizziness, nervousness, weakness, irritability, fainting, trembling, depression, inability to concentrate, indigestion, nausea, palpitations, blurred vision, tiredness, anxiety, crying jags, indecisiveness, hyperactivity, convulsions, headaches, night sweats, confusion, loss of memory, constant hunger, chest tightness, cold extremities, cold sweats and pains in various parts of the body, especially the eyes. Adrenal exhaustion, deficient protein assimilation and poor carbohydrate metabolism are part of hypoglycemia, and candida is often a factor. Taking more sugar when blood sugar levels are low seems logical but worsens the rollercoaster of ups and downs. A woman who is hypoglycemic needs a reduced sugar, low carbohydrate, high fiber and high protein diet, with frequent meals and a significant reduction in stress. Vitamins, herbs and amino acids make a tremendous difference, along with diet control.

Vitamins and Minerals: Along with a quality multiple vitamin and mineral supplement, B-complex vitamins are the most essential. Take a B-complex-50 to -100 daily, with extra B-12 (30 mcg) twice a day, and 500 mg B-5 (pantothenic acid) twice a day. Niacin is a key, and recommendations for it vary from taking an additional 100 mg to an additional 1500 mg per day. If using large amounts, use a time release form and cut back if there is nausea, beginning with lower doses and increasing slowly—use niacinamide to avoid the hotflash sensation. The B-vitamins are important in carbohydrate metabolism and the conversion of glucose to useful energy; pantothenic acid is for adrenal function. Use a calcium/magnesium tablet, 1500 mg calcium to 750 mg magnesium. Most hypoglycemics are deficient in manganese. Chromium (300 mcg daily) is essential for proper insulin function, and can be taken as GTF (Glucose Tolerance Factor) with brewer's yeast and niacin. Use 1000–2000 mg of vitamin C daily, 400–600 IU of vitamin E, and 50 mg of zinc (most hypoglycemics are zinc deficient). Digestive enzymes (pancreatin and proteolytic enzymes) may be helpful for protein digestion, as well as lecithin, or raw adrenal and pancreas glandulars, royal jelly, spirulina and bran. Most hypoglycemics who are over fifty years of age have hypothyroidism—add raw thyroid glandular.

Herbs: A black cohosh, licorice root and passion flower combination (available inexpensively in capsules from Solaray) lowers blood sugar without raising blood pressure and is slightly calmative, or try black cohosh or licorice alone. Licorice is the first choice for lowering blood sugar, but it also raises blood pressure so is off-limits to many women. Hawthorn, ginger or wild yam are helpful, and some women can use dong quai. (If it makes you too nervous switch to black cohosh or something else.) Scullcap or passion flower is calmative and reduces nervous tension symptoms and headaches. Alfalfa is highly nutritious and slows the insulin reaction, as does wheatgrass or spirulina. Instead of sugar, try stevia (available from Sunrider and other companies); it is an herbal sweetener that helps to balance blood sugar. Though on a low sugar diet, avoid chemical artificial sweeteners; they add to the risk of cataracts. Glucomannan, an herbal fiber bulk laxative, also helps to slow insulin reaction. Dandelion root stimulates and cleanses the liver, plus providing B-vitamins and calcium. A Chinese herbal, san-chia-fu-mai-tang, "Decoction of Three Shells to Recover the Pulse," is available through Asian pharmacies.

Naturopathy: Rats fed a high carbohydrate diet develop hypoglycemia. Feeding a high fiber diet with adequate protein controls it, but when returned to a high carbohydrate diet, the rats begin the blood sugar rollercoaster again. Therefore, you can control hypoglycemia with diet, but the diet will not cure it once the dis-ease is there; the diet has to be a permanent change in lifestyle. Fiber slows insulin reaction, and a hypoglycemia diet is also high protein. Eat vegetables, whole grains, seeds, nuts, eggs, yoghurt or kefir, avocados, Jerusalem artichokes, raw cheese, fish or fowl (organic recommended). Use fruit (dried, cooked or raw), fruit juices and vegetable juices only in moderation and with protein (nuts, cheese, yoghurt). In a low sugar reaction, take fiber with protein (crackers with cheese, cottage cheese or nut butter); when sugar is high take fiber alone (crackers, popcorn, oat bran). Avoid sugar, refined flour products, processed foods, alcohol, caffeine, soft drinks, salt, cigarettes, corn, white rice, macaroni and gravies. Eat several small meals a day, including something before bedtime; rotate the diet or do an elimination diet to discover food allergies.

Fasting once a month is extremely helpful to stop the symptoms of hypoglycemia, especially the mental and nervous symptoms and depression. Use spirulina or protein powder supplements in the fast to prevent low sugar reactions, and take lemon juice enemas. Fasts are best done under expert supervision.

Kyolic will also help; use two to six tablets/capsules daily. It stabilizes blood pressure and blood sugar, plus reduces candida albicans over-runs, which may be a high factor. Kelp tablets, fish oil lipids, and chlorophyll also help to balance blood sugar. Kelp stimulates the thyroid.

Homeopathy and Cell Salts: Homeopathic remedies are closely matched to symptoms and emotional states, and are highly individualized. See an experienced homeopath for this, but here are some suggestions. For feelings of emptiness, sinking sensation, headaches and/or indigestion from starchy foods, worse in the early morning and better for eating, try *Sulfur*. Use *Nux vomica* for nausea, headache and nervous irritability, especially if worse after eating or overindulging. Try *Arsenicum* for anxiety, melancholy, restlessness, weakness, exhaustion after the least effort, and with symptoms worse at night. *Aconite* is for the sudden onset of symptoms, with anxiety, restlessness, fears and panic that is better for fresh air and worse for warmth.

Cell Salts: Use *Kali phos.* for headaches, nervousness and stress, *Calc. phos.* for malassimilation, or *Mag. phos.* for spasmodic pains and nerve stabilizing. Also try the Bioplasma combination.

Amino Acids: Twin Labs' predigested liver amino acids combination has made a significant difference for my own hypoglycemia. Single aminos include: L-glutamine (taken with B-6 and vitamin C) to reduce sugar cravings, cystine to block insulin, and carnitine for converting stored body fat into energy.

Acupressure for Hypoglycemia

Do second

Do these two first,
at the same time

On palm below
third finger

Back of hand, base
of little finger

Do First

Do Second

Back of foot, behind little toe

John Thie, DC, *Touch For Health, A New Approach to Restoring Our Natural Energies* (Marina del Rey, Ca, DeVorss and Co., 1973), p. 44 and 80.

Acupressure: Do full foot, hand or ear acupressure twice a day and work the endocrine gland reflexes, particularly the pancreas and pituitary, and the liver point. (See the Immune System Dis-ease section and the body maps.) Two Touch For Health sequences are given in the illustration. A pair of points is done at once in these, and you will need someone's help.

Aromatherapy: Lavender, melissa, peppermint, sage, lemon thyme or rosemary are used in massage oils, baths, diffusers or to inhale.

Flower Essences: Apricot or sugar beet regulates blood sugar levels, mood swings and emotional symptoms. Jasmine is for protein assimilation in hypoglycemia, and banana is a tonic.

Gemstones and Gem Essences: Moss agate or amethyst quartz in essence are used for hypoglycemia. Hold or wear kunzite, lepidolite or chrysocolla for mood disturbances, depression and stress, and/or use malachite, peridot or green tourmaline for balancing the pancreas.

Emotional Healing: Hypoglycemia is a reaction to extreme stress. Stress and trust issues are major work for most women, especially for the many women who have been incested, raped, or abused. Learn to relax and let go, learn to meditate or do yoga and do it nightly, take time to smell the roses and watch sunsets on the beach, and do the Self-Blessing often. You need to trust someone sometime, so start with yourself and the Goddess; it gets easier from there. Be less of a perfectionist, take care of yourself more and others less, and get enough sleep.

Immune System Dis-eases

The immune system is the body's over-all defense against outside interference, and particularly against bacterial and viral infection. When it is functioning at a low or deficient level, infectious dis-eases ranging from the common cold to AIDS results. Other immune deficiency dis-eases include cancer, flu, multiple sclerosis, muscular dystrophy, chronic fatigue syndrome, boils, candida albicans, hardening of the arteries, and any bacterial, fungal or viral infection. These infectious dis-eases may also be the precursors for auto-immune reactions, dis-eases where the body over-reacts and attacks itself. Some of these include allergies, hay fever, asthma, rheumatoid arthritis, or lupus, which may be preceded by mono-nucleosis, strep throats, hepatitis or rheumatic fever. Diabetes onset may occur or worsen after an infectious dis-ease, and cancer seems to be a primary reaction to a weakened immune state. People with AIDS develop such opportunistic dis-eases as pneumonia, cancer, fungus of the blood or skin, candida albicans/thrush, tuberculosis, toxoplasmosis, chronic fatigue and chronic flu symptoms, warts, herpes, wounds that do not heal and a variety of other infections. Homeopaths believe that vaccinating children causes damage to the thymus, resulting in immune dysfunction and dis-eases later on. Exposure to toxins, chemicals and radiation deplete the immune system, and an underactive thyroid reduces immune function. Stress is a major factor, and depression has been proven to deplete the body's resistance to dis-ease.

Immune system dis-eases are present in today's list of dis-eases in a way they were never known before. The concept of immune system dis-ease was first defined in the 1950s, and many dis-eases that are widespread killers today were unknown or rare fifty or a hundred years ago. Everyone's body is under stress, from our high speed-high pressure-high competition lifestyle, from the denutritionalized foods we are left with after refining and processing, and from the pollution and toxins our bodies are forced to drink, breathe, touch and live in daily. That more and more of us get sick from any number of dis-eases is no wonder, since a truly healthy immune system for anyone in this environment is impossible.

Women are generally healthier than men in this picture, but are rapidly catching up. The level of immune system function is the reason why some women in an epidemic or after exposure develop a dis-ease while others do not. Holistic methods are a lifestyle rather than a remedy for maintaining optimal immune system health and function, the best that can be had with what we live under. The pollution that is killing our planet is killing everyone and everything that lives on it, and healing the earth is ultimately our own wellness and survival. Men are not willing to make the changes necessary, and as always it is up to women to save ourselves and our world.

Vitamins and Minerals: A quality multiple vitamin and mineral supplement is a basic start in replacing some of what we've lost nutritionally from food. Use 15,000–25,000 IU of vitamin A as beta-carotene (unless you are diabetic or hypothyroid, then use A itself). The B-complex is essential (50–100 mg per day and more if you are ill). Most women need additional B-6 (100–250 mg) and folic acid (400 mcg), and if you are under great stress use B-5 (500–2000 mg per day total). Vitamin C (1000–5000 mg per day) with bioflavinoids and lots of water is the most significant immune building vitamin factor; with B-complex and calcium/

magnesium even the high doses will cause no problems. Stop at bowel tolerance. Vitamin E (400–800 IU) with selenium (200 mcg) is an important antioxidant and free radical scavenger, a protection against pollutants (with vitamins A and C).

Many women are iron deficient, but try B-complex vitamins first before supplementing with iron. Zinc regulates the immune system; use 25–50 mg per day (don't go over 100 mg). Most women are calcium/magnesium deficient and require a supplement daily to prevent osteoporosis and help menstrual and menopause symptoms. Copper (1–3 mg per day) and boron (1–3 mg per day) are important and may be in your multiple vitamin. Boron prevents the body from losing needed minerals. Germanium or coenzyme Q10 are antioxidants and oxygenate the blood. Essential fatty acids (black currant oil, evening primrose oil, etc.) and acidophilus are useful, as well as combination raw glandulars or raw thymus, lymph, spleen or bone marrow. This is an over-all picture that changes with individuals and individual dis-eases but is basic for immune building.

Herbs: The herbal antibiotics fight infection and build the immune system; these include echinacea, St. John's wort (hypericum), goldenseal, pau d'arco, tea-tree and chaparral. Jason Winter's Tea is a chaparral compound and immune building. Alfalfa, wheatgrass, chlorophyll, oatstraw or horsetail are nutritional and provide minerals, particularly alfalfa that provides all the vitamins and minerals and enhances the assimilation of other vitamins and herbs. Burdock, red clover, yellow dock, yarrow, dandelion or blue violet cleanse the lymphatic system and liver.

Boil a teaspoon of cayenne flowers in a gallon of water for two minutes, then shut off the flame and let cool. Strain and place in a covered jar in the refrigerator. Start small (with a teaspoonful daily) and work up to taking a juice glassful a day. This is *hot* stuff, and may irritate the stomach, but is believed to take over where a weakened immune system leaves off. It will prevent opportunistic infections in AIDS patients, but cannot rebuild the immune system.

Several formulas based on Chinese medicine are available. One called Astra 8 Formula is an energy tonic used for AIDS/HIV patients and is useful in all immune and auto-immune dis-eases. It contains: astragalus, atractylodes, schizandra, ligustrum, ganoderma, eluthero, ginseng, codonopsis and licorice. Another formula called Power Mushroom is a digestive and mild diuretic and is comprised of antiviral mushrooms. It contains ganoderma, lentinus, silver fungus, polyporus and hoelen. Cascade Mushroom Products offer Astragalus Ten Plus for use in chronic fatigue syndrome and Epstein Barr Virus (EBV). It contains: ginseng, astragalus, cistanche, ganoderma, morus fruit, lycium fruit, ophiopogan, ligustrum, licorice, eluthero, schizandra, ho-shou-wu and atractylodes. These are being used at the Quan Yin clinic in San Francisco and are available from ITM Herb Products, 2017 S.E. Hawthorne, Portland, OR 97214, 1-800-544-7504. Bioherb, concentrated *ganoderma lucidum*, is being used in Japan for cancer and myasthenia gravis.[1]

Naturopathy: Begin with a three day juice fast using daily enemas, and reintroduce solid foods slowly, watching carefully for allergic reactions. An elimination and rotation diet for discovering food sensitivities is important. Start and maintain a whole foods diet using raw vegetables, whole grains, beans, fruits, seeds, and some fish. Avoid allergy reacting foods, alcohol, caffeine, processed foods, sugar, soft drinks, animal products, dairy, or fried foods. Eat foods with as few preservatives, additives and dyes as possible. If you smoke or use drugs, stop. Work on reducing stress and depression—meditate daily or learn yoga, take long baths or long walks and get massages. If your job or lover are impossible, change them!

Bee pollen or propolis are major immune builders, and kelp adds minerals and balances the thyroid. As an alternative to kelp, try Edgar Cayce's Atomidine for iodine, or the following: use one drop of Lugol's Solution, one teaspoon of apple cider vinegar, and one teaspoon of honey in a glass of warm or cool water before meals twice a week. Use apple cider vinegar and honey in water (without Lugol's Solution) two or three times a day. If you develop a metallic taste in your mouth, you are getting too much iodine; cut down or stop for awhile. Kyolic, odorless garlic, is an important aid to immune system building. It is antibacterial, antifungal and antiviral, as well as helpful for balancing blood pressure and blood sugar. Take two tablets three times a day.

Toxic metals suppress the immune system and can be defined by hair analysis. Mercury amalgam tooth fillings are immune suppressive; some women have had their mercury fillings replaced with nonamalgam ones and discover that they feel better.

Homeopathy and Cell Salts: An experienced homeopath or homeopathic physician can work with you to find your Constitutional remedy. This is complex work and uses remedies at individually determined potency to remove genetic dis-ease overlays and life-force deep health problems. Layer by layer, dis-ease can be released from the body for greater wellness and increased immuned system strength.

Cell Salts: Take three tablets of each twice a day: *Kali phos.*, *Natrum mur.*, *Ferrum phos.*, *Kali sulph.* and *Natrum sulph.* Combination cell salts, called Bioplasma, is also positive.

---

[1]Moshe Olshevsky, CA, Ph.D, et al., *The Manual of Natural Therapy* (New York, Citadel Press, 1989), p. 245–246.

Amino Acids: A combination free-form or liver-extract amino acids capsule is important in protein, B-complex and many other nutrients and is a free radical scavenger. Single aminos include arginine (3–5 g per day unless you have herpes) or cysteine, methionine, lysine and ornithine (500 mg each twice daily).

Acupressure: Use full foot, hand or ear acupressure massage starting with twice a week and working gradually up to twice daily. Pay particular attention to the endocrine glands, lymphatics, spleen, and liver reflexes. On the hands only are points for the autonomic nervous system and for increasing energy. Also see the body reflex points under AIDS. Try some of the polarity balancing sessions described in *All Women Are Healers* (Diane Stein, The Crossing Press, 1990), as well as reiki sessions, jin shin do, shiatsu, neuromuscular massage or acupuncture.

Aromatherapy: Make a massage oil using 3% each of the following essential oils in a vegetable oil base: bryony, eucalyptus, lavender and rosemary. Other oils to use in massage oils, baths, diffusers or to inhale include: tea-tree, geranium, juniper, St. John's wort, lemon, eucalyptus, niaoli, peppermint, cardamom or lemon thyme. Rose or lavender make wonderful stress reducers.

Flower Essences: Amaranthus is the primary essence for boosting the immune system. Ginseng is for endocrine strengthening and balancing, and lemon is for the lymphatic system. Use hawthorn for cancer, and corn (zea mays) for psychological healing in cancer and leukemia. Use pansy to boost the immune system against all viruses, including the AIDS virus.

Gemstones and Gem Essences: Use any of the following to boost the immune system: emerald, jade, picture jasper, amethyst, blue quartz, rose quartz, ruby, sulfur, blue tourmaline or pink tourmaline. Wear or hold pink tourmaline, blue tourmaline, kunzite or rose quartz.

Emotional Healing: Develop a positive outlook, and realize and release negative emotions. Deal with anger, resentment, fear, hurt and longing. No one is out to get you, life is good and good *for* you. Reduce stress by allowing life its ebbs and flows, and by going along with trust. Care for yourself, for others and the earth, and learn to love.

Acupressure for Immune Dis-eases

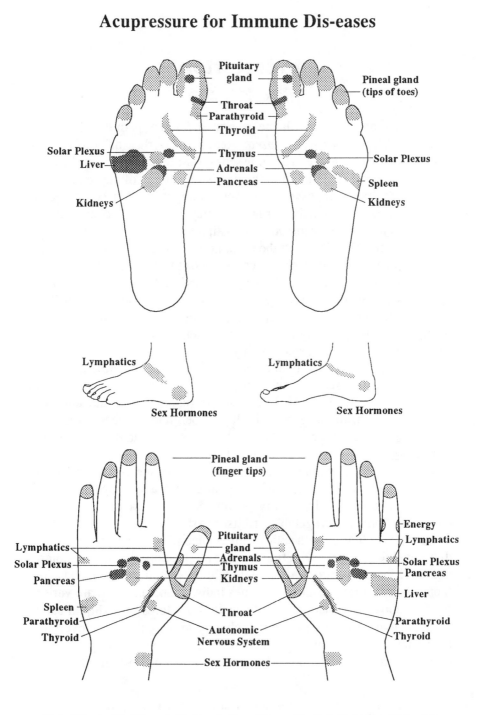

Moshe Olshevsky, CA, PhD., *et. al.*, *The Manual of Natural Therapy* (New York, Citadel Press, 1989), p. 269.

Indigestion

Indigestion includes gastritis, heartburn, abdominal pain or discomfort, irritation, bloating or gas, nausea, vomiting, diarrhea or constipation, general listlessness and/or a burning sensation after eating. It may be acute (immediate) or persistent (chronic), and is a symptom of improper digestion, rather than a dis-ease itself. Acute indigestion can be caused by overeating, eating a food that disagrees with you, poor food combinations, acid foods like citrus or tomatoes, constipation, stress, eating too fast or too frequently, chewing with the mouth open, swallowing too much air, spices including too much salt, or eating foods that are too hot or too cold. The dis-ease is self-limiting. Morning sickness is indigestion in pregnancy.

Persistent or recurrent indigestion may be caused by lack of hydrochloric acid or digestive enzymes, or drinking liquids with meals (which dilutes them). Food allergies, high carbohydrate diets, cooking with aluminum, candida albicans, ulcers, smoking, hypothyroidism, hiatal hernia, or dis-ease of the gall bladder or liver are also causes. Lack of hydrochloric acid (HCL) can be caused by low thyroid, and is particularly common in women over fifty. Low HCL is also prevalent in asthma, allergies, rheumatoid arthritis, osteoporosis, lupus, pernicious anemia, diabetes, systemic candida, eczema, chronic hepatitis, intestinal parasites and vitiligo.[1] Women who consume a lot of milk products may be deficient in HCL also, as digesting the milk dilutes it. Ulcer sufferers have too much.

Diet is usually the cause of acute indigestion and using simple food combining rules will frequently prevent it. Avoid eating together the following: fruits with vegetables, fruits with starches, sugars with proteins or starches, or liquids with solids. Citrus juice with cereals, cherries with dairy products, or miso with fruit are also indigestion/gas-causing combinations. Most people know what foods will upset their stomachs and avoid them. Beans cause gas and sometimes indigestion, and there are various ways to cook them that prevent it. Healthfood stores sell a liquid called "Beano" that's supposed to do the job, and soaking the beans overnight (sometimes with an onion or piece of papaya), then changing the water (and throwing away the onion/papaya) before cooking will help. Other

---

[1]Dr. Ross Trattler, *Better Health Through Natural Healing* (New York, McGraw-Hill Book Co., 1985), p. 225–229.

foods that cause indigestion for many women are green or red peppers, raw onions, cabbage, citrus fruits, tomatoes, spicy foods or fried foods. With hypoacidity (rather than the opposite) more often the problem in heartburn and indigestion, antacid medications do more harm than good. They contain aluminum and sodium, disturb the body's acid-alkaline balance, and longterm use can result in kidney damage. Also avoid taking laxatives when there is stomach pain.

Vitamins and Minerals: If assimilation is a problem, take your daily multiple vitamin and mineral supplement in liquid form. Use a B-complex-50 daily, also in liquid form if needed—the B-vitamins are essential for normal digestion. Folic acid deficiency may be a cause of poor digestion, or B-12 if hypoacidity is the problem. Use vitamin C with bioflavinoids, 1000 mg per day in ascorbic acid form if hypoacid or sodium ascorbate form if hyperacid. Use 400–800 IU of vitamin E daily, particularly if you have ulcers. Calcium/magnesium is an antacid, the safest one to use, but take it between mealtimes. Acidophilus is important for normal digestion and may solve the problem. Try bromelin, pancreatic digestive enzymes, papaya enzyme, proteolytic enzymes, or multi-digestive enzymes. Avoid HCL if you have ulcers. (HCL may be added by using apple cider vinegar and water—see the Naturopathy section). Use a fiber bulk laxative like glucomannan to cleanse the lower bowel (not if there is abdominal pain). For morning sickness, take 400 mg of magnesium in the morning, and 50 mg of B-6 every four hours short-term.

Herbs: Drink pure aloe vera juice, 1/4 cup on an empty stomach in the morning and at bedtime. It helps gastrointestinal symptoms, heartburn and ulcers (do not use if pregnant or nursing), as well as constipation. Catnip, peppermint, fennel or chamomile tea are the best known herbs for indigestion. Others include spearmint, slippery elm, basil, thyme, dandelion, rosemary, ginger, angelica or raspberry. Burdock heals all digestive diseases, as does agrimony; use lovage tea for gas or colic, or a tea made from bay leaves. Dill tea or chamomile are relaxants, catnip helps diarrhea, and meadowsweet is for hyperacidity. Parsley tea or St. John's wort soothes stomach cramps and pain. Use parsley tea, alfalfa and/or balm for healing ulcers, and comfrey and pepsin for ulcerative colitis. Cloves steeped in hot water for five minutes are also helpful for ulcers and stop vomiting. Peppermint, ginger, red raspberry leaf or basil helps morning sickness. For chronic indigestion take one unground mustard seed with water the first day, two the second day, three the third day, adding one each day until you are taking twenty seeds. Then start reducing by one seed a day until you are down to one again. Take them first thing in the morning on an empty stomach.

Naturopathy: To find out if you are deficient in HCL, take a tablespoon of apple cider vinegar or of lemon juice, or a glass of water containing the vinegar or lemon juice. If your indigestion or heartburn goes away, you are deficient; take the lemon or vinegar water daily with meals. If they make the symptoms worse, you are not HCL deficient and should avoid taking HCL or enzyme compounds that contain it. For those whom it helps, the above may be all that is needed.[2]

Fast for two to three days, drinking only apple or pineapple juice four or five times daily. Other fasts include lemon juice and water, carrot juice, carrot and cabbage juice, or slippery elm tea. Use warm water or slippery elm enemas. End the fast with a mono diet of apples, carrots or brown rice for a few days, then reintroduce foods slowly, watching for allergic reactions. Start a diet that avoids problem or allergic foods, refined carbohydrates and sugars, fried, fatty or spicy foods, junkfoods, acid foods, and excess salt. Eat a whole foods diet high in fiber, vegetables and whole grains.

Use kelp tablets or Atomidine if you are hypothyroid. Kyolic capsules aid in digestion and help if candida is present; see the section on Candida Albicans. Drink rice or barley broth for indigestion. In acute cases try charcoal tablets, but not with other remedies; these are not for longterm use. For ulcers, use propolis for internal healing.

Homeopathy and Cell Salts: Use *Nux vomica* for heartburn, gas, bitter taste in the mouth, and heaviness after meals, especially after overindulgence. Use *Arsenicum* for diarrhea and vomiting, restlessness, exhaustion, coldness and thirst for small sips. *Lycopodium* is for heartburn with daily or chronic indigestion, gas and feeling full after eating very little. *Pulsatilla* is for stomach upsets after eating rich foods; there is a white coating to the tongue. *Sulfur* is for gas that smells like rotten eggs. For morning sickness, use *Aconite* and *Bryonia* together in 3X potency.

Cell Salts: *Calc. phos.* is for chronic indigestion, pain after eating and gas. *Nat. phos.,* an acid neutralizer, is for heartburn. *Kali phos.* is for ulcers.

Amino Acids: Use the following single aminos: L-carnitine to break down fats into energy, methionine as a liver detoxifier, or histidine for indigestion and ulcers.

Acupressure: There are a number of acupressure body points for indigestion; see the illustration. Also look at the reflex body maps and work the points for the stomach, gall bladder and liver on the body, hands, ears or feet. For ulcers, see the section on Stress. Use full foot massage with a foot roller.

[2]James Balch, MD and Phyllis Balch, CNC, *Prescription for Nutritional Healing* (Garden City, NY, Avery Publishing Group, Inc., 1990), p. 216.

Acupressure for Indigestion

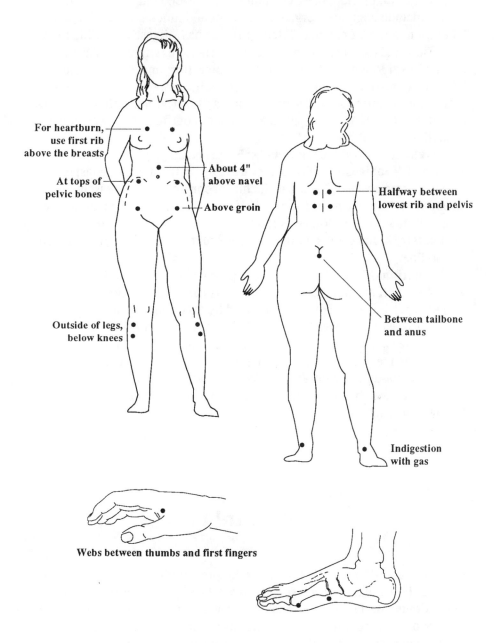

For heartburn, use first rib above the breasts

At tops of pelvic bones

About 4" above navel

Above groin

Outside of legs, below knees

Halfway between lowest rib and pelvis

Between tailbone and anus

Indigestion with gas

Webs between thumbs and first fingers

Pedro Chan, *Finger Acupressure* (New York, Ballantine Books, 1974), p. 17-19; Moshe Olshevsky, CA, PhD., *et. al.*, *The Manual of Natural Therapy* (New York, Citadel Press, 1989), p. 20; Cathryn Bauer, *Acupressure for Women* (Freedom, CA, The Crossing Press, 1987), p.58-59; Iona Marsaa Teeguarden, *Acupressure Way of Health: Jin Shin Do* (New York, Japan Publishing Co., 1978), p. 69, 72-73;

Aromatherapy: Use in a diffuser or place a few drops on the skin for inhaling: basil, black pepper, chamomile and lavender together or singly. Others include angelica, bergamot, cardamom, fennel, ginger, cinnamon, lemon, lemongrass or lovage. Tiferet-Lifetree has a digestive combination.

Flower Essences: For indigestion with nervous stress, use Agrimony (Bach Flower Remedy). Aloe vera is for indigestion, and loquat stimulates HCL and digestive enzymes, and helps in indigestion with nausea. Dill or sage is for assimilation, and sage or cedar is a laxative and colon cleanser. For ulcers use aloe vera, avocado, cedar, comfrey, dill, daffodil or dandelion.

Gemstones and Gem Essences: Beryl and magnesium (mineral) are essences for indigestion. For ulcers use any of the agates or jaspers in essence, or moonstone. Make a malachite or chrysocolla gem essence with the stones left in the water for only half an hour. Hold or wear malachite, green tourmaline, peridot, amber, topaz or amber calcite for indigestion; for ulcers try kunzite, pink tourmaline, rose quartz, dioptase or watermelon tourmaline.

Emotional Healing: When there is peace and security at home and with one's parents and mate, the stomach is calm. Indigestion and ulcers are gut-level fear, dread or anxiety, a need for love and security, and a need to feel successful to be worthy of love. The stomach assimilates nourishment and new ideas; there is a fear of something new or an inability to assimilate it or to change. Ulcers are lack of self-image, a belief that one is not successful enough or good enough. What (or who) is eating at you? Learn to flow with and trust the process of life; you are definitely good enough. Learn to meditate and relax.

Insomnia

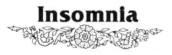

Eight and a half million Americans take prescription sleeping pills and thirty million dollars a year is spent on over-the-counter sleep medications. These drugs interfere with normal sleep patterns if they work at all, or are useless or even contain carcinogenic ingredients. Stress is the cause of most sleeplessness (and eighty-five percent of all dis-ease), and many women have vitamin deficiencies (calcium, B-complex, copper or iron) that cause insomnia. What is enough sleep is also subjective. Some women think they are not sleeping, when in fact they are getting the rest they need by sleeping lightly, and others are unaware of their own body rhythms and needs and are simply sleeping by their own body clocks instead of by the alarm clock. If you are a "night person" or a "day person" honor that and sleep accordingly, and much insomnia will end. Elders need less sleep than younger women, and when menopause begins this decreased need, some women think they are not getting enough though they really are. If you feel well in the morning, you have had what you need, even if you think you haven't slept enough or at all.

The big key for me in overcoming insomnia was my attitude about it. Instead of worrying all night about being awake and not sleeping, I decided to just relax in bed and get what rest I could. I learned to meditate before bedtime nightly, then to lie still and quiet with as cleared a mind as possible. The relaxation was enough to get me the rest I needed, and my sleep gradually became deeper. The same thing works if you wake up during the night. Sleep requirements are individual, and what is enough for you may be too much or too little for someone else. Nightmares, fears or leg cramps can cause sleeplessness, and there are holistic remedies for all of these. The suggestions below are safe, non-carcinogenic and nontoxic, and will not disrupt normal sleep cycles.

Vitamins and Minerals: Use a daily multiple vitamin and mineral supplement that contains copper, iron, manganese, calcium/magnesium and a good amount of B-complex (Schiff's Single Day contains 75 mg of each of the B-vitamins). This with a complete calcium/magnesium supplement (try General Nutrition Center's Calcium Plus) may be enough to end insomnia. It will also end leg cramps and waking up in the middle of the night. Take calcium lactate or calcium chelate (1000–2000 mg) with half the amount of magnesium or more (to 1000 mg), and 30–50 mg of zinc per day. A vitamin B-complex-50 with extra B-5 (pantothenic acid, 500 mg) for stress and B-6 (100 mg, a common women's deficiency), and/or B-3 (niacin, a relaxant) will help. If you are taking a lot of B-complex or B-6 and having nightmares or too vivid dreams, cut down on B-6. A B-complex tablet with two calcium/magnesiums before bed is an effective sleep remedy. Lecithin and brewer's yeast are other helpful B-vitamin sources. If you are iron deficient, the B-complex that transports it may be enough. If there is copper (up to 3 mg) and manganese (1–5 mg) in your multiple, it should be enough. Hair analysis can be used to determine mineral deficiencies. For chronic restless insomnia also try germanium.

Herbs: Try a tea or tinctures of hops, scullcap and catnip singly or together before bed. Valerian is a stronger sedative and pain reliever. Passion flower calms the mind, and feverfew is a physical body relaxant particularly good for women with arthritis or other body pain. Feverfew, scullcap, hops, black cohosh, chamomile, raspberry leaves, rosemary, wild lettuce and rosehips are stress reducers, and alfalfa used with any of these is a nutrient and enhancer of other herbs. California poppy, jasmine, hawthorn, blue vervain, strawberry leaves, lemon leaves, lime blossom or melilot are also calmatives. To prevent nightmares use hops or thyme tea or tinctures. For night fears use passion flower, or passion flower with scullcap. Try a dream pillow of hops for nightmares, or one of mugwort and rose petals to induce pleasant dreams.

Naturopathy: Avoid eating too close to bedtime, and reduce the amount of salt used in your meals. Exclude stimulants after 3 PM (coffee, black or green teas, cola drinks, chocolate, alcohol, cigarettes). Eat a junkfood-free diet, eliminating sugar and refined flour as much as possible. For many women insomnia is an allergic reaction to food additives, dyes or pesticide residues, and women are especially sensitive to the hormones and drugs fed meat and poultry animals. Do not over-eat at dinner. Drink a warm glass of milk with a half teaspoon of nutmeg or two teaspoons of honey in it at bedtime. The amino acid tryptophan is the relaxant in milk, and other tryptophan foods include yoghurt, bananas, figs, dates, tuna, turkey (organic), whole grain crackers or nut butters. A half-grapefruit at bedtime may also help, or drink a half cup of orange juice, a half cup of pineapple juice and a quarter cup of lemon juice together.

Chop a clove of garlic and place it in a glass with just enough water to cover it; put a lid on the glass and allow it to sit all day. At bedtime, fill the glass with warm/hot water and sip slowly. Repeat daily for ten to fourteen days for chronic insomnia. Another recipe is to add three teaspoons of apple cider vinegar to a cup of honey and take two teaspoons nightly before bed. Other foods for insomnia are English lettuce juiced or eaten raw, and celery, also juiced or eaten raw. Cucumbers are calmative and contain calcium. Lettuce is a preventive of nightmares.

Try relaxation exercises, yoga, warm baths with sea salt, foot or body massages, biofeedback or meditation before bedtime. Particularly concentrate on clearing the mind. Masturbation to orgasm relaxes the whole body.

Homeopathy and Cell Salts: Use *Coffea* for insomnia after drinking too much coffee, or when the mind won't shut off. *Ignatia* is for sighing and yawning, and feeling like you will never sleep. Use *Nux vomica* for waking in the middle of the night, usually from 4–7 AM, and especially after drinking alcohol the night before. *Aconite* is for night fears and panic attacks—keep it by the bed; and *Phosphorus* is the remedy if you are having nightmares, and feel tense and fearful about sleeping. Use *Arnica* when you are overtired, aching and the bed feels hard, *Cocculus* for overtiredness and exhaustion after sleeplessness and for jet lag, or *Passiflora* for restless sleep.

Cell Salts: Alternate *Natrum mur.* and *Kali phos.* twice per day. Use *Natrum sulph.* for nightmares or night panics. *Silica* with *Natrum mur. is* for jerking of limbs during sleep, *Natrum mur.* is for anxious dreams. For tiredness in the morning use *Natrum mur.* with *Calc. phos.* Also try the combination Calmes Forte or Bioplasma.

Amino Acids: Tryptophan will be back on the market eventually, and is the amino acid of choice for insomnia. Use GABA for stress and depression. A full amino combination is recommended as a major stress reducer.

Acupressure: Full foot reflexology at bedtime, paying attention to pituitary and adrenals, as well as any other sore spots, is important and positive. There are also a number of body pressure points, shown in the illustration. Look on both sides of the feet, in the sides of the heels where the foot and ankle meet for reflex points, and about three inches above the inner ankles. On the little finger side of both wrists, find a meridian point where the wrist meets the hand. Where the skull and neck meet, find pressure points on both sides of the spine and an inch behind the ears. Work these points for a few minutes each, until they release. See the pressure points under Stress as well.

Aromatherapy: Try a bath before bed containing hops, meadow-sweet or orange blossom essential oils. Other oils to use in baths, massage oils, or a drop on the pillow include chamomile, lavender, jasmine, ylang ylang, rose, melissa, neroli, marjoram or lemon thyme. Tiferet-Lifetree has a relaxing combination for use in insomnia.

Flower Essences: Passion flower essence helps women to let go of the day for a restful sleep, and it also aids dreamwork. Morning glory is for restlessness at night; chaparral is for general insomnia; and forget-me-not is for nightmares and disharmony in dreams. Try Bach Flower Remedy's Rock Rose for nightmares.

Gemstones and Gem Essences: Use the following in essence for insomnia: malachite (leave in water only half an hour if making this at home), amethyst, sulfur, zircon or lodestone. For nightmares, use essence of jet, garnet or chalcedony. Hold kunzite in your hand at night for a restful night's sleep, or aquamarine, amethyst or moonstone. Program a clear crystal for this purpose, or use rutile quartz to stimulate dreams. A boji stone absorbs fears and pain.

Emotional Healing: Insomnia is fear or misplaced guilt, and not trusting the process of life. Leave the day's cares at the bedroom door or turn them over to the Goddess for the night (and day as well). Get to know the Goddesses of the night and moon, and learn to trust the night for her gentle healing.

Acupressure for Insomnia

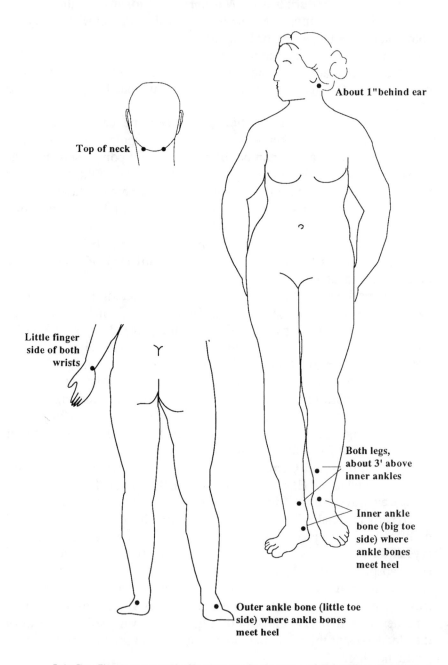

About 1"behind ear

Top of neck

Little finger
side of both
wrists

Both legs,
about 3' above
inner ankles

Inner ankle
bone (big toe
side) where
ankle bones
meet heel

Outer ankle bone (little toe
side) where ankle bones
meet heel

Pedro Chan, *Finger Acupressure* (New York, Ballantine Books, 1974), p. 75-77; Iona Marsaa Teeguarden,
Acupressure Way of Health: Jin Shin Do (New York, Japan Publishing Co., 1978), p. 69-70, 75.

Leg Cramps

Muscle cramps and spasms in the legs and feet at night can make sleeping difficult at best; you wake up to intense pain night after night until you fear going to sleep at all. The calf muscles and feet are usually involved, but night cramps can occur in any of the body's large muscles. The neck, back, abdomen and even facial muscles can have these painful spasms. They can occur in the daytime after heavy exercise, or from using the same set of muscles over and over (writer's cramp or cramped hands in factory workers). Tension and stress as well as cold can add to the problem. Women who suffer leg or muscle cramps are usually from one of three categories; they are young, old, or athletes. The cramps are usually caused by one of three things: mineral deficiencies, poor circulation, or athletic exertion and perspiration. Diuretic drugs for high blood pressure or heart dis-ease can cause muscle spasms by depleting potassium, and night cramps are also a feature of pregnancy.

My first discovery of vitamins and minerals was for the severe nightly leg cramps I had in high school. Another girl told me about calcium/magnesium and it solved the problem after only a few days use. Most night cramps are easily preventable or curable with holistic means, so sleep can be peaceful again. This is one dis-ease healed so readily that there is no need to suffer.

Vitamins and Minerals: Here is where leg cramps are most easily and quickly taken care of. Along with a daily multiple vitamin and mineral supplement, a calcium/magnesium tablet is most often the quickest cure. This is particularly so for night cramps suffered by younger women and those who are pregnant. Use a complete calcium/magnesium formula, 1000–2000 mg calcium to half the amount of magnesium. The trace minerals in a complete calcium are needed for assimilation. For leg cramps while standing or walking, usually caused by poor circulation in elders, vitamin E is the answer. Start with 400 IU per day and increase up to 800–1200 IU, adding 100 IU per week. If you have rheumatic heart dis-ease start with 100 IU per day and stop at 400 IU. For women on diuretics, or women who are athletes and perspire excessively, potassium is usually the remedy; take under 100 mg per day. For exertion with excessive perspiration in hot weather, salt loss can occur, but potassium replacement rather than salt is more usually needed. The B-complex vitamins, particularly B-6 and B-3, are essential in writer's-type cramps and toe cramps and for proper circulation. Vitamin D (400 IU daily) is needed for calcium uptake, and vitamin C with bioflavinoids is needed for proper blood flow/ circulation to the muscles. Vitamin A (25,000 IU), zinc (50 mg), hydrochloric acid (HCL), and/or coenzyme Q10 are all helpful. Boron (3 mg per day) significantly increases assimilation of calcium and other minerals, and some complete calciums include it. The major remedies here are calcium/magnesium, vitamin E, B-6 and/or potassium.

Herbs: Horsetail grass adds silicon and helps in assimilation of minerals. Alfalfa is an all-mineral nutrient that helps in assimilation and enhances the effects of other herbs. Raspberry leaf adds calcium and other nutrients. Chaparral is good for leg cramps, and other herbs include cramp bark, oatstraw, comfrey, elderberry, dong quai, ginkgo biloba or saffron. Antispasmodics include scullcap, feverfew, catnip, valerian, peppermint or wild yam.

Naturopathy: To aid the proper assimilation of calcium and other minerals, sip a warm glass of water with a teaspoon of lemon juice, or a teaspoon each of apple cider vinegar and honey in it, with meals or nightly. This supplements hydrochloric acid, and also is an electrolyte balancer for athletes. For athletic mineral depletion, use one of these or fruit or vegetable juices, rather than salt. Potassium is also replaced by eating bananas or oranges. To increase circulation to the calf muscles make this drink: a teaspoon each of cloves, lemon juice and honey, a tablespoon of ginger wine, and a quarter-pint of boiling water. Steep for twenty-four hours, and then take three tablespoonfuls at night before bed.

For another circulation recipe, simmer two teaspoons of ginger powder or fresh grated root in two cups of water until the water turns yellow. Strain and add to a hot bath to soak in for twenty to thirty minutes. Use mustard foot baths three times a week, using a tablespoon of mustard powder in enough water to cover the feet and splash on the calves. Another foot bath or bath can be made with epsom salts. Take two teaspoons of honey at each meal to prevent leg cramps, and use honey instead of sugar; it helps to retain calcium in the body. Kelp tablets add minerals and iodine.

Massage the affected muscles with dandelion oil. Elevate the feet and legs and slap them with open palms to stimulate the circulation. To release leg cramps in progress, straighten your leg and pull your toes and ball of foot toward your knees. For cramps in the feet, get up and walk. Heat will relieve pain, and neuromuscular massage therapy is recommended.

Homeopathy and Cell Salts: When cramp is a part of general tiredness and overexertion, use *Arnica* (and also Arnica gel externally). *Ledum Palustre* is for pains that start in the feet and work upward into the legs. *Calc. carb.* is for cramp with damp, cold feet, and *Colchicum is* for cramps in the soles of the feet. *Nux vomica* is for night cramps, and *Cuprum metallicum* is for severe cramps. *Rhus tox.* is for pain along tendons and muscles, worse for rest, dampness and getting up in the morning, or with loss of strength in forearms or fingers.

Cell Salts: *Mag. phos.* is the primary remedy for contracted muscles, cramps and spasms, often with profuse sweating. *Kali mur.* is for pains increased by motion or felt only in motion, and pains at night made worse by the warmth of the bed. Use *Silica* and *Natrum mur.* together for jerking of limbs in sleep.

Amino Acids: A combination free-form or liver amino acids provides protein, B-vitamins, antioxidant action and tissue regeneration. All of these are important.

Acupressure: Rubbing the fingers over the cramped muscles with a light feathery touch will release the cramp in the gentlest way. To release leg cramps, massage the cords in the backs of the knees. Find the meridian reflexes on the backs of the thighs, halfway between the knees and hips toward the outside; also find sore reflexes on the sides of the calves near the knees, where the two bones of the lower leg meet.

Aromatherapy: Use chamomile, birch, clary sage or ginger in massage oils, compresses or baths.

Flower Essences: Dandelion essence relaxes the muscles and relieves pain, and is used externally and internally. It also releases mental stress that is held in the muscles of the body.

Gemstones and Gem Essences: Use kunzite, amethyst or lapis lazuli gem essence, or the metal copper in essence. Hold or wear amazonite for absorption of calcium and minerals, and to aid bone and muscle function in the body.

Emotional Healing: Cramps are tension, fear and holding on. In the feet they are lack of understanding of oneself and others, and a fear of moving forward in life. In the lower legs they are not wanting to move forward, or fear of the future and what is to come. Upper leg cramps are holding onto old traumas of the past and childhood. Let go of old pain and move forward into new joys. Relax and flow with change, and progress on your life's path.

Acupressure for Leg Cramps

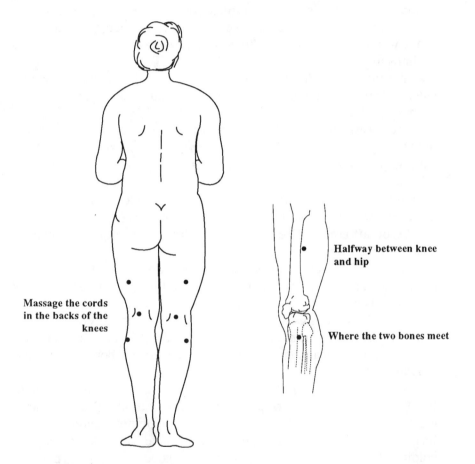

Massage the cords in the backs of the knees

Halfway between knee and hip

Where the two bones meet

Also: rub fingers over the cramped muscle with a light touch.

John Thie, DC, *A Touch for Health, A New Approach to Restoring Our Natural Energies* (Marina del Rey, CA, DeVorss and Co., 1973), p. 118; Iona Marsaa Teeguarden, *Acupressure Way of Health: Jin Shin Do* (New York, Japan Publishing Co., 1978), p. 70-71; Mildred Carter, *Helping Yourself with Foot Reflexology* (W. Nyack, NY, Parker Publishing Co., 1983), p. 160-161.

Liver Cleansing

The liver takes a constant assault from pollutants, heavy metals and chemicals, alcohol and smoking, and medical, street or over-the-counter drugs. It is the organ that filters out toxins, while distributing food through the body. The liver extracts and stores sugars, fats and vitamins, and helps to control blood clotting and produce sex hormones. Bile made by the liver is involved in fat absorption. Early indications of liver congestion are sallow complexion or jaundice, loss of appetite, nausea, vomiting, chronic bowel problems, and spots on the skin. Though the liver is partially self-regenerating, a too-damaged organ cannot support life. The chemicals, poisons, toxins and pollutants that damage the liver surround us daily in ways that no one can fully escape as long as the earth is being polluted and contaminated.

You are exposed to liver damaging toxins if you are exposed to these things or many others: chemicals or paint fumes, pesticides or insecticides, auto exhausts, hair dyes, amalgam dental fillings, canned or frozen foods, deodorants, aluminum or copper cooking pots, aluminum foil, beer or soda in cans, copper water pipes or instant gas hot water heaters, hormone pills, cosmetics, meat, poultry or some fish. If your job requires that you handle these things daily, or many other contaminants and chemicals, you are also in danger. If you smoke, you take into your body a variety of pollutants that are also carcinogens and are particularly poisonous for women. If you use alcohol in excess you are directly damaging the liver, and women are also more susceptible. Many medical, over-the-counter and street drugs contain liver-damaging substances, including artificial sweeteners and acetaminophen (non-aspirin analgesics).

Various contaminants have damaging effects. Lead from auto exhausts may cause everything from intestinal upsets to arthritis, seizures and mental retardation. Lead arsenate is an insecticide used on tobacco. Mercury is found in dental fillings, pesticides, drugs, chemical fertilizers, latex paints and canned fish, and is implicated in birth defects, kidney damage, vomiting, skin eruptions, fatigue and loss of hearing or vision. Aluminum poisoning, from aluminum foil and cookware, beer and soda cans, deodorants and antacids may cause indigestion, skin rashes, brain and motor dysfunction and Alzheimer's dis-ease. Copper toxicity from copper water pipes and heaters, meats (a feed additive), frozen and canned green vegetables (a dye), soft water, copper cooking pots, and hormone pills, can result in mental disorders, anemia, arthritis, hypertension, insomnia, hyperactivity and schizophrenia.[1] We are surrounded by these things everyday, and the effects are cumulative.

For women's health and wellness, occasional liver cleansing is important, and essential if you are exposed to toxins in continuous or concentrated ways. Being aware of and staying away from many toxins is essential, as is eating foods that are as little contaminated as possible. Much of the direction of holistic healing is to establish a lifestyle that reduces pollutants and chemicals through avoiding harmful substances, eating a good diet of unprocessed foods, and using natural methods to decontaminate the body. Naturopaths believe that accumulated toxins are the cause of all body imbalance and dis-ease. The following remedies are suggestions for protecting and cleansing the liver from the pollutants of modern life.

Vitamins and Minerals: Take a multiple vitamin and mineral supplement, particularly one high in B-complex vitamins and containing all the trace minerals. Use a B-complex-50 two or three times a day, and vitamin C with bioflavinoids to bowel tolerance (5000–10,000 mg per day), taken with a calcium/magnesium supplement (1500 mg calcium to 750 mg magnesium per day). Calcium and additional B-complex/B-6 are used with high amounts of vitamin C to prevent kidney stones. High doses of C are essential in hepatitis and chemical poisoning; use calcium and B-complex in fatty liver conditions. Extra lecithin is recommended for chemical poisoning, and B-15 (DMG, dimethyl glycine) helps where there are alcohol cravings. Use 25,000 IU of vitamin A, 400 IU twice daily of vitamin D, and 400–1200 IU daily of vitamin E (with 200 mcg selenium). Vitamins A, E, C and selenium are antioxidants that cleanse the body of toxins and protect against pollutants and primary or secondary cigarette smoke. Additional coenzyme Q10, germanium, or S.O.D. (antioxidants and regenerators) is recommended. Use 30–50 mg per day of zinc, and smokers need B-12 and folic acid.

Herbs: Silymarin, milk thistle extract, is an important antioxidant and tissue regenerator for the liver. This offers high promise in liver cleansing and healing, and for hepatitis and gallstones. Dandelion with alfalfa, and dandelion with kelp tablets, are other herbs of choice for liver cleansing. Use chamomile and/or scullcap when detoxing from alcohol or drugs. Other liver herbs include raspberry leaves, peppermint, strawberry leaves, yellow dock, yarrow, sage, hyssop, rosemary, blue flag, clover, devil's claw or marjoram. Use agrimony, balmony and centaury together

[1]Dr. Ross Trattler, *Better Health Through Natural Healing* (New York: McGraw-Hill Book Co., 1985), p. 329–334.

in a strong infusion, taking two tablespoonfuls two or three times daily. Parsley tea clears liver obstructions, and raspberry or strawberry clears liver congestion. Gentian root and black radish root together stimulate the liver and improve appetite and digestion. Agrimony is helpful with jaundice. Add small amounts of goldenseal to it if there is nausea. The primary herbs are silymarin (milk thistle), and dandelion with alfalfa or kelp.

Naturopathy: Eliminating toxins must be done slowly to not over-tax the body. Follow a three-day apple or citrus mono diet with a raw foods diet that uses cooked beans for protein. Avoid all harmful substances and stop smoking and alcohol. Drink pure apple juice freely, or carrot juice, and a glass of beet juice in the morning once every several days sipped slowly. If detoxing results in skin itching, drink a glass of hot water with the juice of half a lemon in it first thing in the morning. Here is a five-day liver cleansing fast; take no other foods or drinks except water:

Day One:	10 ounces carrot juice, 3 ounces beet juice, and 3 ounces cucumber juice.
Day Two:	10 ounces carrot juice, and 10 ounces spinach juice.
Day Three:	16 ounces carrot juice.
Day Four:	2 ounces coconut juice, 3 ounces beet juice, and 11 ounces of carrot juice.
Day Five:	2 ounces celery juice, 2 ounces parsley juice, and 9 ounces carrot juice.[2]

Use chlorophyll enemas to speed the process. Chlorophyll as a supplement helps to eliminate toxic metals, as does pectin. Kyolic is another powerful detoxifier. Use bran to avoid constipation; drink lots of water, preferably distilled. Aloe vera gel with milk stimulates a sluggish liver and increases bile secretion. Try cleansing baths of a cup of sea salt and a cup of baking soda to a hot tub of water. Cover your body in the water as completely as possible and remain there for twenty-five to thirty minutes. You may feel a period of nausea about half-way, which will lift by the end—stay in the water for the full time. Pat dry then, and go to bed to sweat for an hour or two; you will feel drained for awhile. Do this no more often than every ten days. Try castor oil packs nightly across the abdomen/liver area, for another suggestion.

[2]Mildred Jackson, ND, and Terri Teague, ND, DC, *The Handbook of Alternatives to Chemical Medicine* (Berkeley, CA, Bookpeople, 1975), p. 98.

Homeopathy and Cell Salts: *Podophyllum* is the remedy when the woman is pale, vomits bile, and has constipation with light-colored stools. *Mercurius* is used for upper digestive tract symptoms; the tongue is coated dirty yellow and is swollen, gums are swollen and bleed easily, the liver is tender and swollen and lying on the right side is painful. Stools are light gray or yellow-green, the skin and eyes are yellowed, and there is clammy perspiration. Use *Nux vomica* for liver detox after heavy alcohol or drug use, or when stopping smoking; take it every three or four hours. Use *Chelidonium* when there is tenderness and pain in the liver region that moves to the right shoulder. *China* is used when there is heaviness or fullness in the abdomen, especially after eating. There is bitter, frequent burping, or the burping tastes like the last meal. The liver is sensitive to touch, and there are cravings for cold drinks, coffee or sweets. *Nux* and *Podophyllum* together are used for bilious conditions with dizzy spells, appetite loss, and yellow-coated tongue.

Cell Salts: *Natrum sulph.* is for biliousness and liver conditions of all types.

Amino Acids: Free-form amino acids (combination) are essential for detoxifying and cleansing the liver. Single aminos are those with sulfur action: lysine, cystine, methionine, taken on an empty stomach with juice (not milk).

Acupressure: Do foot or hand acupressure, starting very lightly and only for a few minutes at first. If there is no severe detoxing reaction by the next day, increase the time. Work for only a few minutes twice a week at first, very gradually increasing time and frequency to minimize the detox reactions. Pay special attention to the liver, gall bladder, stomach, pancreas, kidneys, adrenals, spleen and lungs, and the pituitary gland in the pads of the big toes or thumbs. The liver is on the right side and these reflexes will be sore and tender; do not try to release it all at once. The webs between thumbs and first fingers, between big toe and second toe, and meridian points on the thighs are eliminating points. There will be a release of toxins, and you may feel the reaction, so take it very slowly at first.

Aromatherapy: Use in compresses, baths or massage oils: chamomile (any variety), everlasting, lemon, lemon verbena, lime, yarrow or fennel.

Flower Essences: Spruce detoxifies the liver from pollutants and contaminants; lotus is for toxicities and all-healing but is best used with other remedies. Dandelion or ginseng strengthen and regenerate the liver, and eucalyptus is for liver inflammation.

Acupressure for Liver Cleansing

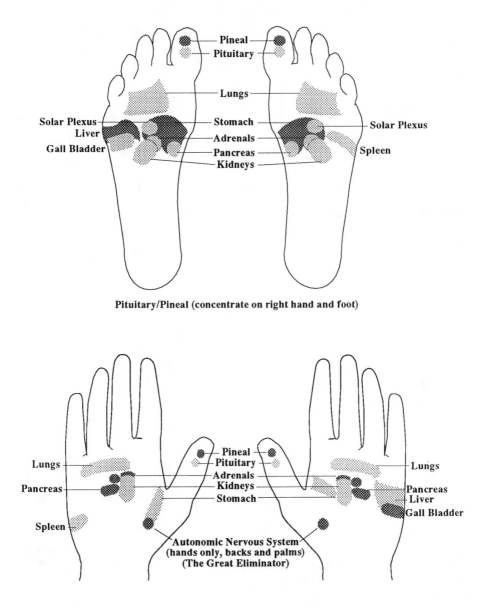

Pituitary/Pineal (concentrate on right hand and foot)

Michael Van Straten, ND, DO, *The Complete Natural Health Consultant* (New York, Prentice-Hall Publishers, 1987), p.194; Mildred Carter, *Body Reflexology* (W. Nyack, NY, Parker Publishing Co., 1983), p. 153-155.

Acupressure for Liver Cleansing

For Toxicity
(physical or
emotional)

For Toxicity

The Great Eliminator (webs between
thumbs and first·fingers)

Webs between
big toes and
second toes

Iona Marsaa Teeguarden, *Acupressure Way of Health: Jin Shin Do* (New York, Japan Publishing Co., 1978), p. 71; Mildred Carter, *Body Reflexology* (W. Nyack, NY, Parker Publishing Co., 1983), p. 153-154; Michael Van Straten, ND, DO, *The Complete Natural Health Consultant* (New York, Prentice-Hall Publishers, 1987), p. 194.

Gemstones and Gem Essences: Any of the following in essence are for detoxifying and the liver: moss agate, azurite-malachite, beryl, calcite, eilat stone, fluorite, diamond, herkimer diamond, ivory, lapis, sugulite, peridot, malachite, moonstone, nephrite, citrine, blue quartz, sapphire, tourmaline quartz, pink tourmaline or turquoise. Hold or wear a natural citrine, topaz or turquoise but clear it often.

Emotional Healing: The liver is the place where anger and primitive emotions are held. Detoxify these from your body and Be-ing; it's time to heal old pain and release the anger and hurt. Do uncording rituals and work on forgiveness (see *Casting the Circle, A Woman's Book of Ritual*, Diane Stein, The Crossing Press, 1990).

Menopause

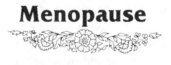

In many nonpatriarchal cultures, menopause is the beginning of a woman's life as a leader of the community. Native American elders of many tribes were (and are) women after menopause, and the Delphic Oracle of Greece could only be a woman over fifty. In Asia, menopause is simply another seven-year cycle of life, one to respect and honor with all of the other cycles. The change of life relieves women from the burdens of childbearing and childraising, freeing her for her own pursuits and service to the community or tribe. Male modern culture degrades the menopausal and postmenopausal woman because it is afraid of her power—or perhaps her realization of it. From that patriarchal degradation comes everything from mother-in-law jokes to estrogen replacement therapy, routine hysterectomies, and the relegating of older women to poverty and obscurity.

The lack of valuation by male culture for older/wiser women has brought about the mutilation of women's bodies in many senseless ways. One in six women over forty-five has her uterus removed. Mastectomies are done less often but are still happening. The insistence on treating women's natural change of life as a dis-ease process has brought about estrogen replacement, which has increased cancer of the uterus and breast from five to twelve times.[1] Estrogen also causes water retention, increases the severity of asthma, heart dis-ease, kidney stones, epilepsy and migraines, and the incidence of strokes. Many of the emotional side effects of menopause are a result of medical drugs and interventions, and no less of patriarchal attitudes toward women. Women reclaiming menopause as a natural process (it is not a dis-ease) are reclaiming women's lives and power. Many women go through menopause in complete comfort (if they do it without the medical system's "help"). Holistic remedies are effective and safe for those who need them.

Vitamins and Minerals: A multiple vitamin and mineral supplement is important for normal hormone function. With it use a B-complex-50 to -100 up to three times a day. You may also need additional B-6 (up to 50 mg three times a day), B-5 (100–500 mg two or three times a day) and/or PABA for adrenal function and stress. B-6 decreases water retention and menopause symptoms, with more needed if you are taking estrogen. B-5 aids adrenal function; estrogen production is shifted from the ovaries to the adrenals at menopause. Vitamin E, along with the B-complex, is the remedy of choice for hot flashes and all menopause symptoms including emotional symptoms. Use it topically for vaginal dryness, and internally start with 400 IU per day, increasing by 100 IU weekly to 800–1600 IU, divided into several doses a day. Stop at the dose that ends the hot flashes. If you have rheumatic heart dis-ease, you are limited to 400 IU per day; if you are on estrogen, you need the higher amounts. A vitamin E with selenium (200 mcg) is recommended. Also for hot flashes, use vitamin C (from 3000 mg per day up to bowel tolerance).

Calcium/magnesium (up to 2000 mg calcium/1000 mg magnesium) helps emotional symptoms and is essential to prevent bone loss. (If this is a problem, add 3 mg of boron; see the section on Osteoporosis.) If you have cervical dysplasia (suspicious Pap smear, too often leading to hysterectomy), B-vitamins including B-6 and folic acid, vitamin E with selenium, vitamin A as beta-carotene (25,000 IU per day), and vitamin D (400 IU) may be enough to change the condition within three or four months for up to seventy percent of women. Also look for low-grade cervical infections in this case. Essential fatty acids (evening primrose oil, black currant oil) act as a sedative and diuretic and aid hot flashes; these are important for estrogen production. Germanium will also help menopause symptoms; use 60 mg twice daily. Insert acidophilus capsules into the vagina at night to help prevent vaginal infections. Enzymes with hydrochloric acid (HCL) help digestion. Primary here are the B-complex, E, calcium/magnesium, and essential fatty acids.

[1]Dr. Ross Trattler, *Better Health Through Natural Healing* (New York, McGraw-Hill Book Co., 1985), p. 435.

Herbs: Dong quai is the women's ginseng, and a Chinese herb that is primary in treating menopause symptoms, including hot flashes. Try it in tablets (which can be made into a tasty tea) or tinctures (a few drops under the tongue will stop a hot flash in progress). It adds energy, lowers high blood pressure, is slightly laxative, and treats profuse menses and vaginal dryness. It is an estrogen precursor (balancer) but is not an estrogen itself. Some women, however, have difficulty in taking dong quai. They experience nervousness like an exaggerated PMS. If this is the case for you, stop it and switch to black cohosh, which does similar things but is a progesterone precursor. For many women, dong quai is the answer, but for most women that cannot use it, black cohosh is. Black cohosh helps to lower blood pressure as well, and is an aid to hypoglycemia, which can be aggravated in menopause. Women with hypoglycemia seem to have more menopause symptoms.

In other herb choices, some women respond well to Siberian ginseng, though it is not considered a women's herb. False unicorn root, licorice root, damiana, mistletoe, gotu kola, motherwort, sage, passion flower, lady's slipper, chastetree (vitex), oats, and squaw vine are other menopause herbs. Use raspberry, lime blossom and pulsatilla together as a relaxant. Use angelica, false unicorn, dong quai, wild yam or licorice root for estrogen, but licorice raises blood pressure. Sarsaparilla is a progesterone precursor, popular in England and helpful to many women. Lady's slipper is for anxiety and insomnia, false unicorn helps menopause depression, and passion flower calms the mind and body and is listed by some sources as the herb of choice for anxiety, insomnia, depression and migraines. Shepherd's purse or nettles, especially if used with alfalfa, help heavy menstruation and breakthrough bleeding, and are good sources of vitamin K. Motherwort helps early menopause symptoms, erratic menstrual cycles, heavy or clotted flows, irritability and hot flashes. If you are coming off estrogen replacement therapy, this is also the herb of choice.

For cervical dysplasia, make vaginal suppositories of chaparral and melted cocoa butter. Also use dong quai for hormone balancing, and red clover, dandelion root and/or burdock for blood and liver cleansing. Drink a pint daily of an infusion made from red clover and blue violet leaf (an ounce of each to a pint of water) for cervical dysplasia, breast lumps, or uterine or ovarian cysts. For cervical dysplasia or ovarian cysts try this recipe. In a quart of water, boil the following herbs for ten minutes, then simmer for half an hour and strain: an ounce each of raspberry leaves, black currant leaves, witchhazel leaves and powdered myrrh. Mix a quarter of a pint of this with a pint of cooled boiled water and use as a nightly douche. With this take internally a tablespoonful three times daily of the following in decoction: one ounce each of dandelion root, comfrey, yellow dock, yarrow and two ounces of licorice root.[2] Keep the bowels moving with senna.

Naturopathy: Dairy products, meat and poultry (estrogen in the feed leaves residues passed on to women who use meat/dairy products) and sugar are the cause of most hot flashes. Cutting down on protein eases heavy bleeding. Use a diet of primarily raw whole foods, grains, seeds and nuts, miso, blackstrap molasses, broccoli, salmon, sardines, yoghurt, kefir or buttermilk, kelp, chlorophyll or seaweed. Fasts or colonics are not recommended in most cases. Eliminate caffeine and alcohol from the diet, and stop smoking. Women who smoke face higher risks of osteoporosis, and cancer of lungs, cervix and uterus after menopause. They reach menopause earlier from toxic effects to the ovaries. If you are hypoglycemic, see that section for diet.

Bee pollen (500 mg, three tablets) per day reduces nervousness and hot flashes for many women. Try it initially for a week, to see if it works for you, or try royal jelly or propolis. Many women's menopause symptoms originate from hypothyroidism. Atomidine or Edgar Cayce's 636, or two to four kelp tablets per day stimulate the thyroid. Also try raw thyroid glandular, or a combination multi-glandular extract for hormone balancing. Single glandulars, besides thyroid, include pituitary, adrenal and ovarian. Lecithin is important for some women, or brewer's yeast for the B-complex vitamins. Cucumbers or licorice stimulate estrogen production and are good for low blood sugar, but licorice also raises blood pressure. For excessive menstrual bleeding during menopause, mix an ounce of grated nutmeg in a pint of Jamaican rum and take a teaspoonful three times a day during the flow. Eat parsley or drink parsley tea for water retention. For uterine, fallopian tube or ovarian cysts or tumors use castor oil packs nightly.

Homeopathy and Cell Salts: *Ignatia* used two or three times a day is the remedy for hot flashes and constipation, or use *Lachesis* for mental irritation and hot flashes that are worse in the morning. *Pulsatilla* is for hot flashes that leave a woman sleepless at night, and for menopause changing temperaments. *Veratrum viride* controls hot flashes. *Sepia* is the remedy for the woman who resents her lack of health and holds other resentments; she feels emotionally burnt out and physically cold, is tired, irritable, and may have chronic constipation. She feels a dragging sensation internally. *Fabiana imbricata* is for sudden sweating, and *Valeriana* for insomnia and irritability.

Cell Salts: For hot flashes, take five tablets of each hourly until the condition improves, then use twice a day: *Kali sulph.*, *Kali phos.*, and *Ferrum*

[2]Richard Lucas, *Common and Uncommon Uses of Herbs for Healthful Living* (New York, Arc Books, 1969) p. 13.

phos. For nervousness and emotional symptoms use the following as above: *Kali phos*. with *Natrum mur*. *Natrum mur*. alone is for fiercely independent women who are hypoglycemic or have adrenal exhaustion, hyperthyroidism or anorexia. They harbor anger, grief and sometimes long-term grudges, have profuse vaginal discharges, and may have headaches near their periods.

Amino Acids: L-arginine (500 mg twice daily) and lysine (500 mg per day) taken on an empty stomach detoxify the liver and aid liver function. These are important in reducing menopause symptoms.

Acupressure: Massage the hand or foot reflexes for the pituitary and ovaries to help hormone production and reduce hot flashes. Foot or hand acupressure for menopause includes these points, plus the reflexes for the thyroid, parathyroids, adrenals, uterus and sex hormones. Meridian points on the back of the hands below the third (ring) finger, the ankle on the big toe side of the feet, at the little toe and top of feet relieve hot flashes. (See illustrations.) For prolonged or profuse menstruation, press the insides of both legs, five inches below the knees, at the same time. This will stop bleeding anywhere in the body within minutes.

Aromatherapy: Use essential oils in baths, compresses, massage oils or diffusers: chamomile, geranium, jasmine, lavender, mugwort, sage or ylang ylang. Use sage to ease tension and balance hormones, and thyme to ease insomnia and improve circulation. Add to baths any of these combinations, three drops of each oil: basil and cypress, thyme or rosemary, or rosemary and basil. Or make a massage oil of three drops of each of the following in an eggcup of vegetable oil: thyme, rosemary, basil and cypress. Chamomile and lavender are relaxants and nervines. For hot flashes take internally two drops of chamomile per day on brown sugar cubes; for depression take one drop each of cypress and fennel.

Flower Essences: Pomegranate is the universal women's remedy for all the stages of women's lives. Use henna for change-of-life identity crisis, or mallow for fear of aging, stress and as a pituitary and endocrine tonic. Use spruce for cervical dysplasia or precancerous states of the breasts or reproductive organs.

Gemstones and Gem Essences: Use the metal gold in essence for hot flashes, or kunzite for hormone balancing. For cervical dysplasia try in essence azurite-malachite, beryl, herkimer diamond, lapis lazuli, moonstone, or blue or pink tourmaline. Wear or hold garnet, moonstone, blue tourmaline, kunzite or pink tourmaline in menopause.

Emotional Healing: There is a fear of no longer being wanted or needed, a fear of aging and a fear of not being good enough. This is the trip that has been laid on women in the patriarchy. Remember that feminist values are very different; there is an honoring of age, wisdom and

Acupressure for Menopause

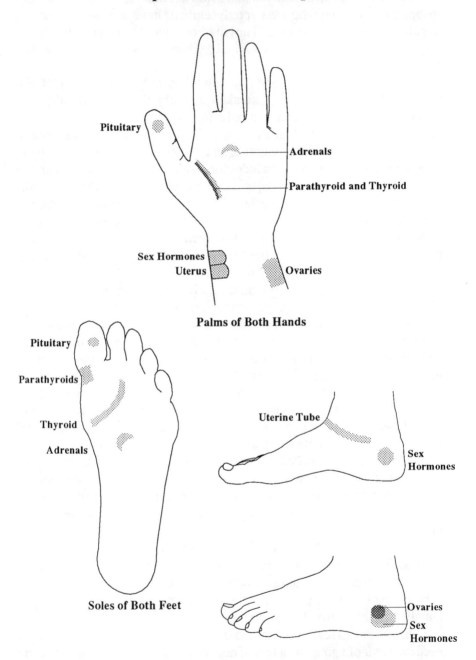

Pituitary

Adrenals

Parathyroid and Thyroid

Sex Hormones
Uterus

Ovaries

Palms of Both Hands

Pituitary

Parathyroids

Thyroid

Adrenals

Uterine Tube

Sex
Hormones

Soles of Both Feet

Ovaries
Sex
Hormones

Moshe Olshevsky, CA, PhD., *et. al.*, *The Manual of Natural Therapy* (New York, Citadel Press, 1989), p. 235.

Acupressure for Menopause
Hot Flash Relief

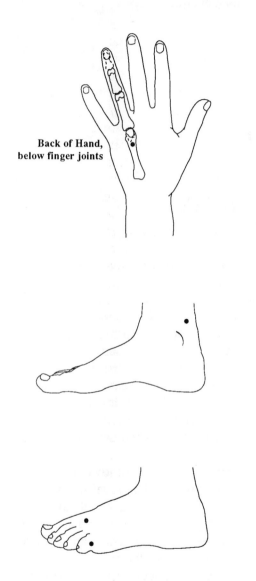

Back of Hand,
below finger joints

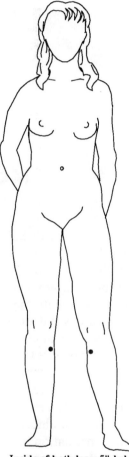

Inside of both legs, 5" below
knees to stop heavy menstrual
bleeding

Cathryn Bauer, *Acupressure for Women* (Freedom, CA, The Crossing Press, 1987), p.115; Mildred Jackson, ND and Terri Teague, ND, DC, *The Handbook of Alternatives to Chemical Medicine* (Berkeley, CA, Bookpeople, 1975), p.74.

experience and a welcoming into the circle of Crones. How long have you waited to join the circle of the wise, to be an elder, a woman respected for her knowledge and abilities to lead? Now is the time, make the best use of it and enjoy it. The time of the Crone is the time of women's greatest power. You are needed now more than ever before.

Menstruation

It is only with Women's Spirituality and the honoring of women's bodies and cycles that menstruation has changed from "the curse" to the pride of modern women's Be-ing. Women bleed and do not die. Women bleed and new life is birthed. Women bleed and learn the power and beauty of being female and living with the cycles of the moon and earth. Five thousand years of patriarchy and misogynist patriarchal religions and attitudes have made women's bleeding and ability to give birth (as well as the ending of bleeding in menopause) something shameful. Women have been told that they (and their blood or because of it) are "dirty," "vessels of sin," and are not to be acknowledged in public. The verdict is changing, as women refuse the propaganda and take back their power. There would be no life without us and our ability to bleed.

Yet, menstruation for many women is not a time of joy but a time of tension and discomfort. Part of this is still from old attitudes that women have been ingrained with, and old attitudes die hard. Much of it, however, is very physical and very much caused by living in a patriarchal culture that degrades women and the earth. Few women today are able to withdraw from activity and give their bleeding time the space of quiet and peace-within that it needs. Most women live under extreme stress and tension—a byproduct of modern living and also of women's place in the patriarchy. Many women are on the contraceptive pill that wreaks havoc with normal hormones by convincing the body that it is pregnant. Most women are meat-eaters and today's meat and poultry is loaded with hormone residues that may be responsible for breast cancer, endometriosis, fibroid tumors and other dis-eases. Many women smoke cigarettes, which are a clear and present danger to women's lives. (Women who smoke are less fertile, have more difficult pregnancies and higher risk babies. Women who smoke reach menopause earlier, and are at a much increased risk for osteoporosis and cancers of the lungs, breast, cervix and uterus.) All women in industrialized America eat food that is polluted with chemicals, pesticides and drugs, and breathe air and drink water that are polluted as well. Heavy metal poisoning is a cause of PMS, along with low thyroid function, candida albicans, food allergies, high fat diets, over-estrogen, hypoglycemia, poor spinal or body mechanics, poor food absorption and vitamin deficiencies. All these things affect women's health and menstruation, and only some of them are avoidable.

Medical drugs for menstruation difficulties add more toxins and hormones to an already imbalanced mix. They worsen symptoms or have side effects that are worse than the symptoms, without touching causes. Too many women have been placed on tranquilizers for PMS, and too many hysterectomies are unnecessary. Holistic healing reaches the causes of menstrual distress while working with instead of against women's bodies. Along with the many remedy choices described below, try acupuncture or spinal manipulation instead of drugs or surgeries. They can make all the difference.

Vitamins and Minerals: Overall nutrition is important; use a quality multiple vitamin and mineral supplement, not something cheap from the supermarket. Add to it a complete calcium/magnesium tablet (General Nutrition's Calcium Plus is good) that contains 1000–2000 mg of calcium and half that amount of magnesium. This can be taken divided into three or four doses a day (including one at bedtime), and taken with water, or sipped with water that has a teaspoon of apple cider vinegar in it for absorption. It can also be taken hourly for acute cramps and pain, with B-6. For some women, this is enough to stop PMS and cramping. To go further, take a B-complex-50 to -100 three times a day. This is especially important for women on the pill or who are smokers. Women on the pill and women who have tension, bloating, premenstrual acne or anxiety need extra B-6 (50–400 mg per day). Vitamins B-5 and B-12 are stress and fatigue reducers, and folic acid (25–50 mg per day)[1] is important for women with suspicious Pap smears (see Menopause section). Use 1000-3000 mg of vitamin C with bioflavinoids or go to bowel tolerance to reduce heavy flows, and 400 IU per day of vitamin D (total) for calcium

---

[1] It may take a doctor's perscription to get this high amount, but it is being used by Atkin's Clinic in New York and by Dr. Ross Trattler, *Better Health Through Natural Healing* (New York, McGraw-Hill Book Co., 1985, p. 442),.with success for cervical dysplasia.

absorption. Chocolate, sugar or salt cravings are deficiencies of calcium, magnesium or zinc.

If you have breast tenderness, smoke or are on the pill, you also need 400–800 IU per day of vitamin E and 25,000 IU per day of beta-carotene/ vitamin A. Selenium with E helps women who are entering menopause. If you have heavy flows you may need vitamin K (usually supplemented in foods and herbs), and/or iron (25–50 mg per day of hydrolized protein chelate or Floradix). For menstrual related headaches and to balance hormones, try essential fatty acids as evening primrose or black currant oil. Lecithin, manganese or chromium (for hypoglycemia) and raw glandulars— thyroid, adrenal or pituitary—can also help hormone balance. Take vitamins and minerals daily, not just while menstruating, but increase the amounts of calcium/magnesium and B-complex in the last three to eight days before the flow starts, with smaller amounts the rest of the month.

Herbs: If dong quai agrees with you, it can be the answer to PMS, cramping, bloating, vaginal dryness, fibroids, heavy bleeding, irregular cycles, and depression. Try it in tablets or tinctures and start slowly; stop if it increases the symptoms. This is the herb of choice for many women; see more about it under Menopause. Black cohosh is useful for ovarian cramps and pain, and for women who are hypoglycemic or near menopause. Try blue cohosh, or raspberry leaf with chamomile in a warm tea for PMS and cramping; raspberry also reduces flow. Motherwort is a menstrual balancer both for lack of periods (amenorrhea) and for premenopausal women, and also helps pelvic inflammation when combined with echinacea or goldenseal. Use cramp bark, wild yam, blue cohosh or squaw vine for difficult periods; squaw vine is especially good at menarche. For heavy or painful periods try cramp bark, red raspberry, strawberry leaf, white oak bark or witchhazel (astringent and for pain). Sarsaparilla is a hormone balancer; accusations of its being a carcinogen have proved to be unfounded.

For pain or tension take a half teaspoonful of valerian tincture (or scullcap, hops, passion flower, feverfew or cramp bark). Raspberry leaf is good for pregnancy, and use false unicorn root to prevent a threatened miscarriage. Shepherd's purse and nettles are sources of vitamin K and help heavy bleeding or hemorrhaging. They are also used after childbirth. To bring on menses, use basil, catnip, angelica, parsley, black cohosh, rosemary, ginger or pennyroyal; do not use pennyroyal for longer than three days and do not use the oil. Siberian ginseng is used for PMS and for menopause, but is not for hypoglycemics; dong quai is more recommended. Motherwort, raspberry leaf, dong quai, wild yam, rosemary, black cohosh and blue cohosh regulate cycles; use blue cohosh for most women under forty, black cohosh for over forty. For nausea with periods use peppermint, or peppermint with chamomile in teas. Pennyroyal increases blood flow, as does blazing star, feverfew, squaw vine or tansy. Parsley, nettles or blue cohosh reduce water retention.

Naturopathy: Use the diet outlined under Hypoglycemia, with high fiber, low fat and adequate protein (mostly from vegetable sources). Eat vegetables, fruit and whole grains, prevent constipation, and use stevia (herbal sweetener) instead of sugar. Reduce or eliminate salt, caffeine, sugar, meat or poultry (unless organic), dairy products, junkfoods, foods with additives and chemicals, and smoking. Eat foods high in calcium and iodine—beans and leafy greens, alfalfa, spirulina and kelp. Drink lots of water.

Bromelin, pineapple enzyme, will help cramps; take two capsules a day between meals for three days before the period. For thyroid function add iodine to the diet as kelp tablets (four–six per day), Atomidine or 636; if you develop a metallic taste in your mouth you are using too much. Alfalfa provides calcium and minerals, and enhances the assimilation of other herbs and vitamins. Chlorophyll, spirulina, or wheatgrass drinks are also positive. One source lists Kyolic (odorless garlic) as a remedy for PMS, and it is also important for ridding the body of candida albicans.

Beet juice will bring on menses. For heavy flows drink the juice of half a lemon in a cup of water twice a day, an hour before breakfast and an hour before dinner. Other choices are 1/8 teaspoon of cayenne in a cup of warm water, or one ounce grated nutmeg in a pint of Jamaican rum; take a teaspoonful three times a day during periods. Bee pollen or propolis are hormone balancers for menstruation and menopause, and help to regulate cycles. For endometriosis or uterine, ovarian or fallopian fibroids or tumors, use castor oil packs nightly. For cramps, apply alternating hot and cold (water) packs to the abdominal area and lower back. Or use ice over the uterus, pubic and sacral regions for heavy bleeding or pain, while applying hot compresses to the legs and feet at the same time. For PMS try herbal agnus castus pills.

Homeopathy and Cell Salts: Use *Nux vomica* for menstrual nerves and tension, when overly sensitive to noise, light or music. Try *Chamomila* when there is irritability, criticalness or anger with severe menstrual cramps that feel like labor pains. Use *Pulsatilla* for depression, moodiness and tears but less anger; there may be cutting pain, dizziness, faintness, chilliness, nausea, vomiting, back pain, diarrhea or headaches, and flow may be late. Use also at menarche for late-starters. If symptoms cease as soon as flow begins, the remedy is *Lachesis*. For painful breasts before and during periods try *Conium maculatum*, or *Lac caninum* when breasts feel full and painful and there is dizziness, irritability, and rage.

Calcarea carbonica is for early, profuse and long lasting menstruation with bearing-down pains. *Urtica urens* is for heavy and prolonged flows. Use *Sabina* for early and too copious flows with bright or dark red clots. For painful menstruation with severe spasmodic pains try *Caulophyllum*, or *Cocculus* for crampy pains, or *Gelsemium* for painful menstruation with headaches. Use *Cimicifuga* for labor-like painful periods with nervousness, restlessness or melancholy and for menopause with restlessness and insomnia; pains seem to move from side to side. *Belladonna* is for cutting pains; the woman is red-faced and congested and her blood feels hot; motion worsens it. Use *Colocynthis* for anger and irritability with relief from curling up and pressing into the abdomen; there may be a lack of periods after anger. Use *Hamamelis* for bleeding midway between periods.

Cell Salts: *Mag phos.* is used when cramping is relieved by warmth and by pressure when bending forward. These are colicky pains helped by curling up with a hot water bottle. *Natrum mur.* is for lack of periods from grief or emotional upset. For heavy pain try *Calc. phos.*; use *Ferrum phos.* if the face is flushed and red and there is nausea or vomiting with menstruation; or use *Kali phos.* if you are anemic or pale with pain and pale menses. The following combination can be taken twice a day: *Mag. phos.*, *Ferrum phos.*, *Kali phos.*, *Natrum mur.* and *Silica* for premenstrual tension and difficult periods. Try Calmes Forte for tension and stress.

Amino Acids: Tryptophan is a calmative and muscle relaxant and will be available again eventually. If you have hypoglycemia or herpes, use 500 mg of lysine starting five days before periods. L-tyrosine (500 mg twice daily) helps with anxiety, depression and premenstrual or menstrual-related headaches. A combination free-form or liver-extract amino acids is recommended for its value as a mood and hormone balancer, calmative, detoxificant, and nutrient.

Acupressure: See the foot reflexology points for Menopause, and the pressure point to stop or slow hemorrhaging or excessive bleeding (illustrated). Meridian points in the webs between thumbs and first fingers will help to bring on menses, as will reflexes in the tongue. Using a tongue depressor or spoon handle, press the tongue as far back as you can without gagging in a firm steady pressure. Hold for two or three minutes, then move the pressure first to one side, then the other side of the back of tongue position. To relieve menstrual pain, do the same thing, holding the spoon or tongue depressor about two-thirds of the way back. Use pressure on the thumbs and first two fingers as well. For body acupressure meridians for emotional symptoms, and for menstrual pain and indigestion, see the illustrations from Cathryn Bauer's *Acupressure for Women*. The tongue information is from Mildred Carter.

Acupressure for Premenstrual Emotions

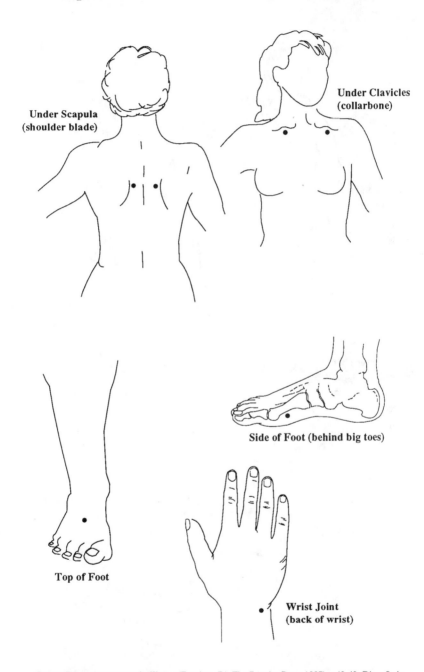

Under Scapula (shoulder blade)

Under Clavicles (collarbone)

Side of Foot (behind big toes)

Top of Foot

Wrist Joint (back of wrist)

Cathryn Bauer, *Acupressure for Women* (Freedom, CA, The Crossing Press, 1987), p.48-49; Diane Stein, *All Women Are Healers* (Freedom, CA, The Crossing Press, 1990), p. 97.

Acupressure for Menstrual Pain and Indigestion

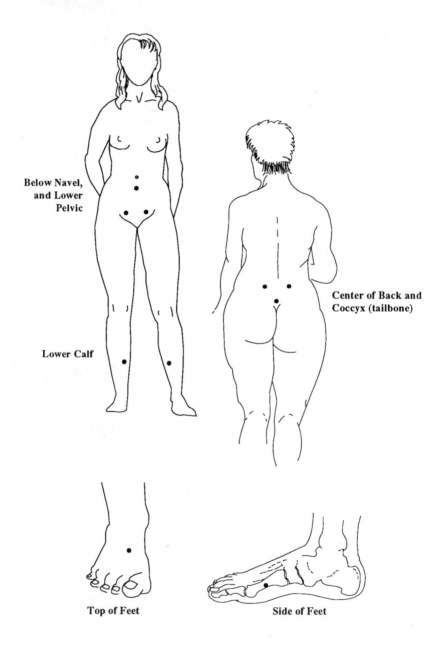

Below Navel, and Lower Pelvic

Center of Back and Coccyx (tailbone)

Lower Calf

Top of Feet

Side of Feet

Cathryn Bauer, *Acupressure for Women* (Freedom, CA, The Crossing Press, 1987), p.58-60; Diane Stein, *All Women Are Healers* (Freedom, CA, The Crossing Press, 1990), p. 96.

Acupressure for Heavy Menstruation

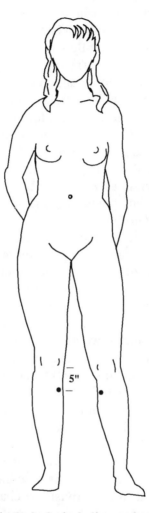

To stop bleeding anywhere in the body, including profuse menstrual bleeding, press both legs on the inside of the leg, five inches below knees and hold for several minutes or until bleeding stops. This is not to be used to stop your periods, but to control hemorrhaging and excessive flows.

Mildred Jackson, ND and Terri Teague, ND, DC, *The Handbook of Alternatives to Chemical Medicine* (Berkeley, CA, Bookpeople, 1975), p.74 and 130.

Aromatherapy: For PMS symptoms, use two drops each of the following in a daily bath while the symptoms occur: chamomile, rosemary, lavender and four drops of lemon. For heavy periods or abnormal bleeding make a massage oil of the following to use on the lower areas of the body: two drops each of cinnamon, juniper, pine, and geranium and five drops of cypress in a vegetable oil base. A massage oil for menstrual pain and discomfort includes the following: two drops of chamomile, five drops of parsley, and a drop of tarragon in an eggcup of vegetable oil. Essential oils to bring on menses and encourage flow include: basil, chamomile, clary sage, hyssop, juniper, lavender, marjoram, myrrh, rose or rosemary. Use chamomile, melissa, lavender, rose or jasmine for premenstrual emotions. Tiferet-Lifetree has a Moontime combination to regulate cycles and reduce heavy bleeding.

Flower Essences: Pomegranate is the universal essence for all women's issues. Use squash as a hormone balancer, and mallow for the emotions of menarche. For pregnancy and fertility, try blackberry or watermelon, and fig for birthing.

Gemstones and Gem Essences: Gem essences for menstruation include beryl, coral, jade, kunzite or pink tourmaline. Hold or wear the following: for PMS, kunzite; for water retention, jade; for cramps and PMS, chrysocolla or turquoise; for menstrual cycle balancing, moonstone; or to bring on menses, garnet.

Emotional Healing: Women who have severe cramps often have sexual abuse in their herstories; women with difficult periods in any way have difficulty with living in a political system that oppresses women. What to do about it? Do moontime rituals that validate you and your body. Do the Self-Blessing on each night of your period, and wear a red gemstone or red underpants or clothing to mark the days as special. Learn the phases of the moon and how your body flows with them, and explore living with that flow. Whatever you do that is woman-affirming at this time, and all the time, will help. Learn to love yourself, and your body and most women's cramps disappear. It is also healthy to get angry at injustices to women, and to do activism to change them. If you were incested or abused, relearn your body as a part of your Be-ing; the hurt is over; release the pain and turn to joy.

Migraines

Seventy percent of the people who get migraines are women, and I have seen migraines in girls as young as seven years old. Most women's migraines end at menopause—a reason to look forward to growing older. Food sensitivities are the source of twenty-five percent of migraines. Other causes include: hypoglycemia, hormone imbalances (too much estrogen, as opposed to progesterone), stress, constipation and digestive disorders, liver malfunction, oral contraceptives, spinal or jaw misalignment, poor circulation, arthritis in the neck and upper spine, sinusitis, environmental toxins, eye strain, abnormal levels of some brain chemicals, PMS, or muscular contraction and tension. High blood pressure, fluid retention, or head or neck injury can cause migraines, as can flickering bright lights, not eating and certain foods. Tyramine-containing foods are most often the source of migraine food allergies and these are: cheese, chocolate, citrus, red wines and coffee. Lesser causes are avocados, plums, alcohol, bananas or raspberries. Different women will have different sensitivities, which can also include gluten, corn, tomatoes, milk products or food additives (especially nitrites and MSG).

A migraine is not a simple headache. It begins at the back of the head and moves to above or behind one eye or one side of the head. There may be nausea, vomiting, blurred vision, diarrhea, tingling and numb limbs, and some women experience periods of paralysis, blackout or seizures. Some migraines are preceded by the migraine aura, involving disturbed vision or speech, weakness, sensory aberrations, flashing lights in front of the eyes, or objects appearing like photographic negatives. This is a disease of the circulatory system, where the blood vessels of the head first expand and then contract abnormally. I have suffered from severe migraines for ten years and have learned to stop most of them at the beginning of the cycle with holistic methods. Use the following remedies at the first sign or aura of beginning migraine, and use them along with regular chiropractic, osteopathic, acupuncture or neuromuscular massage. Do nightly meditation to reduce stress, avoid allergic foods and avoid constipation. Holistic methods are more effective, in my experience, than medical drugs and they have no side effects.

Vitamins and Minerals: Use a multi-vitamin and mineral supplement and a high level B-complex (50–250 mg per day). Start with lower to medium doses of B-complex and raise them if the migraines continue.

Niacin (B-3) is the key here, and there are two philosophies for using it in addition to the full B-complex. One is to supplement with high levels of niacin daily, using up to 800 mg of niacinamide (no hot flush) and 200 mg of niacin daily. The other philosophy is to use less daily and to take a 50–100 mg niacin tablet (not niacinamide or time release niacin) at the first sign of migraine or aura and lie down for a few minutes. In about fifteen minutes you will experience what I call "the hotflash of your life" and the flushing (which dilates the blood vessels to the head and brain) will abort the migraine within a few minutes. If you don't get the flush in fifteen or twenty minutes, take another dose of niacin. Since enough niacin taken daily can prevent them altogether, my suggestion is to experiment and see what works for you, or to try a combination—enough niacin to mostly prevent, with increased doses if an attack begins. If you start to experience nausea on high daily levels, cut back as this is a symptom of toxicity. Once you have taken niacin for a few days and are no longer deficient in it, the flushing will stop, but you need the flush again to stop a beginning migraine and therefore the additional dose. This treatment with niacin will abort ninety percent of migraines if taken early enough in the cycle.

Other vitamins for migraines and migraine prevention include B-6, particularly for women on the pill or for those whose migraines are menstrual related; use up to 50 mg three times a day. Use a vitamin C with bioflavinoids for blood vessel health and as an antioxidant. Rutin, one of the bioflavinoids, removes toxic metals from the body, a possible migraine cause. Use a calcium/magnesium supplement (2000 mg calcium to 1000 mg magnesium per day). Take an additional 800 mg calcium/magnesium tablet hourly during migraine attacks; it relaxes muscle contractions. DMG (dimethyl glysine or B-15) improves oxygen to the brain; take one tablet dissolved in the mouth twice daily. Essential fatty acids, as evening primrose oil, salmon oil or black currant oil, are important in migraine prevention for some women.

Herbs: Feverfew tincture, thirty drops twice a day taken for three months will significantly reduce migraine frequency. Use it also at the early start of the aura and as often as every half hour during the attack. This is a relaxant and has much the same effect as niacin, which you can also use with it. Feverfew and scullcap together (1/3–1/2 dropperful of each) taken early enough can also stop a migraine. Take this every half hour or hour until all symptoms are past. Scullcap taken daily will also reduce the frequency and severity of migraines. Ginkgo biloba increases circulation to the head and brain. Other herbs include valerian for pain and as a sedative, passion flower, blue flag, rosemary, lavender tea, Jamaican dogwood, mistletoe, lady's slipper, or peppermint for nausea and headache. Make an infusion of black horehound with meadowsweet and chamomile for migraine with nausea and vomiting. For menstrual-related migraines, dong quai used daily can be an effective preventive for women who can use it. For prevention also, try a daily tea of hops, scullcap and catnip, or of catnip, scullcap and red clover. Causing vomiting with lobelia tincture will stop a migraine in progress.

Naturopathy: Start with a three-day apple juice fast, or for cleansing the liver a fast using grapefruit juice or lemon juice and hot water. (If you are hypoglycemic, see that section.) Take enemas every other day during the fast—a coffee enema will abort a migraine. Reintroduce solid foods slowly, watching for reactions to any food. Food allergies can be identified this way. Food rotation, not repeating any food more often than every five days, can reduce migraines also. Avoid the tyramine-containing foods listed previously, and eat a hypoglycemia diet. Eat a diet as free of chemicals and additives as possible, low in sugar, with little or no meat, and stop caffeine and smoking. Reduce salt and use sea salt. It is highly important to avoid constipation.

Use odorless garlic (Kyolic), two tablets per day with meals as an antioxidant, and to reduce candida albicans. If you have systemic yeast, work at clearing it; it can be a migraine cause. To abort a migraine, try taking a tablespoonful of raw honey at the first indication; if the migraine isn't gone in half an hour, take the honey again with three glasses of water. Take two teaspoons of honey at each meal as a preventive, or use a teaspoon each of apple cider vinegar and honey in a glass of hot or cold water three times a day to regulate digestion. Propolis or royal jelly can help when migraines are of hormone imbalance origin.

Progest cream, a natural three percent progesterone made from wild yams, will abort a hormone-related migraine. Rub the cream on face, neck, soles of feet and under the arms at first sign. Enzymatic Therapy has a pituitary glandular compound called Neuroplex: Peace of Mind that contains pituitary and brain tissue (bovine) and high levels of niacin and B-complex. I have used this to stop migraines in the same way as the niacin treatment, used early.

Homeopathy and Cell Salts: Use *Aconite* at onset and/or for the emotion of thinking you are dying. *Nux vomica* is for migraine after eating with nausea and vomiting. *Iris* is for right-sided migraine with vomiting; *Spigelia* for left-sided attack, with pressing pain in the eye that feels too large, and palpitations. *Lycopodium* is for right-sided migraines worse between 4 and 8 PM, brought on by irregular eating. *Ignatia* is for band-like pressure headache across the forehead with nausea and dizziness. *Gelsemium* is for right-sided headache worse for movement, light or noise, with visual disturbances and muscle contraction; sleep or urination

Acupressure for Migraines

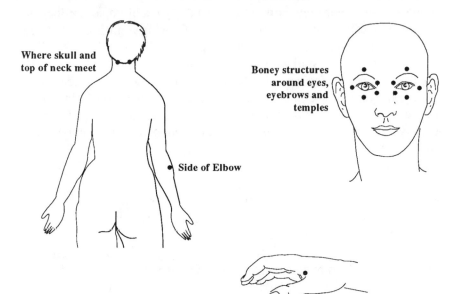

Where skull and top of neck meet

Side of Elbow

Boney structures around eyes, eyebrows and temples

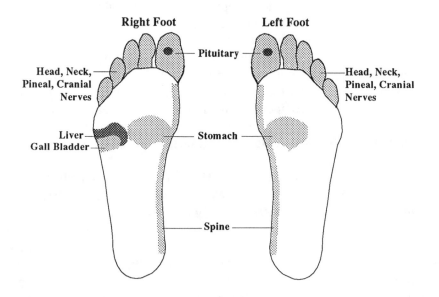

Webs between thumbs and first fingers

Right Foot

Left Foot

Head, Neck, Pineal, Cranial Nerves

Pituitary

Head, Neck, Pineal, Cranial Nerves

Liver
Gall Bladder

Stomach

Spine

Michael Van Straten, ND, DO, *The Complete Natural Health Consultant* (New York, Prentice-Hall Publishers, 1987), p. 201; Cathryn Bauer, *Acupressure for Women* (Freedom, CA, The Crossing Press, 1987), p.87.

Acupressure for Migraines

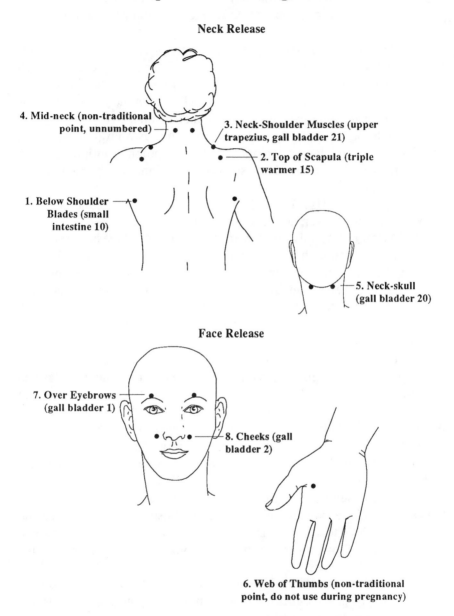

Neck Release

4. Mid-neck (non-traditional point, unnumbered)

3. Neck-Shoulder Muscles (upper trapezius, gall bladder 21)

2. Top of Scapula (triple warmer 15)

1. Below Shoulder Blades (small intestine 10)

5. Neck-skull (gall bladder 20)

Face Release

7. Over Eyebrows (gall bladder 1)

8. Cheeks (gall bladder 2)

6. Web of Thumbs (non-traditional point, do not use during pregnancy)

Press these neck and face release points in order, 1-8.

Iona Marsaa Teeguarden, *Acupressure Way of Health: Jin Shin Do* (New York, Japan Publishing Co., 1978), p.98-99; Diane Stein, *All Women Are Healers* (Freedom, CA, The Crossing Press, 1990), p. 94.

eases it and you want to be left alone. *Sanguinaria* is for the "classic migraines," right-sided, beginning at the back of the head and moving forward with splitting, throbbing, knifelike pain and nausea relieved by vomiting.

Cell Salts: Use *Silica* for right-sided migraine attack, or *Natrum mur.* for blinding headache worse with menstruation. Or take five tablets each of *Ferrum phos.* and *Kali phos.* every half hour until the migraine is over.

Amino Acids: Twin-Labs Predigested Liver Amino Acids, a combination that also contains high levels of niacin and B-12, has made a difference in both frequency and severity of my own migraines. Avoid tyrosine and phenylalanine as single aminos. Tryptophan with B-6, niacin and vitamin E is recommended—such combinations will be back on the market eventually.

Acupressure: Use full foot acupressure paying particular attention to the gall bladder, liver, stomach, spine, pituitary and head/neck/cranial points. Massage and apply pressure to the inside base of the big toes. Look for sore points around the eyes and temples, and especially at the back of the neck. Use the Great Eliminator reflex in the webs between thumbs and first fingers. Other meridians and the Jin Shin Do Neck Release are illustrated. In the Neck Release, start from the lower points and work upward toward the hand—you will be able to reach all but the lowest points yourself.

Aromatherapy: Herbal creams containing oil of wintergreen, lavender, peppermint or ginger are massaged into the forehead, temples and back of neck. Try Sunrider's Sunbreeze for this. Other herbs to inhale or use as above are: basil, chamomile, ginger, lavender, marjoram, melissa, peppermint, spearmint, angelica, rosemary, aniseed or jasmine. Tiferet-Lifetree has a Headache/Migraine combination that eases constricted blood vessels—and it works. Remember that fragrances cancel homeopathic remedies.

Flower Essences: Use green rose for migraines, especially in women who are psychic (as we all are). Grapefruit adjusts the cranial plates and brings more blood to the brain. Don't forget the Bach Rescue Remedy, and whatever Bach Flower Remedy fits your emotional pattern (see the list under Flower Essences).

Gemstones and Gem Essences: Hematite, kunzite, lodestone or amethyst are the gem essences. Carry a boji stone in your pocket, and wear or hold kunzite, turquoise or chrysocolla.

Emotional Healing: Women who get migraines are women who try too hard, or whose competence is stifled by less aware people. They panic at being driven, particularly as they drive themselves to the limits without other's influence, and they are die-hard perfectionists who are often very frustrated and insecure. They feel not good enough and are angry about it, and need to control what happens to them. Stop resisting the flow of life, reduce stress, release anger, and let others make fools of themselves if they have to. Learn to meditate nightly to reduce tension, and learn to be aware of others' games and to be outside of them. Go at your own pace and give yourself less work and more fun. Work on self-image—you are good.

Motion Sickness

Women are affected by this far more often than men; children under two and elders are usually unaffected. It occurs when movement causes the eyes, ears or sensory nerves to send conflicted messages to the brain. Symptoms include nausea, cold sweats, vomiting, excess salivation, sleepiness, dizziness, loss of appetite, vertigo or fainting; the range is from mild to severe. Any form of motion can cause it, from automobiles and airplanes to amusement park rides or boats. Over-the-counter drugs sometimes help but often don't, and the same for prescription medications, which can also cause drowsiness. Natural remedies work as well or better than what the medical system can offer, and natural preventives are effective.

Vitamins and Minerals: Along with the usual multiple vitamin and mineral supplement, take a B-complex-100 the night before travel and the morning it begins. B-1 and B-6 are the target vitamins; take 100 mg of B-6 an hour before travel and two hours later. Take calcium/magnesium tablets daily; besides being essential for women to prevent osteoporosis and premenstrual syndrome, they are muscle relaxants and calm the stomach. Five hundred mg of magnesium taken an hour before travel is a nerve tonic and anti-nausea. Charcoal tablets taken five an hour before travel may help, but do not take with other supplements.

Herbs: Ginger capsules or tinctures are the herbs of choice; take two capsules every three hours, starting an hour before the trip or chew on crystallized ginger or raw ginger root. B-6 is more effective if taken with ginger, and ginger has a better success record than over-the-counter or prescription anti-nausea drugs. Other effective herbs include peppermint, spearmint, catnip or cloves for nausea, or chamomile as a calmative. Use peppermint and chamomile together, and they can be sipped cold. Black horehound is a remedy for nausea and vomiting, and it can be used with meadowsweet and chamomile.

Naturopathy: The day before travel, eat a liquid diet without sugar or salt. If eating solid foods, avoid junk foods, processed foods, sugar or alcohol. Eat a few whole grain crackers before and during the trip. Try to stay cool and to avoid food and smoking odors; do not overeat while traveling. Get as much fresh air as possible, look forward and to the outside, and avoid twisting the neck.

For prevention, beat together an egg white with the juice of one lemon and eat it before leaving home. If you feel nauseated, suck a lemon or drink fresh lemon juice, or lemon juice in water. An eighth teaspoon of cayenne pepper in a glass of water will usually stop nausea, also.

Homeopathy and Cell Salts: *Cocculus* is primary for motion sickness, with nausea, vomiting and dizziness; the sight or smell of food makes things worse. *Petroleum* includes dizziness and nausea when riding in a car or boat; the woman feels faint, looks pale and has cold sweats and excess salivation. She feels better for eating. Use *Ignatia* if the smell of tobacco or gasoline is the cause of the sickness. *Tabacum* is for severe nausea, violent vomiting and retching with the slightest movement. The woman is cold and pale with cold sweat, feels better in open air, and is worse for warmth. *Nux vomica* is the remedy for many women's motion sickness; there is constant nausea, splitting headache and buzzing in the ears. The woman wants to vomit but can't and feels better in fresh air. For nausea with drowsiness, use *Antimonium tart.* Use *Ipecac* for nausea in waves not relieved by vomiting.

Cell Salts: *Natrum phos.* is used for dizziness, nausea or indigestion; there is a dull or full feeling in the head.

Amino Acids: Use a daily free-form or liver extract amino acid combination for its B-complex nutrients, digestive, calmative and antioxidant ability.

Acupressure: Work the stomach, large intestine and pituitary hand reflexes, and the fourth and fifth (ring and little) fingers—especially at the knuckles of the little fingers and the web between. See the illustration for body meridian points; try the one above the wrist for nausea and motion sickness, and the one in the elbow crease to stop vomiting. Find the point where the neck and skull meet about an inch behind the ear. The leg points are about three inches above the ankle bone and about three inches below the kneecaps. The points will be sore; use pressure to release them.

Acupressure for Motion Sickness

About 1" behind ear

Crease of inner
elbow for vomiting

2" above wrist crease
between the two tendons

About 3" below kneecaps

About 3" above ankle bone,
behind the tibia

Pedro Chan, *Finger Acupressure* (New York, Ballantine Books, 1974), p. 85-89; Iona Marsaa Teeguarden, *Acupressure Way of Health: Jin Shin Do* (New York, Japan Publishing Co., 1978), p. 77.

Aromatherapy: Place a few drops of one of these on or near the face or sniff them from the bottle: peppermint, rosewood, spearmint, ginger or lavender.

Flower Essences: Loquat is a remedy for nausea. Star tulip helps inner ear and balance disorders, and French marigold is for inflammation of the inner ear. California poppy is for balance problems originating in the middle ear.

Gemstone and Gem Essences: Use gem essences of coral, rhodolite garnet, spinel, kunzite or turquoise. Hold or wear moss agate or kunzite for nausea.

Emotional Healing: You are afraid of not being in control, and fear for your safety either on the trip or where you are going. Know that you are safe, in control and capable; love and approve of yourself.

Multiple Sclerosis

The medical system has no current answers for this degenerative dis-ease of the spinal myelin sheath that affects so many young women. The dis-ease usually first appears in women between twenty and thirty years of age. There are periods of worsening and of remission. First signs include visual disturbances, double vision, weakness, fatigue, motor uncoordination, dizziness, temporary loss of vision or of bladder or bowel control, emotional disturbance, or stiffness or weakness of an arm or leg. These increase with later active periods, developing with staggering gait, breathing or speech difficulties, tremors, increasing weakness, and paralysis. A progressive dis-ease, MS does not in itself lead to death; most sufferers die of respiratory infections or complications.

Holistic healing has theories for this dis-ease when the medical system does not. The theory on causes includes lead or other heavy metal toxicity, deficiency in the trace mineral gold, glandular malfunction, cumulative reaction to earlier vaccinations, sensitivities to foods, food additives or pollutants that break down the immune system, or activation of miasmatic dis-ease (a homeopathic term referring to an inherited or acquired predisposition to chronic dis-ease). One theory is of an earlier viral infection that lies latent, leading to antibodies that attack the myelin surrounding nerves. This would make multiple sclerosis an auto-immune dis-ease, and most holistic therapies treat it as such. Dr. Lawrence Badgley (*Healing AIDS Naturally*) places MS on a par with AIDS as far as healing techniques. (See the sections on Immune System Dis-eases and AIDS.) Because it is a degenerative dis-ease, healing therapies must be used longterm to have effect. The more nervous system damage that has already occurred, the less likely it is for complete remission or cure. Even in progressed cases, however, holistic remedies can lessen frequency and severity of recurrences and degeneration.

Vitamins and Minerals: Use a daily multiple vitamin and mineral supplement high in B-complex vitamins, and an additional B-complex-50 to -100 three times a day. The B-vitamins regulate nervous system function and most sources list mega amounts of several of them including B-1 (10–15 g per day with 1 mg of B-12), B-3 (500 mg or higher), B-6 (100–250 mg up to three times daily), lecithin (300–600 mg daily), plus folic acid and B-5.[1] These are enormous doses, often given by injection, and should be taken under expert supervision. Use vitamin C to bowel tolerance, vitamin A/beta-carotene (25,000 IU), vitamin D (800–1200 IU), and vitamin E beginning with 400 IU and increasing slowly to 1800–2000 IU per day. Use selenium with vitamin E (200–300 mcg), and a calcium/magnesium tablet (1000–1500 calcium, 500–750 magnesium), manganese (25 mg), zinc (up to 100 mg per day—women with MS are usually deficient), and potassium (300–1000 mg) for muscle weakness and to increase energy. B-13 (orotic acid) may be important, but is not readily available.

Antioxidants are important; therefore the A, D, C, and E. DMG (B-15), a gluconic, is another antioxidant that brings oxygen to the cells. Others are S.O.D. (two to five tablets three times a day), coenzyme Q10 (60 mg per day), and germanium (200 mg—use one of these daily). Acidophilus and/or a multidigestive enzyme may help digestion and food assimilation. Oil of evening primrose, an essential fatty acid (or other EFA source—black currant oil, salmon oil, cod liver oil, Omega-3, etc.) is considered important by several sources; use two to four capsules three or more times a day. Raw thymus extract and/or raw adrenal boost the immune system.

Herbs: The South American bark of the Lapacho tree, pau d'arco, is the herb of choice as an immune system builder, and chaparral is second. Scullcap, a relaxant and anti-stress herb is also a nervous system rebuilder.

---

[1]Dr. Ross Trattler, *Better Health Through Natural Healing* (New York, McGraw-Hill Book Co., 1985), p. 449; and James Balch, MD, and Phyllis Balch, CNC, *Prescription for Nutritional Healing* (Garden City Park, NY, Avery Publishing Group, Inc., 1990), p. 246. These are the highest vitamin doses I have seen.

With these, try alfalfa as a nutrient, detoxifier and high source of minerals, and also for its ability to enhance the effects of other herbs and vitamins. Other herbs include rosemary, damiana, bugleweed, hawthorn (heart and nervous system), motherwort, the cayenne pepper drink described under AIDS, horsetail or Irish moss (for minerals), yellow dock, Oregon grape root, burdock or red clover (detoxifying), myrrh or echinacea (antibiotics), or hops, valerian, catnip, lobelia or scullcap (relaxants and emotional). Lady's slipper is said to repair the myelin sheaths and give relief to both physical and emotional symptoms, and licorice is a natural cortisone.

Naturopathy: Food allergies and hypersensitivities to additives and preservatives are a major concern in multiple sclerosis. Most women with this dis-ease are gluten intolerant—cannot digest wheat products and most other grains except rice and millet. A gluten-free diet is usually considered essential, plus testing to see what other foods may be implicated—allergies to eggs, milk, corn, chocolate or tomatoes are common, but it can be any food/s. The diet needs to be organic—pollutant, additive and chemical free—and free of saturated fats. This is a vegetarian diet without dairy products and usually without yeast. Avoid sugar, caffeine, chocolate, salt or heavy spices, yeast, alcohol, processed foods and junk foods of all types. Avoid constipation. Short fasts with lemon juice enemas are helpful. For a different type of suggested diet, see Linda Clark's *Handbook of Natural Remedies for Common Ailments* (The Devin-Adair Co., 1976), p. 270–274. Most, however, recommend the above.

Kyolic, odorless garlic, is recommended as a sulfur food. Check for candida albicans, which may be a factor in MS. Use the yeast-eliminating methods, described under Candida Albicans if needed. Iodine is also important, as kelp (five to ten tablets per day) or Cayce's Atomidine. Sulfur tablets provide the sulfur amino acids which are anti-bacterial and protect the cells (but can be taken as amino acids, see below). Spirulina, Kyo-green, chlorophyll and other green drinks are recommended; they provide minerals and antioxidants. Bee pollen is a valuable nutrient that helps with hormone balancing, adrenal function, and tissue re-building. All of these are to add optimal nutrition and immune support.

Homeopathy and Cell Salts: An expert homeopath is needed here to release miasms and work with specific symptoms. *Arsenicum album* is a possible remedy, for wasting of muscles and paralysis. One woman worked with *Phosphorus*, for low vitality, weakness and easy exhaustion, and she had good results. Personality types are also involved in choosing remedies.

Cell Salts: *Calc. fluor.* is for muscle weakness, and *Silica* is for paralytic symptoms.

Amino Acids: These are highly important for the nervous system. Use a combination free-form amino acids as well as the following specific combinations: cysteine and cystine (a sulfur-providing amino, also found in onions and garlic), and leucine, isoleucine and valine for muscle absorption of nutrients. Taurine with vitamins A and E is also considered important.

Acupressure: See the illustrations under Immune System Dis-eases and the body meridian points shown under AIDS. Do full foot acupressure, starting slowly and lightly, and working up to three times a week or more. Work the points for the head (on and around the toes) and spine (along the inner length of both feet, big toe sides). Work the points for the endocrine glands, particularly the thymus, adrenals, pituitary and pineal, and the digestive system. Work out any sore spots you find, but don't try to release everything in one session. Don't overdo.

Aromatherapy: Use essential oils in massage oils, diffusers or baths. Oils include: bergamot, cedarwood, cinnamon, lemon, lime, petitgrain, pine, lavender, sage, spruce, tea-tree, marjoram or jasmine. A massage oil containing sassafras and pine in two ounces each of peanut and olive oils with half an ounce of lanolin is suggested; use it to massage along the spine nightly.

Flower Essences: Use California poppy for MS as a gold deficiency dis-ease, and hyssop is positive with it for assimilation of gold. Bo tree essence is specifically for multiple sclerosis, also. Comfrey is a nervous system tonic, dandelion is a stress and muscle system relaxant, and lilac is for the spine. Use redwood for cell regeneration and longevity, or nasturtium for deterioration of the nervous system, especially when the eyes are involved. Bach Flower Remedy's Beech may help emotionally and physically.

Gemstones and Gem Essences: Use gold in essence specifically for this dis-ease. Wear or hold sodalite, lapis lazuli, azurite, azurite-malachite, moonstone or amethyst for the dis-ease, and/or rose-colored stones for love—rose quartz, kunzite, pink tourmaline or rhodochrosite.

Emotional Healing: Reduce stress, negative thinking and the need to control. There is an iron will, mental hardness, hard-heartedness or inflexibility that need to be overcome. These are fear derived, of course— learn to relax, let go and trust. Learn to think and speak positively of situations and people, including yourself. Work on self-love, on being less self-critical and critical of others, and open your heart to universal love and understanding.

Obesity Affecting Health

This is not about dieting but about health. Fat is beautiful, along with every other shape, size or form. The oldest depiction of divinity on earth is the Goddess of Willendorf, a large-breasted, large-bellied clay Mother figure 30,000 years old. She is certainly beautiful, as is the large woman. The issue here is not about fashionable body size, either—the time has long past for women to create their Be-ings and bodies for male fantasies and tastes. What is important in a discussion of obesity is helping the large woman who also has a heart condition, diabetes, liver or kidney dis-ease, or high blood pressure to lose enough weight to stay alive. I am talking strictly about the necessities of health, and use the term obesity only to refer to fat that is health-threatening. Women who are obese are at greater risk for the above dis-eases, which have increased seriousness for them in some cases, as well as for cancers of the uterus and breast.

Malnutrition is the major cause of obesity. The body is not getting what it needs, so is continually hungry looking for what's missing. Most women who are obese were started on the Typical American Diet early, may have had food allergies or were unable to digest the cow's milk and starch they were weaned on, and grew fat rather than well-fed. The problem grows with the child; an adult lacks the physical activity of childhood and the Typical American Diet has also become habit. An abnormal biochemistry develops, with food sensitivities and hypoglycemia. As Adele Davis explains in *Let's Get Well*, too few nutrients are supplied in many women's diets to make fat burning possible. "Fat is only lost when energy is produced, therefore weight cannot be taken off until fat is efficiently burned, a process requiring almost every nutrient."[1] She believed that liver involvement, the inability to produce or activate digestive enzymes due to vitamin deficiencies or allergies, is a central cause of obesity. A further cause is endocrine/glandular imbalance, much of which can also be remedied by full nutrition, and there are many other theories. For the woman who needs to lose weight as a health necessity, reducing diets are not the answer, but good food is—changing the Typical American Diet to give her body what it needs.

---

[1] Adele Davis, *Let's Get Well* (New York, Signet Books, 1965), p. 71.

Vitamins and Minerals: Begin with a multiple vitamin and mineral supplement of good quality; if assimilation is a problem, they come in liquid form. A high level B-complex-50 is next, used twice a day, with additional B-6 (100 mg) for fluid retention and to change stored fat to energy. Additional B-5 (500 mg with each meal) doubles the rate of fat assimilation and boosts the adrenals. Lecithin taken with meals helps the body burn fat, reduces blood cholesterol and prevents or aids high blood pressure and artery dis-ease. These are essential for liver function, as well. Use vitamin C (3000–6000 mg per day) for glandular functions, and vitamin E (400–800 IU per day) doubles the rate of fat metabolism again. Start with 400 IU of E and increase by 100 IU per week; if you have rheumatic heart dis-ease you are limited to 400 IU total daily. Essential fatty acids aid in utilization of fat already in the body, suppress appetite and keep off lost weight. Use as evening primrose oil, salmon oil, black currant oil, or cod liver oil. If you are hypoglycemic, and also to reduce fluid retention, try potassium (90 mg). Chromium (200 mcg) aids weight loss by balancing blood sugar. All women need to be on a calcium/ magnesium supplement; it helps water retention, is a muscle relaxant and slight carminative, and an antacid.

Herbs: Chickweed, cleavers and pokeroot are herbs that stimulate weight loss by helping to burn fat. Raw chickweed can be used in salads with mustard greens, shepherd's purse or pepper grass, or use the dried herb or tincture. Use cleavers as a tea three or more times a day—it will take until the seventh week to notice change, but then the change will be considerable. White ash bark also helps weight loss, and yerba mate or fennel decrease appetite and aid digestion. Saffron is a blood cleanser, as is dandelion (for the liver), and hawthorn is helpful for the heart. Try hawthorn and chickweed together in tincture twice daily for obesity and heart dis-ease or high blood pressure. Stevia is an herbal sweetener that is safe.

Use alfalfa along with other herbs as a nutrient, cleanser and detoxifier that enhances the effects of other herbs and vitamins. Parsley is a diuretic, and senna or cascara sagrada are laxatives. Use glucommanan or bran half an hour before breakfast—it provides fiber, reduces appetite, is a laxative and stabilizes blood sugar. Do not take within an hour of vitamins or medications. Licorice root lowers blood sugar and stimulates the adrenals, but is not for women with high blood pressure; it is an important help for hypoglycemia. Bladderwrack (seaweed) stimulates the thyroid.

Naturopathy: Eat a balanced whole foods diet of citrus, raw veg-etables, vegetarian protein, organic fowl, fish, fiber and unrefined car-bohydrates. (See the diet under Hypoglycemia.) Do not use white flour products, sugar, salt, white rice, junk foods, fast foods, soft drinks, pastries, or foods with additives and preservatives. Avoid animal fats (unsaturated fats), dairy products, ice cream or fried foods. Use unsaturated oils in nuts, avocados, olive oil, or essential fatty acids. Eat whole grains, tofu, lentils, beans and baked potatoes (no topping) moderately. Short fasts with lemon juice or warm water enemas are helpful. Try eating small amounts several times a day instead of three big meals, and neither starve nor overeat. Do not eat between meals. This is a nutrition diet based on unrefined whole foods and adequate protein and fiber:

> When unrefined foods are eaten, nutrients needed for energy production are supplied with every calorie, whereas trash foods both lack these nutrients and tremendously increase the requirement for them.[2]

Drink a half glass of diluted red grape juice before each meal; it decreases appetite. Two ounces of grapefruit juice with an ounce of water will do the same, or a glass of water with a teaspoon of apple cider vinegar in it (recommended). Use one or two drops of Lugol's Solution in water or juice before a meal two or three times a week for iodine and thyroid balance. Other iodine sources are kelp tablets (six to eight a day), or Edgar Cayce's Atomidine. If your mouth begins to taste metallic cut back. Spirulina or other green drinks are a protein source, lower blood sugar, and can be used instead of a meal. Use these fasting if you are hypoglycemic. Raw pancreas, pituitary or thyroid glandulars help endocrine balance.

Homeopathy and Cell Salts: Homeopathy regards obesity as a characteristic, rather than a dis-ease. Work with an expert homeopath for overall healing, but here are some suggestions. Try *Phytolacca Berry* every eight hours on a month's trial. If no response, try *Ammonium bromatum* where there is obesity with chronic mucus congestion, cough, neuralgic headaches, or constrictive pain in head, chest or legs. The woman may bite her fingernails. *Calcarea carb.* is the remedy for obesity from impaired nutrition with pituitary or thyroid dysfunction, increased perspiration, fleeting chest pains, tickling cough, nausea, acidity, and/or easily out of breath. The woman (or child) is pale, sensitive to cold, and has a sour, damp perspiration. Use *Calcarea arsenicosa* for obesity at menopause, where the slightest emotion causes palpitations. There may be edema, chilliness, weak heart, kidney or pancreatic dis-ease, and symptoms are worse for the slightest exertion.

Cell Salts: *Natrum. sulph.* is for obesity and water retention.

---

[2]Ibid., p. 73

Amino Acids: These are important for easy-to-assimilate protein and B-vitamins for obesity and hypoglycemia; use a free-form combination. Single aminos include DL-phenylalanine as an appetite suppressant (100–300 mg per day); avoid high amounts if you are diabetic or have high blood pressure. The combination of arginine, ornithine and lysine (500 mg of each) decreases body fat; avoid for diabetics and children. Carnitine aids fat assimilation and weight loss.

Acupressure: Massage the full ear flesh on both sides for endocrine balancing and see the points for appetite suppression and hormones in the illustration. Body points for water retention are also illustrated. Do full foot or hand acupressure, working slowly up to daily or twice a day. Pay particular attention to the following organs: pituitary, pineal, parathyroid, thyroid, pancreas, adrenals, kidneys and sex hormones.

Aromatherapy: Use any of the following in baths or massage oils: angelica, birch, fennel, citrus, red thyme, or lemon. Sage, marjoram and rosemary improve elimination of toxins and tone intestinal tissues.

Flower Essences: Apricot and banana essence are for obesity due to hypoglycemia, and paw paw is for malassimilation of nutrients and eating disorders. Use redwood for obesity from endocrine imbalance or pituitary dysfunction, and sunflower dissolves fatty tissue.

Gemstones and Gem Essences: Coral, fluorite or ruby essence are used for weight loss. Hold or wear citrine, amber, topaz, malachite or peridot.

Emotional Healing: You are insecure and vulnerable, afraid to show your power or your fear. Food is a hiding place, a substitute fulfillment, and weight is a protection. There is a small, scared child inside who needs your love; take care of her, protect her, and allow her real feelings to emerge. There is a powerful woman inside with the child; let her throw her weight around and take up space. You are strong and competent and good. You don't need to hide behind fat or food. You are loving and lovable—love yourself. You are safe.

Acupressure for Obesity

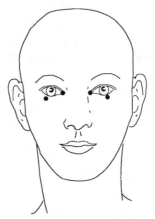

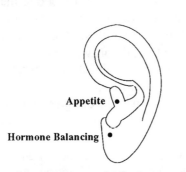

Appetite

Hormone Balancing

Acupressure ear point for hormone balance and appetite suppression. Also massage the whole ears for endocrine balancing.

Corner of eyes and under eyes for water retention

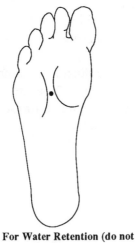

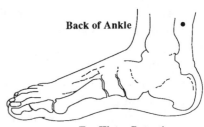

Back of Ankle

For Water Retention

For Water Retention (do not use during pregnancy)

Cathryn Bauer, *Acupressure for Women* (Freedom, CA, The Crossing Press, 1987), p.51; Moshe Olshevsky, CA, PhD., *et. al.*, *The Manual of Natural Therapy* (New York, Citadel Press, 1989), p. 7-8.

Acupressure for Obesity

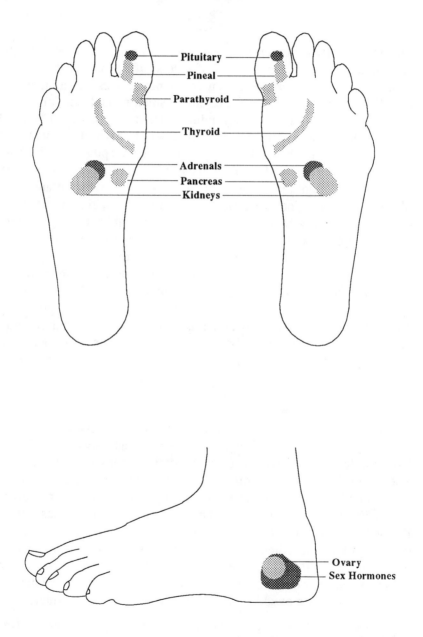

Osteoporosis

This is primarily a women's dis-ease (seventy percent of those having it are women) and a great crippler of elders, affecting one fourth of all women past menopause. Estrogen deficiency, a lack of calcium or the inability to assimilate it, prolonged stress, smoking and alcohol, anorexia nervosa, heavy metal toxicity (aluminum in particular), many childbirths, lactose intolerance, fluoridated or soft water, thyroid or parathyroid imbalance, birth control pills, high phosphorus/phosphate additives diets, and vitamin-mineral deficiencies have all been implicated as causes. Some medical drugs, including antibiotics, steroids, and anti-inflammatories like ibuprofen, surgical gastrectomies, and overuse of bicarbonate of soda (baking soda) may be other causes. The medical system's solution of estrogen replacement therapy risks cancer, and does no more than vitamin therapy can, while vitamins and minerals are perfectly safe. When minerals are deficient, the body draws them from the bones, causing bone weakening and thinning; these minerals and vitamins include calcium, magnesium, phosphorus (in balance), vitamins D and C, protein and boron. Symptoms include back pain, loss of height, spinal curvatures (kyphosis), pain on weight-bearing, muscle spasms and spontaneous fractures in hips, lower back, legs or vertebrae, usually in women over fifty. Women who are vegetarians are less at risk, with average bone loss at seven percent, compared to thirty-five percent for meat-eaters.

The bone thinning of osteoporosis is not apparent until it is too late; it doesn't show on x-rays until thirty percent of bone mass has been lost, and many women's first knowledge of this dis-ease is with a broken hip. One in sixteen women will die from the complications of such hip injuries. The following women are more at risk: women who are of fair complexion, are thin and small-boned, have gone through a natural early menopause, have never been pregnant, have family heredity of the dis-ease, smoke, live sedentary lifestyles, drink alcohol, soft-drinks or caffeine in excess, eat high protein meat diets that are high in phosphorus but low in calcium, use cortisone, anticoagulants or anti-seizure drugs longterm, have liver or kidney dis-ease or overactive endocrine glands, have digestive disorders or their ovaries removed.[1] Many or most of us live in fluoridated water

---

[1]James Balch, MD, and Phyllis Balch, CNC *Prescription for Nutritional Healing* (Garden City Park, NY: Avery Publishing Group, Inc., 1990), p. 256.

systems, and fluoride drains calcium from the bones. This is another disease of modern society, and a clear and present danger to all women. Healing for osteoporosis must begin early, long before menopause, to prevent it.

Vitamins and Minerals: Begin with a multiple vitamin and mineral supplement and a complete calcium/magnesium for all women from the teenage years on. Calcium need increases with age. Use 1000–2000 mg of calcium daily with half the amount of magnesium, and the trace minerals found in complete calcium formulas (vitamins A, D, C, iron, zinc). Some include bromelain for assimilation. For women closer to menopause or with the dis-ease, add silicon and boron (3 mg per day of boron, no more). Both increase calcium utilization, and boron reduces calcium loss by forty percent, magnesium loss by a third. Digestive enzymes and/or HCL may be important for assimilation. Add to these vitamin C (1000–3000 mg per day for younger women or 3000 mg and up for elders—C deficiency has been linked to osteoporosis). Use 400–1000 IU of vitamin D (total), or A and D together in dry form (25,000 and 400 IU), and vitamin E (400–800 IU). Cod liver oil is an A and D source, but it is not for diabetics. Elders will benefit from an E with selenium (200 mcg). Zinc (50 mg) and sulfur (in tablets or garlic, onions or amino acids) are important for calcium uptake. Use a B-complex-50 at least once a day, for younger and older women both. Essential fatty acids are important, and if you have bone pain try germanium. If you already have osteoporosis, the above will prevent new fractures and lessen pain.

Herbs: The most positive single herb is alfalfa, which contains all the minerals and vitamins and enhances the assimilation of any others you are taking. Horsetail grass or oatstraw are high in silicon and calcium. Feverfew contains minerals and vitamins, and reduces pain, menopause symptoms and migraines. Nettles or comfrey are also high in minerals. See kelp under Naturopathy.

Naturopathy: A diet high in green leafy vegetables and vegetable protein is best, using fruits, whole grains, beans and legumes, tofu, sprouts, kefir and yoghurt, and nuts. Milk products are not high in assimilable calcium and many women are lactose intolerant. Eat fish, particularly salmon with bones and sardines. Caffeine decreases bone minerals (coffee, tea, soft-drinks), and foods with phosphate additives upset the balance of phosphorus/calcium/magnesium causing mineral loss. Eat a diet as free of additives and chemicals as possible. Stop smoking, and avoid sugar, refined flour and salt. Some foods (spinach, beet greens, wheat and oats) have been considered negative for calcium deficient women because of oxalic and phytic acid. Nutritionists are rethinking this; the loss is no more than the amount in the food itself and therefore is very minimal. Use caution with these foods but there is no need to avoid them. Drink spring water, rather than fluoridated tap water or nutrient-depleted distilled bottled waters. Exercise, sun and sea bathing are recommended. Avoid cooking with aluminum cookware.

To aid in digestion and assimilation of minerals, and to add potassium and other minerals to the body, use a glass of water with a teaspoon of apple cider vinegar and a teaspoon of honey in it two or three times a day with meals. Replace sugar use with honey, also. Kyolic, garlic or onions add sulfur, which helps in calcium uptake. Kelp is important for minerals and iodine and to balance the thyroid and parathyroid—use six to eight tablets per day; it is especially positive used with alfalfa and helps with heavy metal detoxification.

Homeopathy and Cell Salts: *Phosphorus* is the remedy for degenerative bone dis-ease, bone fragility, fractures, weak spine, joints that suddenly give way, and shooting pains. The woman is worse for exertion, change of weather, evening, and getting wet in warm weather, and better for darkness, cold open air, washing in cold water, and sleep. *Ruta grav.* is for spine and limbs that feel bruised, weak lower back and pain in bones. The woman feels worse lying down and in cold wet weather. Use *Arsenicum album* for degenerative changes, weakness in the small of back, drawing in of shoulders, kyphosis, burning pains in the back, or spasms, and weakness or heaviness of extremities. She is restless, has great thirst, is worse late at night, is exhausted after the slightest exertion, and feels better for heat.

Cell Salts: Use *Silica* for dis-eases of bones or weak spine caused by imperfect assimilation and defective nutrition. The woman is cold and chilly, worse in winter, and seeks warmth. *Calc. phos.* is for bone problems and defective nutrition, and is especially useful to elders. These can be used in alternation. *Calc. flour.* is for the coverings of bones.

Amino Acids: DL-phenylalanine, taken on an empty stomach with vitamins B-6 and C helps bone pain; do not use in pregnancy or with high blood pressure. Use lysine and arginine together for calcium absorption. Methionine and leucine are other single aminos, and a combination free-form amino acids is recommended.

Acupressure: Use full foot acupressure, increasing gradually to daily use or to ten minutes per day with a foot roller. Pay particular attention to painful spots along the spine reflexes, as well as to the pituitary, thyroid and parathyroid, ovaries and sex hormones (sides of feet), and to the other endocrine/chakra glands. See the body maps and the section under Immune Dis-eases for endocrine gland locations. For pain see the pain relief maps under Cancer. Additional meridians are shown in the illustration. The massage must be done daily and longterm.

Acupressure for Osteoporosis
Bone Health

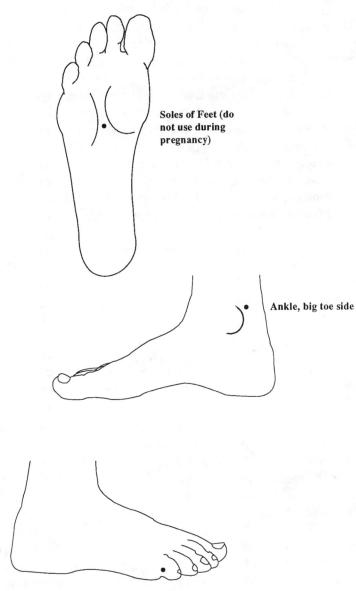

Soles of Feet (do not use during pregnancy)

Ankle, big toe side

At first joint of little toes

Cathryn Bauer, *Acupressure for Women* (Freedom, CA, The Crossing Press, 1987), p.122.

Aromatherapy: Use chamomile, cardamom, marjoram or lavender in compresses, baths or massage oils. In diffusers also, chamomile or lavender are relaxants and pain relievers. Tiferet-Lifetree has combinations for pain and joint relief.

Flower Essences: Take the following with germanium (mineral) for vitamin and mineral assimilation: banana, dandelion, peach or nettles. Sunflower is for the spine and bone degeneration, lilac is for the spine, and peach is for degenerative dis-ease from poor absorption. Use dandelion for pain. The major essences here are sunflower, peach or banana.

Gemstones and Gem Essences: Use platinum, gold, silver or pyrite in essence, or essences of ivory, coral, pearl, opal, sapphire, lodestone, lapis lazuli or moonstone. Hold or wear amazonite, turquoise or chrysocolla, and use kunzite for mineral balance and for pain.

Emotional Healing: The bones are the foundation and support of the body; how is your foundation crumbling? Do you feel unsupported, or unable to meet the requirements for support of others? Let the Goddess do the supporting; flow with and trust in your life.

Psoriasis

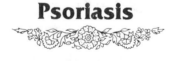

Psoriasis is a skin dis-ease, in which the skin's outer layer grows too fast, forming patches of silvery scales or red areas on the body. Legs, knees, arms, elbows, ears, scalp and back are most frequently involved, and finger and toenails develop ridges and pits. The skin may crack and bleed in some cases, or ooze and itch. There are periods of worsening and remission; the dis-ease comes and goes and usually is better in the summer months. It is not contagious. Women from fifteen to twenty-five years of age are more often affected, and attacks can be triggered by stress, viral or bacterial infections, sunburn or poison ivy, cuts, surgery and some drugs. Women who have psoriasis commonly also have arthritis in the smaller joints, leading to the consideration of psoriasis as an auto-immune dis-ease. The medical system has no causes or cures.

Homeopaths and naturopaths connect this dis-ease to vaccination, which they believe compromises the immune system, and Edgar Cayce named it a dis-ease of the thinning of the walls of the small intestines. Other considerations include liver and kidney malfunction, food allergies, constipation and poor elimination, copper excess and zinc deficiency, acid/alkaline imbalance, excess meat eating and poor diet, and assimilation problems of essential fatty acids. Adele Davis suggests that reducing blood cholesterol levels with lecithin is the answer. This is a persistent disease that comes and goes, and medical system drugs used for it are highly toxic. Holistic methods will do as much as medical drugs or more and do it safely.

Vitamins and Minerals: Along with the usual complete vitamin and mineral supplement and a calcium/magnesium tablet, adding essential fatty acids is considered the most important remedy. Use a capsule three times a day of evening primrose oil, or any other essential fatty acid form—salmon oil, black currant oil, Omega-3, linseed oil, cod liver oil, or olive oil—and these can also be used externally on lesions. Take four to eight tablespoons of lecithin daily; Adele Davis reports that no new lesions form after a week on this, with complete remission within five months. It removes cholesterol from the blood. Take a B-complex-50 two or three times per day, with 75 mg of folic acid, B-1, B-6, and sublingual B-12. Add PABA (30–100 mg three times daily). Use 25,000 IU per day of vitamin A, 400–1000 IU of vitamin D and 800 IU of vitamin E. Use 50–100 mg per day of zinc, and vitamin C with bioflavinoids (2000–10,000 mg daily or to bowel tolerance). Proteolytic enzymes taken between meals help assimilation and are important, and/or hydrochloric acid (HCL) with meals. A germanium cream may be used externally.

Herbs: Liver and blood cleansing is the goal here with burdock, red clover, dandelion, yarrow, blue violet, mullein, saffron, sarsaparilla, chamomile, bloodroot or yellow dock. Herbal antibiotics are used for inflammation: chaparral, pau d'arco, goldenseal (not for hypoglycemics), echinacea, or Oregon grape root. Externally, use poultices of yellow dock, comfrey, thyme, sarsaparilla, calendula, dandelion, or aloe vera, and also use aloe vera juice internally as a cleanser and laxative. See the herbs and remedies listed under Blood Cleansing and Liver Cleansing, particularly for the liver. Use blue violet and red clover together, or red clover with burdock. Another combination is red clover, burdock, blue flag and sassafras to drink as a tea twice daily. Or drink a pint of burdock infusion daily as a cleanser. Milk thistle extract, silymarin, is excellent for liver cleansing.

Naturopathy: Start with a three-day fast (or seven to twenty-one days with expert supervision) using carrot juice and spirulina, as well as teas of mullein, slippery elm and saffron. Take enemas or colonics during and after in a series. Start a diet of fifty percent raw foods, also eating fish, seaweed, green and yellow vegetables, soybeans, tofu and whole grains. Avoid saturated (animal) fats totally, dairy products, tomatoes, citrus, red meat, sugar, alcohol, soft drinks, refined flour foods, junk foods and processed foods (additives). Avoid constipation, eliminate candida albicans if that is a problem (see Candida Albicans), and check for hypothyroidism. Test for food allergies and use a rotation diet, not repeating use of any food more often than every five days.

To aid digestion and assimilation, drink a glass of water with a teaspoonful of apple cider vinegar and a teaspoonful of honey with meals. Drink three cups of cranberry juice per day as a cleanser, using the natural unsweetened type from healthfood stores. Use kelp tablets, four to six per day, for thyroid balance, and take Kyolic (odorless garlic), four to six per day to add sulfur and reduce yeast; both kelp and garlic are blood cleansers. Use spirulina or other green/chlorophyll drinks.

Apply castor oil packs to the lower abdomen nightly—these can make a tremendous difference—and apply castor oil externally to lesions. Or pat garlic oil on patches nightly. Make a solution of half a cup of sea salt in a gallon of water and soak the lesions several times a day; if you live near the ocean, swim often. Sunbathe but avoid sunburn. Ultraviolet lamps are frequently used. It is important to avoid burning.

Homeopathy and Cell Salts: *Psorinum* in a large single dose is available from homeopathic physicians. For general, acute or chronic psoriasis use *Arsenicum*; there is restlessness, thirst and burning, worse at night. Use *Sulfur* where the patches are itching, hot and burning and made worse by the warmth of being in bed; standing and water are uncomfortable and the skin is dry. For psoriasis behind the ears or on the palms or backs of the hands, use *Graphites*. External Calendula lotion can be soothing.

Cell Salts: Use *Silica* with pus, *Kali sulph.* with scaling, *Calc. fluor.* with cracked skin, or *Calc. sulph.* for the minor cases. Use a combination of the following four times per day for a month: *Natrum sulph.*, *Natrum mur.*, *Silica*, *Ferrum phos.*, and *Kali mur.*

Amino Acids: Use a combination free-form amino acids for detoxifying, antioxidizing, nutrients, tissue regeneration, and for sulfur and B-complex.

Acupressure: Use the pressure points and program described under Liver Cleansing.

Aromatherapy: Bergamot oil sensitizes the skin to ultraviolet light; apply the oil to lesions, then expose them to the sun or a UV lamp. Be very careful not to burn. Lavender in a vaporizer or diffuser helps to regenerate the skin cells. Other oils to use as compresses, in baths or as massage oils include patchouli, sage, palmarosa or fennel.

Flower Essences: Aloe vera, luffa, redwood and angelica are all skin cell regenerators; luffa and redwood are primary.

Gemstones and Gem Essences: In gem essence, use agates of any kind, azurite, azurite-malachite, aventurine, coral, emerald, garnet, lodestone, pearl, spinel, star sapphire or pink tourmaline. Also see the gemstones listed under Liver Cleansing. Hold or wear rose quartz, kunzite or pink tourmaline for the skin and the emotions.

Emotional Healing: You are afraid of being hurt and feel obstructed and ostracized. There is a deadening of the senses and the self, and a refusal to accept responsibility for your feelings. What are you ashamed of? What are you hiding from yourself or others? The skin lesions are something you use to hide behind, so you don't have to face others with your emotions or shame. Deal with yourself and your emotions and feelings, and end your need for the dis-ease.

Sinusitis and Allergies

Sinusitis is an inflammation of the mucous membranes in the spaces of the skull above and below the eyes. There is congestion and nasal discharge, drainage into the back of the throat, headache, pain in the sinus areas, forehead or cheekbones, or pain behind the eyes. There may be loss of sense of smell, sneezing, earache or toothache, general malaise and occasionally a fever. Acute sinusitis is usually caused by colds or viruses; chronic sinusitis may be caused by smoking, exposure to irritants or pollutants, growths in the nose, injury to the nasal bones, hay fever, food or other allergies, or a diet high in refined starches and dairy foods. If the mucous is greenish or yellowish an infection is present; clear mucus without a cold is probably allergies. Drainage and mucus are also signs of elimination of toxins, from toxins and chemicals or from constipation. Children (or adults) living in homes where there is a smoker have double the incidence of sinusitis, ear and respiratory problems, including colds, pneumonia, allergies and bronchitis, even if they do not smoke themselves. Sinusitis can also be brought about by dry environments, as in closed-up heated homes in northern winters. The feces of the common housedust mite is a frequent allergy.

Vitamins and Minerals: Use a complete vitamin and mineral supplement, particularly one high in B-complex vitamins. Add to it mega doses of B-complex, using a B-complex-100 twice daily, with extra B-6 (100 mg twice a day) and B-5 (500 mg twice a day). Use vitamin C with bioflavinoids (2000–10,000 mg per day or to bowel tolerance). In acute sinusitis attacks, take 1000 mg hourly with B-6 or a calcium/magnesium tablet. C is an anti-inflammatory, and anti-fungal and anti-bacterial; the B-6 or calcium prevent megadoses of C from causing kidney stones. Take 25,000 IU daily of vitamin A in dry form or beta-carotene, or take as much as 100,000 IU daily for up to one month, then cut back to 25,000 IU. A is a nutrient for the mucous membranes. In chronic cases, coenzyme Q10 (60 mg) or germanium (100 mg daily) increase oxygen to the cells, are free radical scavengers, and boost the immune system.

Herbs: For sinus infections use echinacea tincture three times a day for two weeks, about 1/3 eyedropperful doses. You must stay on echinacea for the full two weeks, though symptoms will clear sooner. Or use an echinacea and goldenseal combination (unless hypoglycemic), or echinacea with white willow bark, or echinacea, white willow and hyssop, or goldenseal with myrrh. Ephedra (Mormon tea, Brigham tea, squaw tea or ma huang) is another sinus herbal; as ma huang it is stronger, so use a fourth less. Fenugreek with thyme or comfrey is also a popular remedy. Use ground ivy where there is nasal congestion with headache; horehound and lobelia are expectorants. For chronic sinusitis use blood cleansing herbs: red clover with burdock, a pint of burdock tea taken daily, or dandelion, nettles or yellow dock. Alfalfa is also a good cleanser and relieves allergies, or drink aloe vera juice daily. Other herbs include mullein, eyebright, marshmallow, sarsaparilla, elder or cayenne. A strong infusion of melilot herb poured over the head after hairwashing clears the sinuses.

Naturopathy: Naturopaths credit sinusitis to diet, especially a high starch, refined carbohydrate diet with excess milk and dairy products and lacking in raw vegetables. Start with a three-day fast or three-to-five day mucous cleansing diet. A vegetable juice fast could include:

Day One:	6 ounces spinach juice and 10 ounces carrot juice.
Day Two:	Eat a pint of horseradish with a whole lemon.
Day Three:	10 ounces carrot juice, 3 ounces each of beet and cucumber juice.
Day Four:	Drink a pint of carrot juice.

With this drink at least three eight-ounce glasses of water a day. After the fast, eat horseradish once a week with fish and rice. Horseradish is a strong anti-histamine. Avoid milk products totally.[1]

A mucous cleansing diet consists of citrus fruits for breakfast, a plate of boiled or steamed onions with an orange for dessert for lunch and dinner, and carrot juice in between meals, used for three to five days and followed by a raw food diet for another three to seven days. Reintroduce other foods slowly, avoiding coffee, tea, alcohol, spices, salt, sugar and smoking, as well as dairy products, refined flour foods and junk foods. Watch for allergy reactions, and eliminate those foods (wheat, corn, citrus, milk, tomatoes or chocolate are common problems). Take two garlic capsules three times a day with meals.[2]

Bee pollen and garlic are highly important; start with one or two tablets of bee pollen daily, increasing slowly to the amount where symptoms disappear. This is especially positive with hay fever or other allergies; the pollen does not have to be local. Chew comb honey at the start of hay fever attacks; it will stop them. Take two Kyolic (odorless garlic) tablets, or garlic perles, or garlic and parsley capsules three times a day. Garlic is a natural antibiotic, cleanser and antihistamine, and helps with primary or secondary cigarette smoking poisoning. Another choice is onion syrup, cooked onions or raw onions used in the same way as garlic. A glass of water with a teaspoon of apple cider vinegar and a teaspoon of honey in it taken three times a day will also help to clear sinus congestion.

Foods that reduce mucous include horseradish eaten or sniffed (eat a teaspoonful an hour before breakfast mixed with lemon juice), blueberries, carrots, cucumbers, or apple, grape or cranberry juice. Camphor salves like Tiger Balm or Sunbreeze rubbed on the face or temples will also clear congestion. Take five or six drops of castor oil internally once a day for allergies. Chlorophyll in water may be used as a nosedrop, or garlic, sea salt or goldenseal and water.

Homeopathy and Cell Salts: Try *Allium cepa* for watery discharge with burning in nose, mouth, eyes or throat, sinus headache with face pains, sneezing or cough, or nasal polyps. The symptoms are worse in the evening in warm rooms, and better for cold and open air. *Thuja* is for chronic nasal congestion and sinusitis, particularly when nasal polyps are the cause. Use *Ignatia* for a hoarse, hacking cough that irritates the throat, with headache and cramping pains at the root of the nose. The woman cannot tolerate tobacco. *Kali bichromicum is* for colds, hay fever, sinusitis, postnasal drip, and sore throat; there is a tough, stringy discharge and

[1]Mildred Jackson, ND, and Terri Teague, ND, NC, *The Handbook of Alternatives to Chemical Medicine* (Berkeley, CA: Bookpeople, 1975), p. 44.

[2]Dr. Ross Trattler, *Better Health Through Natural Healing* (New York: McGraw-Hill Book Co., 1985), pp. 518–519.

shifting symptoms. *Pulsatilla* is for colds, hay fever, congested runny nose, itchy, runny, teary eyes, and dry cough in the morning, loose cough in the evening. Use *Sulfur* when other remedies are not effective.

Cell Salts: *Ferrum phos.* is the remedy for acute sinusitis with pain, fever, flushed face and rapid pulse. *Kali mur.* is for thick white discharge and stuffed head. *Natrum mur.* is the remedy for watery discharge, nasal obstruction and loss of sense of smell. Use *Silica* for chronic thick mucous discharge, and with bad odor use *Calc. flour.* For thick yellow discharge, use *Kali. sulph.* or *Natrum sulph.*, and *Mag. phos.* for hay fever. Take any of these hourly until there is relief.

Amino Acids: Use a combination free-form or liver-based amino acids. Single aminos include lysine, histidine and tyrosine.

Acupressure: Look for sore points around the sinus area, along the bony structure rims around the eyes, on the face and around the eyebrows. Massage the full ears, and look for sore spots behind the earlobes, first on the bony section, then in the hollow behind and below. Look for sore points on and below the collarbone. On the feet, work the toes and bases of toes, especially the bottom of the second and third toes; find the point on the sole for the ileocecal valve. (See illustrations.)

Aromatherapy: Take two drops of eucalyptus oil in a teaspoonful of honey nightly before bed. Inhale eucalyptus essence twice a day for three weeks, and massage the sinus area and temples with lavender in vegetable oil twice a day. Other aromas include marjoram, cajuput, myrtle, naiouli, cypress, peppermint or yarrow. Tiferet-Lifetree has a respiratory combination positive for sinusitis.

Flower Essences: Use jasmine, manzanita, eucalyptus, or snapdragon for sinus congestion, luffa or green rose for allergies, or corn for food allergies.

Gemstones and Gem Essences: Sulfur in essence is the remedy for sinusitis; essence of moss agate, picture jasper or silver (metal) is for allergies. Hold or wear moonstone, azurite or lapis lazuli.

Emotional Healing: The irritation is from someone close to you; who are you allergic to? Allergies are denying your own power.

Acupressure for Sinus and Allergies

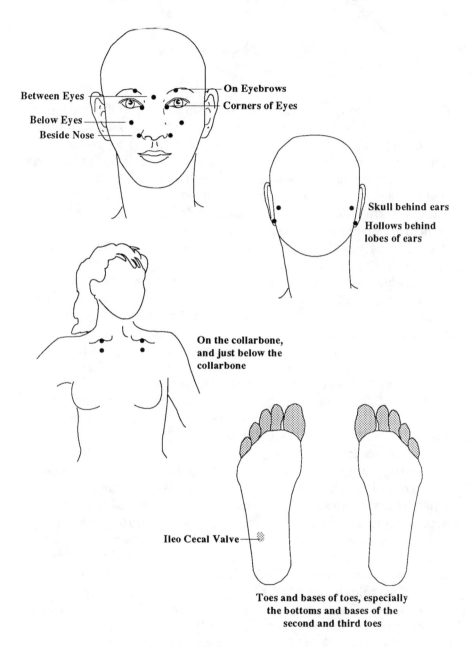

Between Eyes

Below Eyes

Beside Nose

On Eyebrows

Corners of Eyes

Skull behind ears

Hollows behind lobes of ears

On the collarbone, and just below the collarbone

Ileo Cecal Valve

Toes and bases of toes, especially the bottoms and bases of the second and third toes

Cathryn Bauer, *Acupressure for Women* (Freedom, CA, The Crossing Press, 1987), p.83; Pedro Chan, *Finger Acupressure* (New York, Ballantine Books, 1974), p. 101-103; Mildred Carter, *Body Reflexology*, *Helping Yourself to Foot Reflexology* (W. Nyack, NY, Parker Publishing Co., 1983), p. 49 and 90-91.

Skin Dis-eases

The skin is the body's largest organ of elimination, as well as the largest organ of the body. It is subject to reactions from the outside or inside environment. From the outside, dermatitis is caused by contact with metals, perfumes, cosmetics, rubber, medications, or plants such as poison ivy. From the inside, women with asthma or hay fever, allergies, stress or food intolerances may suffer eczema, a chronic dermatitis with itching, scaling, flaking, thickening, cracking and dryness of the skin. Young women, usually from ages twelve to twenty-four, may develop acne from blocked sebaceous glands; the Typical American Diet is often the cause, along with vitamin deficiencies (B-6 and zinc), and imbalanced hormones. Adult women on the contraceptive pill, under stress, with menstrual problems, vitamin deficiencies (B-6 and zinc), or eating refined food diets are also subject to acne and blackheads. Poor elimination, malfunctioning liver and gall bladder, constipation, food allergies, or endocrine imbalances are involved. Skin cancer has become a subject of great concern in the last few years for women of all ages, as the thinning ozone layer allows more ultraviolet rays to reach the earth. The sun has become deadly, and incidence of skin cancer has quadrupled. Women also experience oily skin, dry skin, combination skin and changes in hair and fingernails, all related to skin dis-eases, diet and skin care.

Vitamins and Minerals: Women with any form of skin dis-ease need a daily multiple vitamin and mineral supplement, a B-complex-50 to -100, a complete calcium/magnesium tablet (1000–2000 mg calcium and half as much magnesium), and zinc. Add 50–250 mg of B-6 for acne, menstrually related acne, and eczema; B-3 (100 mg up to three times daily) for skin cancer and stress; PABA (under 400 IU) for eczema and as a skin cancer protection; and sublingual B-12 (300–1000 mcg) for skin cancer and stress. Eczema may be a PABA deficiency dis-ease. Use a vitamin C with bioflavinoids for all skin dis-eases (1000 mg per day and up, to bowel tolerance for skin cancer). Dry form vitamin A or beta-carotene is important for any skin dis-ease; use up to 100,000 IU daily for as long as a month, then cut back to 25,000 IU per day. Nausea and stomach upsets indicate too much; stop for a week, then start again at lower amounts. Use vitamin D (400–800 IU), vitamin E (400 IU and up-1000 IU daily with skin cancer), and add selenium to the E (100–200 mcg) with high zinc use, skin cancer or for elders. For acne in young women, take 50 mg of zinc and for adults take up to 100 mg total daily (not over).

Evening primrose oil (essential fatty acids) is vital for healing skin dis-eases. Use two capsules two or three times a day for acne, eczema, dermatitis or skin cancer. This can also be applied topically. Other forms of essential fatty acids include: salmon oil, cod liver oil, black currant oil, Omega-3, sesame seed oil or linseed oil. The above will aid itching, sores, eruptions or other symptoms, prevent scarring and regenerate the skin. With skin cancer, add an antioxidant such as S.O.D., coenzyme Q10 (100 mg), or germanium (200 mg) daily. Chromium reduces skin infections, and acidophilus helps digestion. If vitamins seem not to help, add HCL or digestive enzymes; it may be an assimilation problem.

The fingernails can be an indication of what vitamins you are deficient in. Ridges indicate protein or vitamin A deficiency, and wash-board ridges deficiencies in calcium, iron or zinc. Thin, brittle nails are lack of iron, calcium, vitamin D or hydrochloric acid, while splitting nails are deficient in the sulfur amino acids. Peeling nails need vitamin A and pale nail beds are anemia. White spots indicate deficiencies in zinc, hydrochloric acid or a thyroid deficiency. Poor nail growth usually means lack of zinc.[1]

Herbs: These are primarily for blood cleansing; try burdock with red clover, yarrow, sassafras, Oregon grape root, alfalfa or parsley internally. For skin cancer use red clover with blue violet internally, and blue violet externally, or pau d'arco, chaparral, echinacea, or goldenseal internally. For eczema use the blood cleansing herbs as above, or comfrey, dandelion or myrrh. Use purple loosestrife internally to heal broken, cracked skin, while blackberry leaf tea dries the skin and elder eases dermatitis and eczema. Externally, try aloe vera gel, comfrey ointment, chickweed or calendula ointment, or goldenseal mixed with vitamin E.

For acne, use blue flag, barberry, burdock, alfalfa, dandelion, echinacea, red clover, yellow dock, birch bark or Oregon grape root. Make a poultice of chaparral, dandelion and yellow dock, or a steam sauna using red clover, lavender and strawberry leaves. For oily skin, use saunas with licorice root, lemon grass and rose buds, and for dry or combination skin use lavender peppermint and chamomile. Blue violet leaf in tea or tincture is good for all skin disorders; use three times a day. Comfrey or alfalfa will also clear many skin dis-eases. For all skin dis-eases make the following tea: two ounces red clover, an ounce each of burdock and blue flag, and half an ounce sassafras in a pint of cold water. Allow to stand overnight;

[1]Dr. Ross Trattler, *Better Health Through Natural Healing* (New York, McGraw-Hill Book Co., 1985), p. 450.

in the morning bring to a boil and simmer for fifteen to twenty minutes. Cool, strain, and drink 1-1/2 ounces three times a day for as long as needed.

Naturopathy: Start with a three day fast using noncitrus fruit juice or vegetable juice and enemas every other day of lemon juice, lobelia herb or warm water. See the information under Blood Cleansing. Begin a diet free of saturated (animal) fats, gluten (wheat and other grains except rice and millet), dairy products, red meat, sugar, salt, refined flour, alcohol, processed foods and junk foods, chocolate, fried foods and caffeine. Eat a diet high in raw noncitrus fruits, vegetables, salads, seaweeds, nuts, tofu, yoghurt or kefir, sprouts, fiber, fish and organic fowl. Add grains one by one to check for allergies, and watch for reactions to other foods. This is particularly important in eczema. In acne the goal is primarily a diet with no saturated fats but high in fiber, vegetables, grains, seafish and essential fatty acids. The diet listed under Blood Cleansing is a good skin healing diet; it clears the body of toxins and aids elimination. Check for allergies, thyroid function and candida in eczema and dermatitis, and for thyroid function in acne.

Kelp tablets (four to six per day) are positive for all skin dis-eases, and Kyolic, odorless garlic (two capsules taken three times a day), is for all skin dis-eases including skin cancer. To aid digestion and add hydrochloric acid and potassium, drink a glass of water with a teaspoon of apple cider vinegar in it and a teaspoon of honey with meals. Foods for acne include apricots and watercress, and eat a green pepper, a carrot and a stalk of celery daily for lunch. Drink cucumber juice and also apply it externally for skin eruptions; raw potatoes (eat two a day) help to clear eczema. Castor oil rubbed into skin lesions (including acne and skin cancer) daily will help to heal them, as will garlic oil with vinegar (half and half), or strawberries steeped in white vinegar. Simmer a sliced medium onion in half a cup of honey until the onion is soft; mash into a paste and apply cool to pimples; rinse after an hour and repeat nightly. For eczema, soft-boil three eggs, keep the yolks warm and rub drops of yolk on the lesions several times a day; results begin in about a week. Drink three cups of unsweetened cranberry juice a day for eczema and skin cancer; for acne or skin cancer drink three glasses of carrot juice daily.

Homeopathy and Cell Salts: For eczema use *Rhus venenata* 3x every six hours; if there is an aggravation, change to 30x. Use *Oleander* for scalp eczema, *Arsenicum* for chronic dry eczema, or *Urtica urens* for burning, stinging, itching eczema. *Lycopodium* is for eczema with violent itching, worse for heat or in the evenings at bedtime. *Alumina* is for dry, irritative eczema with constipation, and *Mercurius sublimatus corrosivus* is for severe, stubborn weeping eczema.

For acne in youth, *Carbo veg.* is used in the acute stage. *Hepar sulph.* is for pimples on the forehead and face, painful to touch and seeming to disappear in open air; there is pus. *Hydrastis canadensis* is for many small pustules, and *Veratrum album* is for pustules on the face that feel abraded when touched. Use Sulfur for eczema or acne when other remedies fail.

Use *Graphites* for general dermatitis when there is oozing of sticky fluid; *Petroleum* with painful cracks in the skin of toes or fingers; *Rhus tox.* for itching and blisters; or *Sulfur* for dry dermatitis.

For skin cancer when the ulceration is angry, irritable and increasing use *Hydrastis canadensis* internally, and hydrastis ointment. Where there is bleeding, use *Sanguinaria*, and locally Hamamelis lotion. Boracic acid ointment or Ruta ointment are also recommended. See a homeopathic physician.

Cell Salts: For acne, try *Silica* for eruptions on chin, pus or scarring, *Calc. sulph.* for boils that never erupt, or *Silica* and *Kali mur.* together. For eczema, use the following combination twice a day—*Kali mur.*, *Kali sulph.*, *Calc. sulph.* and *Silica*. For skin cancer, use *Silica*, or *Kali mur.* with exhudations.

Amino Acids: Take a free-form amino acids combination for eczema, acne, dermatitis or skin cancer. Single aminos for all skin dis-eases are L-cysteine and methionine together as detoxifiers and antioxidants, or taurine for skin cancer to rebuild tissues.

Acupressure: See the acupressure points under Blood Cleansing and Liver Cleansing, as well as Immune System Dis-eases (for skin cancer). Use full foot acupressure to work the points for the endocrine glands, lymphatics, spleen, liver, gall bladder and kidneys. Use the Great Eliminator/autonomic nervous system point on the hands. Additional points are shown for acne and for itching, as well as foot reflexes for acne and eczema. Check digestive system reflexes and work out any sore spots.

Aromatherapy: For acne, make a massage oil of juniper (10%) and lavender (2%) in an olive oil base. Massage the skin for ten minutes nightly, then wash with 2% lavender water and apply a lavender cream. Other essential oils for acne include bergamot, chamomile, everlasting, geranium, rosemary, rosewood, tea-tree, lemon thyme, linden or fennel. For eczema, massage daily with chamomile in an olive oil base. Others include bergamot, myrrh or palmarosa. For dry, chapped cracked skin make a massage oil of patchouli, sandalwood, rose or clary sage in olive oil. Palmarosa or sandalwood are for cellular regeneration (skin cancer), or use tea-tree. For other dermatitis, use benzoin, carrot seed, tea-tree or everlasting in an oil massage base. Essential oils can be mixed with vitamin E oil.

Acupressure for Skin Dis-eases

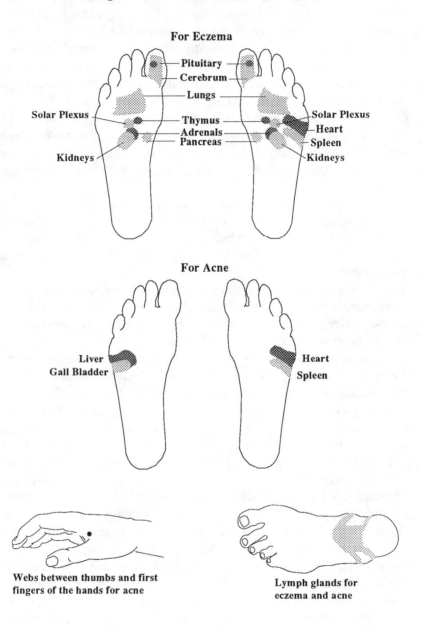

For Eczema

Pituitary
Cerebrum
Lungs
Solar Plexus
Thymus
Adrenals
Pancreas
Kidneys
Solar Plexus
Heart
Spleen
Kidneys

For Acne

Liver
Gall Bladder
Heart
Spleen

Webs between thumbs and first
fingers of the hands for acne

Lymph glands for
eczema and acne

Check digestive system reflex points for soreness

Moshe Olshevsky, CA, PhD., *et. al.*, *The Manual of Natural Therapy* (New York, Citadel Press, 1989), p. 171 and 174.

Acupressure for Skin Dis-eases

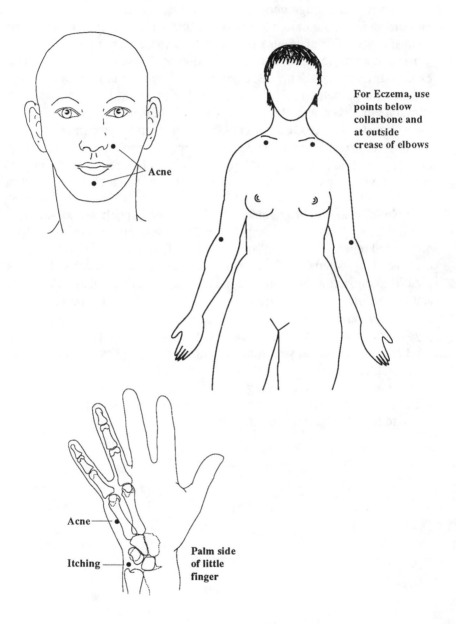

For Eczema, use points below collarbone and at outside crease of elbows

Acne

Acne

Itching

Palm side of little finger

Cathryn Bauer, *Acupressure for Women* (Freedom, CA, The Crossing Press, 1987), p.69; Michael Van Straten, ND, DO, *The Complete Natural Health Consultant* (New York, Prentice-Hall Publishers, 1987), p. 153; Iona Marsaa Teeguarden, *Acupressure Way of Health: Jin Shin Do* (New York, Japan Publishing Co., 1978), p. 76 and 78.

Flower Essences: For eczema, angelica knits together skin, banana is used where there is sugar imbalance, and bloodroot is for the emotional aspects and heart chakra. Use saguaro externally, or eucalyptus for skin and lung dis-eases together. For skin cancer, use aloe vera, angelica or bloodroot; apply saguaro externally for tumors. Luffa eliminates toxins from the skin. For acne, use banana where there is a sugar imbalance, ginseng for hormonal imbalance, or redwood for scarring. Use petunia externally over scars, lemon as a lymphatic cleanser and also for scarring, and luffa eliminates toxins. Use onion for most skin dis-eases and to stimulate the liver, and aloe vera essence for cuts and ulcers.

Gemstones and Gem Essences: Use in essence agate (all varieties), aventurine, azurite, azurite-malachite, dioptase, garnet, hematite, ivory, picture jasper, lodestone, pearl, spinel or sulfur. Hold or wear citrine for acne, amber for eczema (clear it often), or gem rhodochrosite for skin cancer.

Emotional Healing: Acne: There is a need for self-acceptance and self-love. Work on self-image; do the Self-Blessing nightly. Stare in a mirror and repeat "I love you" over and over for five minutes—don't stop or look away when emotions come, let them come. Eczema: There is breath-taking antagonism and mental eruptions, perhaps also reflected in asthma or allergies with this dis-ease. Work on healing the anger and resentment, release the emotions and learn to live in peace. Emphasize the joys in life, not the hurts. Skin cancer: Deep hurt, hatred, resentment or grief are eating away at you. Release it now before it goes deeper; learn to let go and forgive, work on self-image and self-blessing. Others: The skin is the body's protection and biggest elimination organ. What (or who) is getting under or through it? Work on releasing anxiety and fear; you are safe and loved. Heal your heart.

Sprains and Strains

Trauma to any joint can result in a sprain or strain. A sprain is injury to the ligaments connecting muscle to bone, and a strain is when a muscle knots up from over-use or over-lifting. Either results in rapid swelling, pain and bruising of the soft tissues. Sprains can happen in any joint, though ankles, back, fingers, knees and wrists are the most common, and strains can occur in any muscle. These may be sports injuries, falls or household accidents and are common first aid situations. Use standard first aid: take all weight off the injury and apply ice for the first twenty-four to thirty-six hours, as long as swelling continues. Use an ace bandage making sure that circulation is not impeded (no blue toes). The joint or muscle must have complete rest, no weight or mobilization, for the twenty-four to forty-eight hours it takes for pain and swelling to subside. Keep ice packs (or use a bag of frozen peas) on the injury for twenty to thirty minutes, and take it off for twenty minutes before applying again. Elevate the injured joint and wrap it snugly. Be careful not to reinjure it when starting to return to use. Where sprains are severe, or where there is any doubt, have an x-ray to make sure no bones are broken.

Vitamins and Minerals: Use your normal daily vitamins. The following are specific for sprains, strains or other muscle injuries. Take 3000–5000 mg of vitamin C as soon after the injury as possible; then take 1000 mg of C with a calcium/magnesium tablet hourly while the pain is acute. Use a C with bioflavinoids, if possible. Vitamin C prevents swelling, bruising and inflammation, and the calcium/magnesium is a muscle relaxant and pain reliever. Use the two together to prevent problems from the high doses of C as well. In the calcium/magnesium supplement, the magnesium can be of larger amount than the calcium. Use proteolytic enzymes (three tablets a day taken between meals) or bromelain (two or three tablets, three or four times a day) to protect against free radical damage from the injury. Take a high potency B-complex (100 mg daily) with additional B-5 (up to 2000 mg per day) for stress and tissue repair. DMG or topical DSMO oxygenates the blood. With severe pain use germanium (200 mg per day).

Herbs: Poultices of several herb choices are beneficial. These include: comfrey leaves, witchhazel, slippery elm, yellow dock, marjoram, mullein or burdock. Also drink comfrey or burdock teas three or four times a day. Use ginger as a poultice and add the tea to bathwater to soak in.

For muscle spasms, use poultices of peppermint. To relieve pain, use valerian, scullcap and catnip alone or together, or hops, passion flower or white willow. To add needed minerals for healing drink alfalfa tea or use the tablets; horsetail grass, oatstraw and Irish moss add calcium and needed silicon.

Make the following liniment and keep it available for emergencies; it takes a week or two to make. To two cups of vodka add four tablespoons of cayenne pepper and three tablespoons each of powdered myrrh and goldenseal. Place in a dark bottle with a tight-fitting lid, shake well, and store it out of sunlight. Shake it once or twice a day for one or two weeks. On the last day, don't shake it; pour out the liquid (leave the sediment) into another dark bottle, close and keep stored away from light.[1] Use externally.

Naturopathy: Massage on alternate days as follows: day one with equal parts of olive oil and myrrh, and day two with apple cider vinegar and sea salt. Drink a glass of water with a teaspoon of apple cider vinegar and a teaspoon of honey in it to add minerals and potassium; use this three times a day to reduce swelling. Use massages of peanut oil, or castor oil massages and packs. Make a poultice of marigold (calendula) steeped in apple cider vinegar or in milk. Or make a paste of turmeric (cooking spice) and hot water and apply it to bruises or injured areas to reduce swelling. Raw onions or onions roasted with honey or salt make an inflammation-reducing poultice for sprains or strains. Heat may be used in poultices after the swelling subsides (twenty-four to thirty-six hours); then alternate hot and cold compresses or packs.

Homeopathy and Cell Salts: These have great effectiveness. Start with *Arnica* 30x immediately after the injury, and use Arnica lotion or salve externally. This can make a real difference in the amount of bruising and swelling, so do it as soon as possible. Use it hourly for a few hours if there is much swelling and bruising, or if the strain is in the back. After the immediate injury and first aid switch to *Rhus tox.* for strains or sprains, every six hours for a few days. Use *Ruta grav.* every six hours for ligament injuries, or bruised pain in bones. *Calc. carb.* is for the last vestiges of weakness and pain in an old injury.

Cell Salts: Use *Ferrum phos.* immediately, and *Calc. flour.* for muscle injuries. *Mag. phos.* is for pain.

Amino Acids: A combination free-form amino acids complex offers protein for tissue repair, and is important for healing sprains or strains. Single aminos are lysine, valine, arginine or cystine; take arginine only with lysine.

[1]Joy Gardner, *The New Healing Yourself* (Freedom, CA: The Crossing Press, 1989), p. 28.

Acupressure for Sprains and Strains

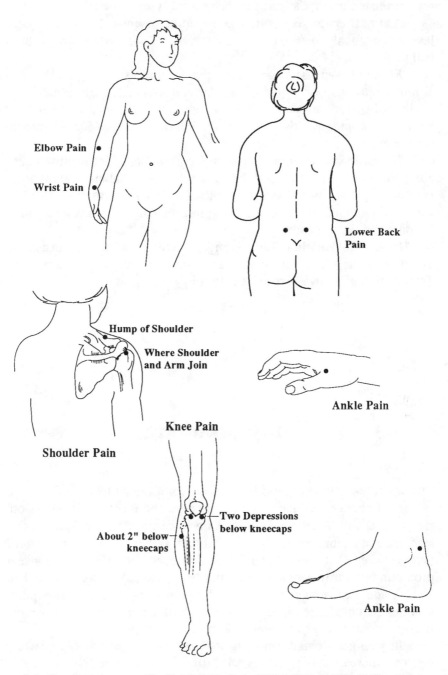

Elbow Pain

Wrist Pain

Lower Back Pain

Hump of Shoulder

Where Shoulder and Arm Join

Ankle Pain

Knee Pain

Shoulder Pain

Two Depressions below kneecaps

About 2" below kneecaps

Ankle Pain

Pedro Chan, *Finger Acupressure* (New York, Ballantine Books, 1974), p. 20-21, 48, 78-80, 99-100 and 122.

Acupressure: The illustrated points are for pain in commonly injured joints. Never use pressure on swollen tissue. Also see the pain reflexes listed under Cancer; they are for all types of pain.

Aromatherapy: Bay, birch, peppermint, rosemary, nutmeg, myrrh, lavender or eucalyptus are used in compresses (dilute with olive oil) or in baths.

Flower Essences: Angelica regenerates torn tissue, and bottlebrush eliminates toxins from injured muscles and tissues. Comfrey increases neurological response and heals nerve endings; it is especially good for back strains and sprains. Use Bach's Rescue Remedy for all trauma situations.

Gemstones and Gem Essences: Gem essences for the muscles include: apatite, coral, diamond, herkimer diamond, kunzite, labradorite, lazulite (sugilite), pearl, sapphire, sulfur or black tourmaline. Hold or wear herkimer diamond, Kunzite, sugilite, malachite or black tourmaline for pain and tissue healing.

Emotional Healing: There is anger and resistance to the process and direction of one's life. You do not want to move in the way you have to go. Trust in life and move forward easily. Flow with change.

Stop Smoking

The women's movement has been at the forefront of much radical and important change. We have worked on rape and incest, fat oppression, racism and ablism, alcoholism, and on releasing drug addictions. But smoking is a major source of harm to women's lives and health that is still being ignored. Patriarchal big business is making billions of dollars a year promoting death to women, particularly youth and minorities, and to already addicted women who have to keep on using. The smoker population has become increasingly female in the last thirty years and women have even more to lose than men do by a nicotine addiction.

In younger women, smoking reduces fertility, and smoking while pregnant increases miscarriages, stillbirths and premature deliveries, plus complications of pregnancy for the mother with low birth weight and higher mortality for infants. Infants of smoking mothers go through withdrawal symptoms, and nicotine passes through breastmilk. Children in smoking homes suffer far more respiratory ailments, earaches and allergies, miss more school, and are likely to become smokers themselves. Women who smoke reach menopause early due to tobacco's effects on the hormones and ovaries, and smoking is either a direct cause or clear aggravation of osteoporosis. In older women, the smoker may be at higher risk for lung cancer than are men, and lung cancer is now the leading cause of cancer deaths in women. Eighty-five percent of lung cancer and eighty-five percent of chronic cardiopulmonary dis-ease are directly smoking related. All forms of cancer and dozens of other dis-eases are caused by nicotine. Cigarettes contain over four thousand poisonous toxins, and each cigarette smoked lessens life by eight minutes. A two-pack-a-day smoker can lose twelve to sixteen years from her life, and much more from her quality of life. Everyone in the room with a smoker suffers from cigarette smoke poisoning. I could give more statistics and reasons but aren't these enough? I would like to see nonsmoking support groups with the frequency of today's twelve step networks. Women need to quit.

The following remedies are help to the smoker, the woman who is exposed to her smoke, and to women in the process of quitting. Smoking is as much an addiction as cocaine or crack. Nicotine as a drug acts much like cocaine in the bloodstream. After you quit, it takes time for each organ to detoxify, and you will go through a number of periods of withdrawal after the initial one. Detoxification is complete when the liver is clear, which takes from six months to two years depending on the amount of toxicity. Be aware that you are still in withdrawal when cravings periodically hit—awareness helps in holding out. Cravings to light up generally last no more than five minutes, so wait them out and they become less frequent. You may experience coughing with phlegm, stomach cramps and upsets, a bad taste in your mouth, headaches, irritability, anxiety, impatience and depression; these will last a few weeks initially, then reappear from time to time for shorter periods less and less often. Use the information in the Liver Cleansing section to speed the process of quitting and of removing the chemicals from your body. Acupuncture, hypnosis or aversion therapy can help tremendously. Once you quit, you must realize that with even one cigarette you are addicted again; it needs to be a permanent commitment to life.

Vitamins and Minerals: Smokers suffer depletion in a number of vitamins and minerals, so start with a quality multiple vitamin and mineral supplement. Use a B-complex-50 to -100 in time release form up to three times a day with meals; additional B-1 (50–100 mg), B-3 (100–1000 mg two–three times a day), B-12 and folic acid. Use vitamin C with bioflavinoids (3000–10,000 mg per day or to bowel tolerance) to detoxify nicotine from the body; up to 30 g are used intravenously daily for withdrawal. With each dose of vitamin C, or at least four times a day take either a B-complex capsule, B-6, or a calcium/magnesium tablet. Calcium is one of the things leached from the bones by smoking and it is a nervous system relaxant (as is B-3 and B-complex) to aid in withdrawal symptoms. Use vitamin A as beta-carotene up to 100,000 IU per day for up to one month, then cut back to 25,000 IU per day; it heals the mucous membranes, is an antioxidant, and protects the lungs from cancer. Starting with 200 IU of vitamin E per day, increase by 100 IU per week until you are taking 800–1200 IU daily, preferably with selenium (200 mcg). Vitamins A, E and C are antioxidants and help the liver and other organs to detoxify. Zinc (50–80 mg per day) boosts the immune system, and coenzyme Q10 (30 mg) or germanium (30 mg) are other powerful antioxidants. Chromium is important to reduce nicotine cravings and balance blood sugar; take 300 mcg per day— cigarette withdrawal is an induced hypoglycemia. Essential fatty acids, black currant oil or fish lipid oils, may help.

Herbs: Use liver and blood cleansing herbs to speed the release of toxins from the body—alfalfa, chaparral, dandelion, red clover, burdock or pau d'arco. Use relaxants to help with withdrawal—scullcap, valerian, hops, catnip, passion flower, lady's slipper or chamomile. Wood betony cleanses the spleen and is a calmative, and black cohosh balances blood pressure, clears the lungs and is calmative. A drop of stevia, peppermint oil, or licorice root extract placed on the tongue will stop cravings, or lozenges of licorice and zinc. Suck on a small clove when cravings hit, start a new one every hour or two, or chew chamomile flowers or gentian root. Try aversion therapy: chew a piece of calamus root or take five to fifteen drops of lobelia tincture and then smoke; nausea will result. If you must smoke something, smoke coltsfoot herb rolled into a cigarette; it helps to clear the lungs. Silymarin, milk thistle extract, is extremely important in cleansing the liver and breaking addictions, and it helps to stop cravings.

Naturopathy: Start with a three-day vegetable juice fast, or as long as twenty-one days with supervision, to detoxify quickly. Take enemas every other day, and start a series of colonics. Eat a whole foods, high fiber diet with adequate protein—see the diet listed under Hypoglycemia. High amounts of vegetables, citrus and carrot juice help the body detoxify and speed withdrawal. Other foods to emphasize are asparagus, broccoli, brussels sprouts, cabbage, cantaloupe, cauliflower, spinach, sweet pota-toes and turnips. Drink large quantities of water and take steam baths or saunas to help flush the liver and the bloodstream. Increase exercise. Alfalfa and/or kelp tablets, and spirulina or other chlorophyll drinks add important nutrients and aid in detoxifying, as well. If you drink a lot of coffee, reduce it gradually; it will have a toxic effect now. Raw thymus extracts help to boost immune function.

Homeopathy and Cell Salts: A homeopathic physician can provide a preparation of Nicotine as a remedy. *Caladium seguinum* modifies tobacco cravings and the physical damage of nicotine. Try *Nux vomica* every four hours, and when there are cravings chew a homeopathic *Camphor* pellet. To reduce or stop cravings in women who are nervous, with gas and dyspepsia, use *China.* For chilly, restless women with great thirst for cold drinks, and with nausea or vomiting use *Arsenicum.* For cravings with nervous headaches, impatience, quarrelsomeness, and changeable and contradictory moods, *Ignatia* is indicated. Caladium and Nux are primary, and Nux deals with irritability and anxiety, as well.

Cell Salts: Take five tablets of each every hour until cravings stop, then take three times a day: *Ferrum phos., Natrum mur., Calc. sulph.* and *Calc. fluor.* For a raw throat from smoke, take *Calc. phos.*

Amino Acids: A complete free-form amino acids combination helps with nutrition, detoxification, free radical scavenging, and tissue repair. Single aminos include taking cysteine with vitamin C, or methionine, cysteine and cystine together.

Acupressure: There is a stop-smoking point on the cartilage pads at the entrance to each ear; use pressure on both of these for five minutes to stop cravings. Use the autonomic nervous system point on the hands, in the indent where the bone of the thumb joins the bones of the rest of the hand. In foot or hand reflexology, pay particular attention to the pituitary, adrenals, kidneys, and liver while doing full foot or hand massage. Use the detoxifying point on the backs of the thighs. Also see the sections on Liver Cleansing and Hypoglycemia.

Aromatherapy: Chamomile and everlasting are liver cleansing essential oils, and chamomile, lavender, marjoram or rosemary strengthen the nervous system. Use rose, eucalyptus and fennel together in baths, diffusers or massage oils, and in drops on brown sugar cubes internally to quit smoking. Pine, eucalyptus, niaouli or lavender improve oxygen supply to the tissues and aid the heavy smoker.

Flower Essences: In the Bach Flowers, Crabapple is for addiction cleansing, and Cerato is for confidence in the process. In other essences, morning glory is a tonic and cleanser for the entire nervous system, and aids in breaking addictions. It also helps in the emotional side effects of cigarette withdrawal.

Acupressure to Stop Smoking

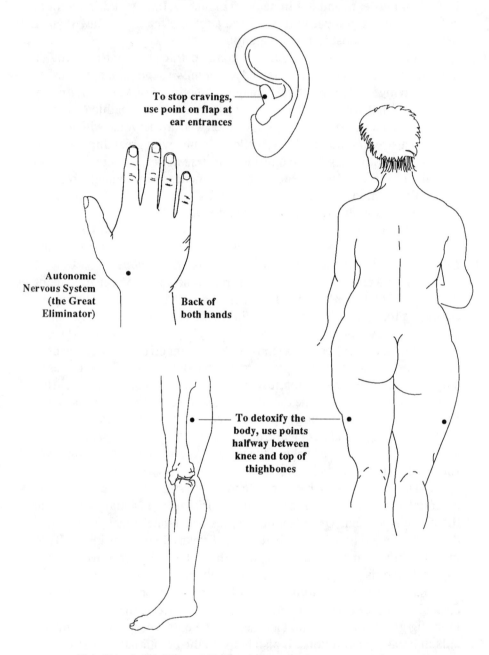

To stop cravings, use point on flap at ear entrances

Autonomic Nervous System (the Great Eliminator)

Back of both hands

To detoxify the body, use points halfway between knee and top of thighbones

Moshe Olshevsky, CA, PhD., *et. al.*, *The Manual of Natural Therapy* (New York, Citadel Press, 1989), p. 303; Iona Marsaa Teeguarden, *Acupressure Way of Health: Jin Shin Do* (New York, Japan Publishing Co., 1978), p. 71.

Gemstones and Gem Essences: Botswana agate is the gemstone essence, and hold or wear smoky quartz.

Emotional Healing: Smoking is a form of suicide; you know the risks but continue. Nicotine is also an emotional suppressant. While you smoke the issues are repressed and don't have to be dealt with. Stop smoking and return to life; no problem is so difficult it can't be faced or solved, and no problem (or person) is worth dying for. Emotional healing is part of the withdrawal; you can do it.

Stress

Women live in a society where stress is a fact and factor of our daily lives. It is the cause of eighty-five percent of all dis-ease. We work twice as hard for half the pay, and others (men) get most of the recognition, power, promotions and perks. We then come home to work a second job—homemaking, child raising, cooking and cleaning—for ourselves and/or our families. If we are the single heads of households we worry constantly about how the bills will get paid and how to accomplish everything that needs doing by ourselves. Too many of us are in poverty, homeless, in jeopardy of losing jobs in a failing economy, and barely able to manage financially. If we are nonwhite, ill, disabled, fat or elders, the stress is worse, the jobs and pay are less and often the exertions and responsibilities are greater. There is little time for fun, recreation, entertainment, creativity, or just to be ourselves. If we are caught in dead-end jobs with longings (and often educations) for better lives or more fulfilling work, we are even more under stress. This is the situation of many women. If we are single parents, we worry for ourselves and for our children's lives and futures.

Add to our own situations the condition of the planet, the pollution, lack of peace in the world, the struggle to find clean air, food and water, the constant threat of violence against women, the economic situation, racism, and the daily news, and stress goes even higher. We live in a fast-paced world where people care little for each other, and where there is no time-out for rest or recuperation. If for some reason we can't take care of ourselves either temporarily or permanently, there are few places to turn. All we can do is to take things day by day, creating worlds that emphasize hope and positive magick, good energy, caring, peace and healing from within. This goes a long way towards reducing stress.

Every woman lives under stress, and some women even thrive on it. The remedies below list suggestions for how best to keep mind and body healthy while we cope. For some basic suggestions, learn to meditate or do yoga and do it daily even if only for a few minutes before bed. Get enough regular exercise and get enough sleep (see the section on Insomnia if this is a problem), get a massage occasionally, take time out for fun or just to relax, and take time for yourself. Avoid stimulants, caffeine, drugs or alcohol, don't miss meals, and eat as quality a diet as you can. The results of longterm stress are in every dis-ease of this book—learn to relax.

Vitamins and Minerals: Use a quality daily vitamin and mineral supplement as a foundation. Add to it a B-complex-50 to -100 one to three times a day with meals, and additional B-5 (pantothenic acid-100–500 mg three times a day or as high as 2000 mg each day). Use vitamin C with bioflavinoids in time release form, from 1000 mg per day up to bowel tolerance, as an immune system builder, antioxidant and anti-stress agent. Use 25,000 IU of vitamin A as beta-carotene daily, 400–800 IU of vitamin E with selenium, and 50 mg of zinc. A complete calcium/magnesium supplement (1000–2000 mg calcium with half the amount of magnesium) is a relaxant and nerve calmative, and is essential for all women to prevent osteoporosis and PMS; the chelate form assimilates best. Other supplements that help are lecithin, brewer's yeast, raw glandulars (hypothalamus, adrenal, thymus), chromium, and/or essential fatty acids (evening primrose oil, fish lipid oils, EPA, flaxseed oil, salmon oil, GLA, etc.). Germanium may be especially helpful; use 100–200 mg daily.

Herbs: A number of herbs are relaxants and anti-stressors, among them scullcap, feverfew, hops, catnip, chamomile, motherwort, passion flower, valerian, rosemary, sage, peppermint or black cohosh. Try scullcap, catnip and hops together in a tea as a major relaxant. Horsetail grass adds needed calcium and silicon, as does oatstraw, and alfalfa is especially recommended as a nutrient and cleanser with other herbs. Lemon balm is a mood raiser and relaxant, as is vervain, and lady's slipper is good for anxiety. Gotu kola, ginseng or dong quai are balancers and tonics, as are sarsaparilla or dandelion. Juniper berries, chia seeds, or ginkgo biloba strengthen the nerves and brain, St. John's wort is a sedative, and mistletoe is a nerve nutrient. A drop or two of lobelia tincture added to other herbs makes a powerful relaxant—don't add too much or it becomes an emetic. Feverfew is a migraine preventive and also a good relaxant, and wood betony is a mild relaxant, also helpful for tension headaches and migraines. (See the sections on Headaches and Migraines.)

The Holmes-Rahe Stress Scale[1]

If your score rates over 300, you have a 79% chance of becoming seriously ill

Death of Spouse   100
Divorce   73
Marital Separation   65
Detention in Jail   63
Death of Close Family Member   63
Major Injury or Illness   53
Marriage   50
Being Fired from Job   47
Marital Reconciliation   45
Retirement   45
Major Change in the Health or Behavior of a Family Member   44
Pregnancy   40
Sexual Difficulties   39
Major Business Readjustment   39
Major Change in Financial State—Better or Worse   38
Death of a Close Friend   37
Change to a Different Type of Work   36
Change in the Number of Arguments with Mate—Better or Worse   35
Taking Out a Mortgage or Other Major Loan   31
Foreclosure on Mortgage or Loan   30
Change in Responsibilities at Work   29
Child Leaving Home   29
In-Law Troubles   29
Outstanding Personal Achievement   28
Mate Beginning or Ceasing Work   26
Beginning or Ending of Formal Schooling   26
Major Change in Living Conditions   25
Revision of Personal Habits   24
Troubles with Boss   23
Major Change in Working Hours or Conditions   20
Moving   20
Changing Schools   20
Change in Recreation   19
Change in Religious Activity   19
Change in Social Activities   18
Lesser Mortgage or Loan   17
Major Change in Sleeping Habits   16
Major Change in Number of Family Get-Togethers   15
Major Change in Eating Habits   15
Vacation   13
Christmas   12
Minor Violations of Law   11

[1]Marc S. Hoffman, Ed., *The World Almanac and Book of Facts, 1990* (New York: World Almanac Inc., 1990), p. 175.

Naturopathy: Eat as quality a diet as possible, avoiding sugar, refined flour foods, junk foods, caffeine, alcohol, fried foods, and colas. Dairy products may be a cause of stress; they are common food allergies. Try a diet without them for a few weeks and see, then add them back slowly and watch for reactions. Other foods, particularly wheat/gluten, corn, chocolate, tomatoes, eggs or the additives in processed foods or meats may be allergens. If you eat meat or poultry, stop lunchmeats totally and use organics—the additives, antibiotics, dyes and hormones can be part of the problem. Change sugar or artificial sweeteners to honey or stevia—sugar makes you nervous and Nutrasweet is implicated in cataracts and cancer. If you are hypoglycemic, try the diet described under that section; it can make a tremendous difference. Eat a whole foods diet high in raw vegetables, fiber, whole grains, fish, tofu, yoghurt and fresh fruits.

Kyolic, odorless garlic, helps to build the immune system. Take two tablets one to three times daily with meals. Raw or cooked garlic and onions are sedative in effect and immune builders. Bee pollen, propolis, royal jelly and comb honey are stress protectors and build the immune system. Iodine added to the diet in the form of kelp tablets, Atomidine or Lugol's Solution aids the thyroid. Drink a glass of water with a teaspoon of apple cider vinegar and a teaspoon of honey in it one to three times daily, and add a drop of Lugol's Solution to it twice a week. This adds potassium, iodine and minerals, plus hydrochloric acid for digestion and assimilation; do not use if you have ulcers.

Several foods are calming. Drink apple, pineapple, prune, grape or cherry juice; use them natural and unsweetened, and sip them through the day at room temperature. Add an egg yolk to a glass of cherry juice, or eat celery or strawberries (without toppings). Before bed, drink a half cup of orange juice, a half cup of pineapple juice and a quarter cup of lemon juice mixed together—it helps you to relax and sleep. Take warm epsom salt or sea salt baths.

Homeopathy and Cell Salts: Use *Nux vomica* for premenstrual stress, irritability, weakness, loss of appetite and constipation that are stress related. The woman works hard and plays hard, may smoke or drink too much and eats on the run—a typical Type A personality. *Ignatia* is for women of sensitive, nervous temperaments; stress is worse in the mornings, in open air, and increased by coffee or smoking. *Magnesia carbonica* is for overwrought, nervously run-down women, *China* is for debility from overwork or anxiety, and *Pulsatilla* is for stress in women of light coloring and changable moods. *Strychninum nitricum* is for nervous exhaustion. Use Calmes Forte, a homeopathic combination for reducing stress, calming and insomnia.

Cell Salts: Try combination cell salts (Bioplasma) for general calming and nervous system building. Use *Calc. phos.* for exhaustion after overwork or over-worry, *Ferrum phos.* for stress and a tired feeling in the brain, or *Mag. phos.* for nervous headaches. *Kali phos.* is the remedy for nervous exhaustion, stress, tension, and nervous headaches or indigestion.

Amino Acids: Take a combination free-form or Twin Labs Predigested Liver amino acids; they are a major stress reducer. Single aminos include GABA (750 mg with niacin and inositol) as a tranquilizer, tyrosine (with B-6 and C on an empty stomach), or methionine (an anti-stress agent). Tryptophan is a major anti-stress supplement; it will be back on the shelves eventually.

Acupressure: Do full foot acupressure, starting twice a week and increasing slowly to twice daily, or ten minutes with a foot roller daily, for releasing pain and tension in every part of the body and mind. Pay particular attention to the pituitary and endocrine gland reflexes, or work the following reflexes twice a day: pituitary, parathyroid, thyroid, adrenals, liver, and thymus for two minutes each, and the autonomic nervous system point in the hands for five minutes. Also look for sore spots where the neck meets the skull, where the shoulder joins the neck, and in the hollows at the tops of the shoulder blades. (See illustrations.)

Aromatherapy: Use any of the following essential oils in baths, massage oils or diffusers: geranium, lavender, marjoram, melissa, neroli, orange, rose, tangerine, ylang ylang, chamomile, clary sage, cedarwood or pine. As a muscle relaxant and for pain use a massage oil with dandelion. Tiferet-Lifetree has a relaxing combination that contains lavender, ylang ylang, melissa and bergamot, and can also be used as a perfume.

Flower Essences: Chamomile is the primary essence, for emotional tension, stress, insomnia and nervous indigestion. Also use dandelion as a muscular relaxant, bottlebrush for physical exhaustion, ginseng for endocrine strengthening and the immune system, or hyssop to overcome guilt and emotional blocks. Lotus eases all emotional states, aids in meditation, and helps to assimilate all forms of healing; use it with other essences.

Gemstones and Gem Essences: Apatite, chrysocolla, diamond, sugulite, or opal are used in essence, as is the metal gold. Hold or wear kunzite, rose quartz, amber, amethyst, smoky quartz, turquoise or chrysocolla.

Emotional Healing: There is fear, anxiety, tension, struggle and rushing. Get more in contact with the Earth and Earth Mother and learn to relax. Trust the process of life. You are not alone.

Acupressure for Stress

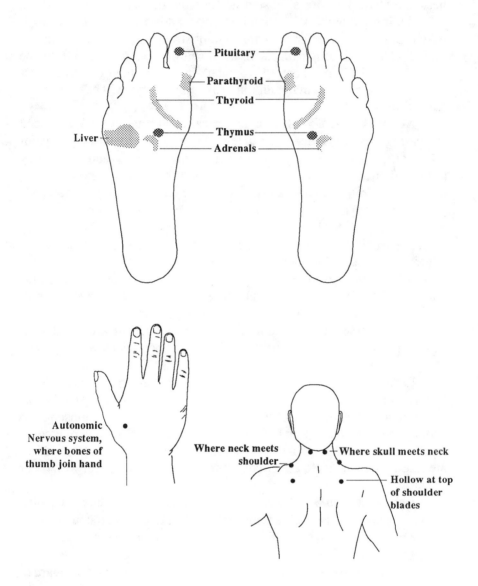

Moshe Olshevsky, CA, PhD., *et. al.*, *The Manual of Natural Therapy* (New York, Citadel Press, 1989), p.300; Iona Marsaa Teeguarden, *Acupressure Way of Health: Jin Shin Do* (New York, Japan Publishing Co., 1978), p. 73-75.

Vaginitis

This is a vaginal irritation and inflammation with redness, odor, discharge, itching and painful sex. If trichomonas (a protozoa) is the cause, there may be a frothy, thin discharge, burning, itching and a rash; if candida albicans (yeast, thrush, monilia) is the cause, the discharge is curdy and profuse, with odor, itching and inflammation. Leukorrhea is a watery, white vaginal discharge with the same causes as above, and hemophilus (non-specific vaginitis) is the cause when there is a creamy white, yellowish or greyish discharge, possibly with some blood, and cramps, lower back pain, and swollen glands in the abdomen and inner thighs. Trichomonas can be stubborn to treat but will usually respond to holistic methods, and holistic methods almost always work for the other varieties. Flagyl, the antibiotic of choice for vaginitis, can cause birth defects, gene mutations and cancer. Any alternatives are more positive.

The use of antibiotics for cystitis or other infections is often the cause of candida vaginitis, and adding more antibiotics to cure it only starts a vicious cycle, resulting in systemic candida over-run and the triggering of multiple allergies. Other causes of vaginal infections include the contraceptive pill, cortisone or steroids, tight underwear, stress, pregnancy, diabetes, miscarriage or abortion, menstruation when the body's acid/alkaline balance is affected, postmenopausal hormone changes, immune deficiency, dry vagina during intercourse, or nutritional deficiency (B-6 and B-complex). A diet high in sugar and white flour products encourages vaginitis. (See the section on Candida Albicans.) Since discovering some very simple remedies many years ago (vinegar and water douches), I have not needed to use doctors for vaginitis; the remedies work. Make sure that it is really a vaginal infection you are treating; if there is fever or lower abdominal pain, get a diagnosis. Also make sure that venereal dis-ease is not involved. With these ruled out, the remedies below will do the trick, even for most women with trichomonas.

Vitamins and Minerals: Along with a daily multiple vitamin and mineral supplement, take a B-complex-100 two or three times a day, with additional B-6 (50–100 mg) and B-5 (100–500 mg two or three times a day). If you are on the contraceptive pill or taking estrogen the additional B-6 is most important. A deficiency in B-2 can cause vaginal itching, and for longterm vegetarians a B-12 deficiency can cause vaginitis. Use vitamin C with bioflavinoids (1000–5000 mg per day or to bowel toler-ance) to acidify the environment. Take high doses of vitamin A (dry form or beta-carotene-50,000–75,000 IU daily short term, then decrease to 25,000 IU) and vitamin E (400–800 IU) daily. These reduce vaginal inflammations and uterine infections.

Important minerals include a calcium/magnesium supplement (1000–1500 mg calcium with half the amount of magnesium), 1000 mg daily of vitamin D (total), and a high dose of zinc sulfate—220 mg twice daily if you have trichomonas vaginitis. Use acidophilus, one teaspoon or two capsules three times a day—essential for regulating intestinal flora, particularly where vaginitis accompanies taking antibiotics or is caused by candida or hemophilus. A tablespoon of acidophilus to a quart of water makes a douche; alternate with apple cider or white vinegar and water (see below), or insert two acidophilus tablets into the vagina nightly at bedtime. If you are taking antibiotics, as soon as you stop them, begin taking two acidophilus tablets or a teaspoon or two of the liquid half an hour before meals for a week—this will prevent vaginitis. See the infor-mation on garlic/Kyolic below. For external itching, use vitamin E oil topically. Essential fatty acids can be helpful, especially evening primrose oil, for hormone balancing.

Herbs: A number of herbs are used as douches for vaginitis; choose among the following. For trichomonas, all vaginitis and cervicitis, use a douche of two teaspoons each of powdered myrrh and goldenseal and a half teaspoon of ginger (optional) to a pint of water. Echinacea or echinacea and goldenseal are also positive. Boil, strain, cool, and use daily until healed; make a fresh batch each time. Take a goldenseal capsule by mouth daily, with vitamin C and yoghurt, along with the douches.[1] Three tablespoons of chickweed to a quart of boiled water is also for trichomonas, or pau d'arco, or oatstraw to drink, bathe and douche with. For yeast infections use goldenseal and myrrh, St. John's wort, bayberry bark, comfrey, sage, yarrow, black walnut or oatstraw. Drink oatstraw tea daily for a month; use it as a douche only once a week, and lie down for half an hour after using it to saturate the tissues. For leukorrhea, use slippery elm as a douche or suppository (make it stiff with a little water), blue cohosh, lavender, white oak bark, red sage, pau d'arco or blue flag. For nonspe-cific/hemophilus vaginitis use goldenseal or goldenseal with myrrh again, calendula as a douche, witchhazel, bayberry, or a combination of an ounce of uva ursi, and half an ounce each of poplar bark and marshmallow boiled

---

[1]Joy Gardner, *The New Healing Yourself* (Freedom, CA: The Crossing Press, 1989), p. 209; and Cobra, "Remedies for Vaginitis," in *Goddess Rising*, Issue 20, Spring, 1988, p. 9. Many of the herbal remedies are from these two sources.

for twenty minutes in a pint of water. Cool, strain, and dilute with two parts water before using as a douche.

Herbs to take internally while using the douches include blue cohosh, comfrey or raspberry leaf, goldenseal and echinacea together, pau d'arco, or oatstraw. For itching of the vulva dab on goldenseal with witchhazel liquid, chickweed ointment, or calendula lotion or ointment. If you don't know what type of vaginitis you have, use the goldenseal/myrrh/echinacea douche and take the capsules internally, or use oatstraw or pau d'arco. For chronic uterine problems use St. John's wort. To restore the proper acid balance to the vagina, important in all forms of vaginitis, use a douche to a quart of white vinegar—this must steep for two weeks before using, so make it in advance and keep it handy.

Naturopathy: Follow the diet for candida albicans (see that section). For at least two weeks eat a diet that is eighty-percent raw vegetables/salads, and acidify the urine by drinking three or four glasses of unsweetened cranberry juice daily. After the two weeks, eat a diet of vegetables, whole grains, sea vegetables, and fish. Avoid sugar, unsaturated fats, white flour, processed foods, fermented foods and alcohol. Eat a lot of garlic and onions at all times, and yoghurt or kefir. If yeast is the cause of the vaginitis, eat a diet without yeast foods (no brewer's yeast) and make sure your vitamins are yeast-free (most are).

Kyolic, odorless garlic, taken two capsules or tablets per meal to start, then decreasing to two per day for prevention will stop many women's yeast infections and vaginitis completely. This is especially important when vaginitis recurs cyclically or frequently. Also use a raw clove of peeled but unnicked garlic in the vagina for infections, wrapped in gauze or with a string of dental floss, and changed daily. After the third day use a white vinegar douche, two tablespoonsful to a pint of water. This works for yeast infections, trichomonas, and all other vaginal infections, but stop if the garlic irritates.

Douches of white vinegar described previously can be alternated with yoghurt (two or three tablespoons of plain yoghurt to a quart of warm water), garlic or acidophilus douches. Some sources recommend apple cider vinegar, while others use white vinegar—I have had good results with white vinegar for this. Combined with Kyolic this is often the only remedy needed. Use it two or three times a day and continue for a few days after the symptoms are gone. Iodine, Atomidine or Betadine douches can be used for trichomonas. Put boric acid into 00 gelatin capsules and place two a night into the vagina at bedtime for two nights; for the next week use one capsule per night, then use it once a week as a preventive. Acidophilus capsules can be used along with the boric acid capsules. For itching, dab on a weak apple cider vinegar solution (same strength as for a douche). For a sore in the vagina use honey on it, or douche with slippery elm and water. Cottage cheese or farmer's cheese on a menstrual pad will aid itching and draw out vaginal infections; change it every few hours. Castor oil packs over the lower abdomen are also positive. Take twenty-minute warm baths with three cups of apple cider vinegar or half a cup of sea salt in the bathwater, and allow the water to enter the vagina. Never use chemical douches, they are irritants and unnecessary; the vagina doesn't need cleaning. Douches are for infections only, and if you really want to use them at other times use vinegar and water.

Homeopathy and Cell Salts: *Calcarea carb.* is for thick white or yellow discharge with intense itching that may come in gushes; it may be needed by young girls. *Graphites* is the remedy for a thin, white, burning discharge, tending to occur in sporadic gushes, worse for walking and in the morning. Use *Pulsatilla* for white discharge, mostly in women of light complexion. *Fagopyrum* is for yellow discharge with itching; *Sepia* is for thick or profuse greenish discharge with odor; or use *Alumina* for irritating, burning white discharge and raised itchy spots in the vagina before or after periods. For yellow discharge with an acrid odor, and itching or burning of the vulva, the remedy is *Kreosotum*—the first remedy to consider when there is irritation of the external genitalia. Use these four times a day.

Cell Salts: *Natrum mur.* is for watery discharge, *Natrum phos.* is for yellowish creamy discharge with acrid or sour odor, *Kali mur.* is for white nonirritating discharge, and *Kali phos.* is for burning, acrid yellowish discharge with nervousness. *Silica* is the remedy for pus-like yellow discharge and vaginitis.

Amino Acids: Use a free-form or liver-extract amino acids combination.

Acupressure: Do full foot or hand reflexology on both feet or hands twice a day. Pay particular attention to the meridian points for the female organs and the autonomic nervous system. Also work the points for the endocrine glands, particularly the pituitary.

Aromatherapy: Use tea-tree essential oil, a tablespoon to a quart of warm water as a douche, or use it in baths. This is particularly effective with trichomonas vaginitis. Or use a daily bath with the following: four drops each of bergamot and eucalyptus and two drops of lavender oil. Other baths include fir, pine or juniper. Stay in the water for twenty minutes, allowing it to enter the vagina. Two drops of juniper or two drops of lavender in baths are also recommended for yeast vaginitis.

Acupressure for Vaginitis

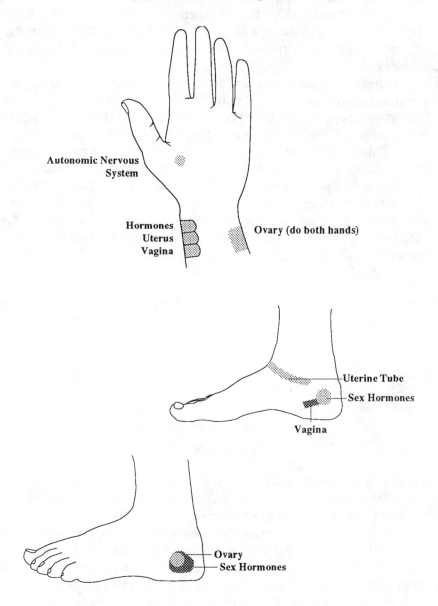

Autonomic Nervous System

Hormones
Uterus
Vagina

Ovary (do both hands)

Uterine Tube
Sex Hormones

Vagina

Ovary
Sex Hormones

Do both hands and/or both feet

Moshe Olshevsky, CA, PhD., *et. al.*, *The Manual of Natural Therapy* (New York, Citadel Press, 1989), p. 211 and 222.

Flower Essences: Bach's Crabapple is for cleansing, or use pomegranate essence for any women's issues emotional and physical. Pomegranate increases the blood flow to the organs, and helps leukorrhea, yeast infections and nonspecific vaginitis. Bells of Ireland is for the vaginal fluids and for vaginal tissue regeneration, and ginseng is for all vaginal dis-eases.

Gemstones and Gem Essences: The metal silver in essence is for vaginal healing, and use magnesium (mineral) for the uterus. Use garnet, rose quartz or pink tourmaline in essence for trichomonas infections. Hold or wear garnet, rose quartz or pink tourmaline for all vaginitis.

Emotional Healing: Many women with recurrent or acute vaginal infections are emotionally depressed; there may be anger at a mate, sexual guilt, or sexual punishment of oneself. You may be avoiding making love. All acts of love and pleasure are the Goddess' rituals, when lovemaking is an act of love and pleasure. Validate who you are as a woman. Your sexuality is a thing of goodness and beauty. Heal the sexual hurts of the past, take your power sexually now, and release the need for healing of your sexual self.

Varicose Veins

Four times more women than men are affected with varicose veins, and they affect about half of middle-aged Americans. These are enlarged, swollen veins in the legs, often bluish and bulging. There may be leg sores, ulcers or skin eczema in advanced cases, and leg cramps, swollen ankles, sore calf muscles, and a general feeling of heaviness and fatigue in the legs. Spidery red veins close to the skin surface cause little problem, but varicosities in deeper veins or varicose ulcers can be a serious circulatory disorder leading to blood clots, heart embolisms, or strokes. Hemorrhoids are varicose veins of the rectum (see that section). Varicose veins involve weakness in the vein valves that move blood from the legs back to the heart. This weakness can be hereditary, but is commonly caused by standing or sitting in one place (particularly with crossed legs) for prolonged periods, as at a job. It is also caused by obesity, pregnancy, constipation, lack of exercise, poor spinal or body mechanics, poor circulation, fatty liver, refined carbohydrate diets, or vitamin deficiencies (E and C). This is another dis-ease of civilization, with its sedentary lifestyle, and white sugar/white flour junk food diets. Constipation is a major cause and controlling it is a large part of the cure; see the section on Constipation in this book.

Vitamins and Minerals: In addition to a daily multiple vitamin and mineral supplement, take a B-complex-50 two or three times a day. Folic acid, B-6 and B-12 are important for healing. Take liquid lecithin (one to two tablespoons) with meals for circulation. Use 1000–6000 mg daily or to bowel tolerance of vitamin C with bioflavinoids (rutin is most important here), to promote healing, reduce bruising and prevent or dissolve blood clots. Use vitamin A (25,000 IU per day), and vitamin E starting at 400 IU and increasing slowly (add 100 IU per week) to 1000–1200 IU daily. Take a complete calcium/magnesium supplement (1500 mg calcium to 750 mg magnesium), 1000 IU of vitamin D, and 50–80 mg of zinc. Manganese, silicon and selenium should be in your daily multiple. Essential fatty acids (evening primrose oil, salmon oil, fish lipid oils, black currant oil) are helpful, plus proteolytic enzymes (bromelin), and up to 100 mg of potassium daily. Vitamins E, C, rutin and bromelin appear to be the most important supplements, along with enough B-complex. Use bran to prevent constipation.

Herbs: White oak bark, centella, horse chestnut, butcher's broom, pau d'arco, black walnut, marshmallow, oatstraw, stone root, or mullein are used as teas or tinctures internally, as well as cayenne, ginger, rue or prickly ash to increase circulation. Use yarrow, parsley or dandelion for ankle swelling (edema). Buckthorn, oatstraw, hawthorn, white oak and horse chestnut contract and tonify the blood vessels and are primary. A number of herbs are used externally as compresses or poultices on the swollen veins. These include: witchhazel, tansy, calendula (marigold), sage (apply hot), mullein compress or oil (relieves pain), wood sorrel, white oak bark, horse chestnut, oatstraw, bayberry, stone root, sassafras, marshmallow or black walnut. Horsetail grass adds needed minerals, and cascara sagrada, rhubarb and aloe vera are for constipation. If there are skin ulcers use goldenseal, echinacea, chaparral or pau d'arco, or poultices of slippery elm or comfrey externally to soothe. Also use calendula infusion in warm baths.

Naturopathy: See the section on Constipation and use the diet described there. Start with a three-day fruit juice fast and nightly enemas, or a three-day apple and apple juice mono diet. Take one or two tablespoons of olive oil (laxative) on the third evening. Take twenty-five drops of cascara sagrada herb tincture four times a day for a period of four to six weeks, gradually decreasing the number of times per day as bowels become regular. Use a high-fiber diet, with large amounts of citrus and raw vegetables. Except when fasting, take a tablespoon of raw bran with a glass of water three times a day, on a permanent basis. After the fast and enemas used with it, no further enemas or laxatives are to be taken.[1] The goal here is regular elimination without constipation, as constipation puts pressure on the veins. Increase exercise; start by taking walks.

Foods to eat include fish, fruits and raw vegetables, complex carbohydrates and unsaturated (nonanimal) fats. Berries—hawthorn, cherries, blueberries, blackberries—are high in bioflavinoids and strengthen the blood vessels. Garlic and onions are important. Drink enough water, but no fluids are taken with meals. Avoid animal fats and animal protein, dairy products (cheese and ice cream), junk foods, processed and refined foods, sugar, fried foods, smoking, alcohol and salt. Take kelp tablets (four to six per day) and/or chlorophyll/spirulina drinks. Kyolic, two tablets three times a day helps blood pressure and the blood vessels, circulation, and prevents infections if there are ulcers.

Elevate the affected leg whenever possible, including raising the foot of your bed by four inches. Lying with the chest lower than the hips allows the veins to drain. Alternate hot and cold leg sprays, sitz baths or showers. Lightly massage the legs in an upward direction, not directly over bulged veins, using warm olive oil with myrrh. Massage the feet in the fluid from used coffee grounds and apply this over the affected veins. Apply apple cider vinegar compresses to the legs, and also drink a teaspoon of apple cider vinegar (with a teaspoon of honey) in a glass of water twice a day. Wear support stockings or wrap bandages, being careful not to constrict circulation. Avoid crossing the legs, heavy lifting or putting pressure on the legs and veins. Wear clothing that does not restrict blood flow, take walks, and take times to elevate the legs frequently. A cold foot bath to the knees followed by brisk walking increases circulation. To tighten red spider veins use a compress or Swedish Bitters nightly.

Homeopathy and Cell Salts: Hamamelis tincture, lotion or ointment is applied externally, and may be used every three hours internally in pellet form. Use *Carbo veg.* for sluggish circulation, constipation and/or varicose ulcers. *Fluoric acid* is for varicose veins without ulcers, where there are "knots" in the veins. Use *Lachesis* for bluish veins mainly on the left side. *Arnica* is the remedy for veins that feel bruised, and *Mercurius* is for ulcerated veins with infection, pus and discharge with odor. *Pulsatilla* is for varicose veins during and after pregnancy.

---

[1]Dr. Ross Trattler, *Better Health Through Natural Healing* (New York: McGraw-Hill Book Co., 1985), pp. 568–569.

Acupressure for Varicose Veins

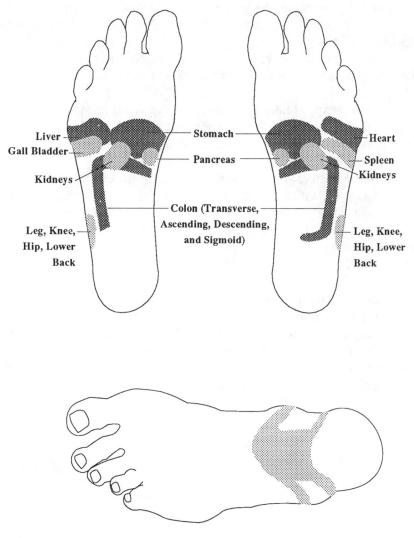

Liver
Gall Bladder
Kidneys
Leg, Knee, Hip, Lower Back

Stomach
Pancreas
Colon (Transverse, Ascending, Descending, and Sigmoid)

Heart
Spleen
Kidneys
Leg, Knee, Hip, Lower Back

Lymphatics

Moshe Olshevsky, CA, PhD., *et. al.*, *The Manual of Natural Therapy* (New York, Citadel Press, 1989), p. 135-136; Mildred Carter, *Helping Yourself with Foot Reflexology* (W. Nyack, NY, Parker Publishing Co., 1983), p. 99.

Amino Acids: Phenylalanine strengthens the blood vessels and lysine aids circulation; arginine is for the veins (take with lysine), and methionine, histidine and cystine cleanse and detoxify. A full combination amino acids is recommended.

Acupressure: Massage the whole hands or feet three times daily, then follow by working the reflexes for the heart, spleen, kidneys, pancreas, liver, gall bladder, stomach, leg/knee/hip/lower back, and colon (transverse, ascending, descending and sigmoid). Work the lymph gland reflexes on the tops and sides of the feet as well. Never use pressure over bulged, ulcerated or varicose veins themselves. Also see the section on Constipation.

Aromatherapy: Make a massage oil of olive oil and the following essential oil aromas: calendula, lavender and rosemary, singly or together. Use cypress or lemon for lymph drainage, also in a massage oil base. These aromas can be used in baths.

Flower Essences: Use hops or redwood for the circulatory system and blood vessel elasticity. Mallow is for the circulatory system and for skin and tissue regeneration, particularly for women at or after menopause.

Gemstones and Gem Essences: Gem essences of clay, coral or the metal copper are used for varicosities. Hold or wear amber or citrine for cleansing the lymphatic system, or bloodstone for the blood vessels and veins.

Emotional Healing: Who do you want to kick? You are "standing" in a situation you hate, feeling discouraged, overworked and over put-upon. What you give out is not returning fast enough, or not returning. Release the anger by kicking a pillow until it is gone. What you send out comes back to you; give without thought of return and the return will come all the sooner. Do you need to make some changes in your life?

Warts

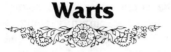

Common warts are small noncancerous skin growths ranging in size from the head of a pin to a size of a pea. They often appear first at adolescence, when the glands are developing and frequently occur in areas exposed to friction, and on the hands, feet, knees, forearms, or face. They can usually be left alone and will eventually disappear although warts that receive constant friction or on the feet may cause discomfort and need special attention. They are highly contagious. Touching or rubbing them can spread them, so care must be taken. They incubate for several months before appearing on the skin. Plantar warts are warts on the bottoms of the feet, causing discomfort in walking, and warts can sometimes occur on the vocal cords causing hoarseness. Venereal warts are cauliflower-like growths around and in the vagina, vulva and groin area. They are more serious for women than common skin warts, as they are indications of an increased risk for cervical cancer. Women who have these need frequent Pap tests. These warts are spread easily by sexual contact, primarily heterosexual. All warts are caused by viruses, and their appearance indicates that immune system building is needed. Rather than using the cutting, freezing and burning of medical technology, try healing the immune system to get rid of them. See the section on Immune System Diseases. Warts are also easily susceptible to hypnosis and affirmations: nightly declare them gone by a specific date, and they will be.

From Dr. Cindy Brown:

> I'd like to do a little rap about genital warts and cervical cancer, because the boys have tried to keep a lid on this for a long time. Genital warts are caused by the Human Papilloma Virus (HPV) and are highly transmissible from men to women during sex. In men, they don't cause much, if any problem. Warts on the penis may or may not be visible, and doctors are very reluctant to treat them in men because the treatment is painful. In women, the evidence is very strong that they cause cervical cancer, although (surprise) this has never been adequately studied. Except for one very poor study by Planned Parenthood in the early '80s, there has been no study of the use of barriers (condom, diaphragm) to prevent transmission.

Cancer of the cervix is virtually unknown in populations of women who do not ever encounter penises socially—nuns, lesbians. Trouble is, the cervical mucosa seems to be most sensitive to the carcinogenic influence of HPV during the teenage years, and we are currently seeing a virtual epidemic of cervical dysplasia/cancer in teenagers and young women. While it's usually diagnosed early enough not to be fatal, the women lose their reproductive capacity as a result of treatment, be it surgery or radiation therapy.

Infected men are carriers, literally. There's one study that suggests that as many as ten cases of cervical cancer occurring in a cluster in a housing project in Atlanta could possibly be traced to one man. Another study showed that if a man's first wife dies of cervical cancer, his second wife has four times the normal chance of getting it. This info has been around since the '70s, a pretty closely guarded secret.[1]

Vitamins and Minerals: Use a daily multiple vitamin and mineral complex to begin immune building. Deficiencies of vitamins A, C and zinc are implicated in warts, so take up to 100,000 IU of dry form vitamin A for as long as one month, then cut down to 25,000 IU per day. Pierce a 25,000 IU vitamin A capsule with a pin, and use the oil topically three times a day; keep the warts covered if possible. Take 2000–10,000 mg of vitamin C per day, or to bowel tolerance, as an antiviral, and 50–100 mg of zinc to boost the immune system. Powdered vitamin C can also be used topically; make it into a paste with water. These are essentials. Other important vitamins include a B-complex-50 two or three times a day, with additional B-6 (50 mg twice a day). Use 600–1200 IU of vitamin E internally, and also apply it topically three times a day—it should get rid of the wart in about two months.

Herbs: Rub the wart daily with juice from the stalk of the dandelion or greater celandine plant, protecting normal skin. Use the juice or tincture of mullein, milkweed, plantain, chickweed, aloe vera, marigold (with turpentine), buckthorn, or comfrey topically. Try a poultice of nettles for half an hour daily, then remove it and apply castor oil to the wart. Black walnut tincture, sassafras oil or tormentil oil applied daily will dissolve warts in a few weeks. Make a paste of apple cider vinegar and cayenne powder and apply daily, covering with a bandaid. For plantar warts use plantain tincture or poultices, and for genital warts apply mandrake

---

[1]Cindy Brown, MD, Personal Communication, August 12, 1991.

tincture twice daily, protecting surrounding skin from the liquid. Immune building tinctures or teas taken internally are particularly useful for genital warts; these include chaparral, echinacea, pau d'arco, goldenseal, or Oregon grape root. (See the information on cervical dysplasia under Menopause and Cancer). Drink chamomile tea to reduce lime in the system, three or four cups a day.

Naturopathy: Use the diet described under Immune System Diseases. Building the immune system helps the body shed the wart viruses. Eat more whole foods and raw vegetables and less white flour, junk foods, saturated fats and sugar. With genital warts avoid hot peppers and red meat. Acidify the system by drinking three or four glasses of unsweetened cranberry juice daily. Dr. Ross Trattler suggests taking twenty to thirty drops of orthophosphoric acid in water daily, also to acidify the system and particularly when there are many warts on the body. Include barley and daikon (a Japanese sea vegetable available dried in healthfood stores) in the diet. Eat four tablespoons of mashed canned or frozen asparagus twice a day.

Any number of home remedies are available for warts; they take from a week to two months to work. Rub the warts two or three times daily with castor oil, or use the nettles poultice with castor oil described above. Mix castor oil and baking soda into a paste and apply it at night, and cover. For genital warts, rub them twice daily with the inside skin of a pineapple (bromelain enzyme), or apply a used teabag to the area for fifteen minutes a day (tannic acid). For all warts, apply lemon juice twice daily, followed by chopped raw onion left on for fifteen minutes. The onion can also be mixed with salt (not recommended for the genitals). Other foods include grated carrots combined with olive oil and left in place for half an hour twice a day, or the same with crushed figs. Tape a piece of raw potato to the wart overnight every night; if the wart isn't gone in a week, replace the nightly potato with a clove of garlic.

Take Kyolic, odorless garlic, two capsules three times a day with meals, and rub the warts twice a day with a clove of raw garlic. Or use a slice of garlic as a continuous poultice. Garlic is an anti-viral, immune system booster, and provides needed sulfur.

Homeopathy: *Causticum* is for fleshy warts, warts on stalks, and especially for warts on the face, eyelids, arms, hands or near the fingernails. Use *Dulcamara* for warts on the backs of the hands, on the fingers or face; they are large, smooth and flat. *Antimonium crudum* is for horny hard warts with a smooth surface; this is the remedy for plantar warts. *Thuja* is particularly for warts on the genitals, anus or chin, but for warts in other places as well; these are soft warts that may be painful or bleeding. Also use Thuja ointment topically. Genital warts often respond to *Nitric* *acid*, and so do warts on the anus or lips; these are soft warts, often painful and bleeding.

Cell Salts: Use *Kali mur*. for warts on the hands, or any with a burning sensation. Take it internally twice a day and apply it as a paste with water topically. Use *Natrum mur*. for warts on the palms of the hands and for dry warts. *Silica* is for genital warts, and warts that bleed or ooze.

Amino Acids: Aminos are important for their sulfur content, B-vitamins, immune building, and as antiviral and antioxidants. Take a full amino combination. Single amino acids include: L-cysteine as a sulfur source, and/or taurine, lysine and glutamine.

Acupressure: Do full foot reflexology twice daily, or ten minutes twice daily with a foot roller to stimulate the entire immune system. Pay particular attention to the endocrine glands, and work the autonomic nervous system point in the webs between thumbs and first fingers. See the section on Immune System Dis-eases and the illustration.

Aromatherapy: Dab niaouli or tea-tree oil onto the warts twice daily, protecting surrounding skin. Make sure these are pure essential oils, and use them for genital warts as well. Lemon, melissa or oregano are also positive, used topically and in diffusers or massage oils to boost the immune system. For general immune system boosting, use the following oils together in an olive oil base as a massage oil: bryony, eucalyptus, lavender and rosemary.

Flower Essences: Ginseng is for boosting the endocrine system, and is useful combined with essential oils for genital warts. Pomegranate is for all women's dis-eases, including cysts, growths and warts, particularly those involving the reproductive organs. Use sweet corn in a salve with other remedies topically, or amaranthus for the thymus and pituitary and to repel viral inflammations.

Gemstones and Gem Essences: Picture jasper or sulfur in essence are used to boost the immune system; use moss agate, amber, peridot or obsidian for viral inflammations. Hold or wear rose quartz, kunzite or pink tourmaline to heal the skin and boost the immune system, and for the emotional aspects of the dis-ease.

Emotional Healing: Warts are "little hates" and a belief in one's ugliness; plantar warts are feeling stepped on; and genital warts indicate sexual fears with a new partner or the wrong mate. Let go of little hates and hurts and learn to say no, and the warts will disappear. Work on self-love; you are beautiful.

Acupressure for Warts
Immune Building

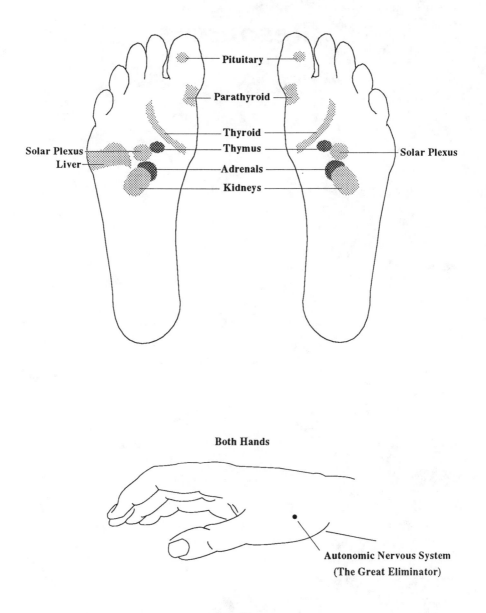

Pituitary

Parathyroid

Thyroid

Solar Plexus — Thymus — Solar Plexus
Liver — Adrenals

Kidneys

Both Hands

Autonomic Nervous System
(The Great Eliminator)

Moshe Olshevsky, CA, PhD., *et. al.*, *The Manual of Natural Therapy* (New York, Citadel Press, 1989), p. 269.

Resources

Women and General

American Holistic Medical Association
4101 Lake Boone Trail, #201
Raleigh, NC 27607
(919) 787-5146

Boston Women's Health Book Collective
240-A Elm Street
Somerville, MA 02144
(617) 625-0271

Federation of Feminist Women's Health Centers
6221 Wilshire Blvd., #419A
Los Angeles, CA 90048
(213) 930-2512

National Women's Health Network
1325 G Street, N.W.
Washington, DC 20005
(202) 347-1400

American Chiropractic Association
2200 Grand Ave.
Des Moines, IA 50312

American Osteopathic Association
142 E. Ontario St.
Chicago, IL 60611

Herbs

Herbal Research Foundation
P.O. Box 120006
Austin, TX 78711

Mail Order:
Coyote Moon
Theresa Finkbeiner
P.O. Box 312
Gainesville, FL 32602
(904) 377-0765

Spider Herbs
22 Radnor Ave.
Pittsburgh, PA 15218
(412) 829-2893

Goldenseal
1917 Murray Ave.
Pittsburgh, PA 15217

Frontier Cooperative Herbs
P.O. Box 69
Norway, IA 52318

Nature's Herbs
281 Ellis St.
San Francisco, CA 94102

STAMPS Apothecary
33 Van Buren
Eureka Springs, AR 72632

No Common Scents
King's Yard
Yellow Springs, OH 45387

World Wide Herbs, Ltd.
11 St. Catharine's East
Montreal 129, Quebec
Canada

Global Health, Ltd.
Box 18, Site 1, RR 2
Tofield, Alberta T0B 4J0
Canada

Miah Le Croy
35 Beck Ave.
Greenville, SC 29605
(803) 235-3670

Chinese herbs & immune-building formulas
ITM Herb Products
2017 S.E. Hawthorne
Portland, OR 97214
(503) 233-4907
(800) 544-7504

Naturopathy

Edgar Cayce Products:
PMS
P.O. Box 3074
Virginia Beach, VA 23453

Heritage Store
P.O. Box 444
Virginia Beach, VA 23458

Naturopathic Remedies:
Naturopathic Formulations
3363 S.E. 20th
Portland, OR 97232

Orthophosphoric Acid and Other Products:
VM Nu-ri Inc.
1012 Hort Dr.
P.O. Box 286
Lake Geneva, WI 53147

Schools:
National College of Naturopathic Medicine
11231 S.E. Market St.
Portland, OR 97216
(503) 255-4860

John Bastyr College
144 N.E. 54th
Seattle, WA 98105

Associations:
American Association of Naturopathic Physicians
P.O. Box 33046
Portland, OR 97233

Canadian Association of Naturopathic Physicians
P.O. Box 4143 Station C
Calgary, Alberta
Canada T2R 5M9

Hospitals and Clinics:
American Biologics
Mexico S.A. Medical Center
15 Azucenas St.
Tijuana, B.C.
Mexico
(800) 227-4458 or (619) 429-8200
Live Cell Therapy and Nutritional Treatment for Degenerative Diseases

Wildwood Sanitarium and Hospital
Wildwood, GA 30757
(404) 820-1493
Fasts, Diet, Water Therapy, Stress Therapy

Homeopathy

Physician Referrals:
International Foundation for Homeopathy
2366 Eastlake Ave. E. #301
Seattle, WA 98102
(206) 324-8230

National Center for Homeopathy
1500 Massachusetts Ave. N.W.
Washington, DC 20005

Homeopathic Educational Services
2124 Kittredge St.
Berkeley, CA 94704

Homeopathic Pharmacies:
Beckett Apothecary
1004 Chester Pike
Sharon Hills, PA 19079
(800) 727-8188
(215) 586-3100

Boericke and Tafel, Inc.
1011 Arch St.
Philadelphia, PA 19107
(800) 272-2920
(215) 922-7467

Standard Homeopathic Co.
P.O. Box 61067
Los Angeles, CA 90061
(213) 321-4284

Acupressure and Acupuncture

American Association of Acupuncture and Oriental Medicine
National Acupuncture Headquarters
1424 16th St. N.W., #501
Washington, DC 20036
(202) 265-2287 (12-4 p.m. EST)

American Acupuncture Association
5473 66th St. N.
St. Petersburg, FL 33709

Shiatsu Education Center
52 W. 55 St.
New York, NY 10019

Reflexology:
International Institute of Reflexology
P.O. Box 12642
St. Petersburg, FL 33733-2642

Reflexology Tools and Correspondence Course:
Stirling Enterprises, Inc.
P.O. Box 216
Cottage Grove, OR 97424
(503) 942-4622

Applied Kinesiology:
International College of Applied Kinesiology
P.O. Box 680547
Park City, UT 84068

Touch for Health Foundation
1174 N. Lake Ave.
Pasadena, CA 91104

Aromatherapy

Flower Essence Society
P.O. Box 1769
Nevada City, CA 95959
(800) 548-0075
(916) 265-0258

Tiferet-Lifetree
210 Crest Dr.
Eugene, OR 97405
(503) 344-7019

Atlantic Institute of Aromatherapy
2590 E. Bearrs
Tampa, FL 33612
(813) 977-4116

Great American Bulk Foods
4121 16th St. N.
St. Petersburg, FL 33707
(813) 521-4372

Correspondence Course:
Pacific Institute of Aromatherapy
P.O. Box 606
San Rafael, CA 94915
(415) 459-3998

Mail Order:
Aroma Vera Inc.
P.O. Box 3609
Culver City, CA 90231
(800) 669-9514

Herbal Endeavors
3618 S. Emmons Ave.
Rochester Hills, NY 11101
(313) 852-0796

L & H Vitamins
37-10 Crescent St.
Long Island, NY 11101
(718) 937-7400

The Ol'Factory Sensation
Miah LeCroy
35 Beck Ave.
Greenville, SC 92605
(803) 235-3670

Publications:
American Aromatherapy Association
P.O. Box 1222
Fair Oaks, CA 95628
Common Scents Magazine

Flower Essences

Bach Centre
Mount Vernon
Stowell
Wallingford
Oxon OX10 OPZ
England

Ellon Bach USA, Inc.
644 Merrick Road
Lynnbrook, NY 11563

Gurudas
PO Box 868
San Rafael, CA 94915

Pegasus Products, Inc.
PO Box 228
Boulder, CO 80306
(800) 527-6104

Flower Essence Society
PO Box 1769
Nevada City, CA 95959
(916) 265-0258
(800) 548-0075

Heal Thyself
Kathleen Harms
3914 Leona St.
Tampa, FL 33629
(813) 837-6212

Gemstone Essences

Gurudas
PO Box 868
San Rafael, CA 94915

Pegasus Products, Inc.
PO Box 228
Boulder, CO 80306
(800) 527-6104

Gemstones for Essences:
High Peak Crystal Co.
1272 Bear Mt. Court
Boulder, CO 80303

Heartsong Crystals
3318 Bay to Bay Blvd.
Tampa, FL 33629
(813) 832-3255

Emotional Healing

Louise Hay Books and Tapes
Hay House, Inc.
PO Box 2212
Santa Monica, CA 90406

Bibliography

Bach Centre. "The Bach Flower Remedies." Woodmere, NY: The Bach Centre, 1983 (pamphlet).

Badgley, Lawrence, MD. *Healing AIDS Naturally*. San Bruno, CA: Human Energy Press, 1987.

Balch, James, MD, and Phyllis Balch, CNC. *Prescription for Nutritional Healing*. Garden City Park, NY: Avery Publishing Group, Inc., 1990.

Bauer, Cathryn. *Acupressure for Women*. Freedom, CA: The Crossing Press, 1987.

Bethel, Mary. *The Healing Power of Herbs*. North Hollywood, CA: Wilshire Book Co., 1968.

Boericke and Tafel, Inc. *The Family Guide to Self-Medication (Homeopathic)*. Philadelphia: Boericke and Tafel, Inc., 1988.

Brennan, Barbara Ann. *Hands of Light*. New York: Bantam Books, 1988.

Buchman, Dian Dincin. *Herbal Medicine: The Natural Way to Get Well and Stay Well*. New York: Gramercy Publishing Co., 1980.

C.C. Pollen Co. *Is Honeybee Pollen the World's Only Perfect Food?* Phoenix, AZ :C.C. Pollen Co., 1984 (pamphlet).

Carter, Mildred. *Body Reflexology*. W. Nyack, NY: Parker Publishing Co., 1983.

Carter, Mildred. *Hand Reflexology: Key to Perfect Health*. W. Nyack, NY: Parker Publishing Co., 1975.

Carter, Mildred. *Helping Yourself with Foot Reflexology*. W. Nyack, NY: Parker Publishing Co., 1969.

Chan, Pedro. *Finger Acupressure*. New York: Ballantine Books, 1974.

Clark, Linda, MA. *Linda Clark's Handbook of Natural Remedies for Common Ailments*. Old Greenwich, CT: The Devin-Adair Co., 1976.

Clark, Linda, MA. *Get Well Naturally*. New York: Arco Publishing, Inc., 1965.

Clarke, John, MD. *The Prescriber*. Essex, England: Health Science Press, 1972.

Cobra. "Remedies for Vaginitis." In *Goddess Rising*, Issue 20, Spring, 1988.

Crook, William G. *The Yeast Connection*. New York: Vintage Books, 1983.

Cummings, Stephen, FND, and Dana Ullman, MPH. *Everybody's Guide to Homeopathic Medicines*. Los Angeles, CA: J.P. Tarcher, Inc., 1984.

Davis, Adele. *Let's Get Well*. New York: Signet Books, 1965.

Flower, Sidney B. *The Biochemistry of Schuessler*. Nokelumne Hill, CA: Health Research, 1970; Original 1921.

Gardner, Joy. *The New Healing Yourself*. Freedom, CA: The Crossing Press, 1989.

Gerber, Richard, MD. *Vibrational Medicine: New Choices for Healing Ourselves*. Santa Fe, NM: Bear and Co., 1988.

"Germanium." In *Nutrition News*, Vol. X, no. 11, 1987.

Global Health Ltd. *The Vitamin Herb Guide*. Tofield, Alberta, Canada: Global Health Ltd., 1990.

Griffin, LaDean. *Herbs to the Rescue*. Provost, UT: Biworld Publishers, 1978.

Gurudas. *Flower Essences and Vibrational Healing*. San Rafael, CA: Cassandra Press, 1989 revised.

Gurudas. *Gem Elixers and Vibrational Healing, Vol. I*. Boulder, CO: Cassandra Press, 1985.

Hay, Louise. *You Can Heal Your Life*. Santa Monica, CA: Hay House, 1984.

Hay, Louise. *Heal Your Body: The Mental Causes for Physical Illness and the Metaphysical Way to Overcome Them*. Santa Monica, CA: Hay House, 1982.

Hoffman, Marc S., Ed. *The World Almanac and Book of Facts, 1990*. New York: World Almanac, Inc., 1990.

Jackson, Mildred, ND, and Teague, Terri, ND, DC. *The Handbook of Alternatives to Chemical Medicine*. Berkeley, CA: Bookpeople, 1975.

Jarvis, D.C., MD. *Folk Medicine: A New England Almanac of Natural Health Care From a Noted Vermont Doctor*. New York: Fawcett-Crest Books, 1958.

Kamen, Betty, PhD. *Germanium: A New Approach to Immunity*. Larkspur, CA: Nutritional Encounter, Inc., 1987.

Kaminski, Patricia. *Aromatherapy As a Healing Art*. Nevada City, CA: Flower Essence Society, 1989 (pamphlet).

Keith, Velma, and Gordon, Montene. *The How-To Herb Book*. Pleasant Grove, UT: Mayfield Publishing, 1984.

Lavabre, Marcel. *Aromatherapy Workbook*. Rochester, VT: Healing Arts Press, 1990.

Locke, Steven, MD, and Colligan, Douglas. *The Healer Within*. New York: Mentor Books, 1986.

Lucas, Richard. *Common and Uncommon Uses of Herbs for Healthful Living*. New York: Arc Books, 1969.

McGarey, William, MD, *The Edgar Cayce Remedies*. New York: Bantam Books, 1983.

Mills, Simon, MD, and Finando, Steven J., PhD. *Alternatives in Healing: An Open-Minded Approach to Finding the Best Treatment for Your Health Problems*. New York: American Library, 1988.

Mindell, Earl. *Earl Mindell's Vitamin Bible*. New York: Warner Books, 1985.

Murray, Michael T. "A Natural Approach to Varicose Veins." In *Health Store News*, August, 1990.

O'Connor, Tom. *Living With AIDS*. San Francisco: Corwin Publishers, 1987.

Olshevsky, Moshe, CA, PhD, Schlomo, Noy, MD, Zwang, Moses, PhD., and Burger, Robert. *The Manual of Natural Therapy: A Practical Guide to Alternative Medicine*. New York: Citadel Press, 1989.

Potts, Billie. *Witches Heal: Lesbian Herbal Self-Sufficiency*. Ann Arbor, MI: DuReve Publications, 1989, Original, 1981.

Reynolds, Barbara, and Benedetto, Wendy. "Inquiry: Topic Breast Cancer." In *USA Today*, Thursday, May 16, 1991.

Rota, Francine. "50 Ways to Better Women's Health." In *East/West Journal*, November, 1990.

Ryman, Daniele. *The Aromatherapy Handbook*. London: Century Publishing, 1984.

Serinus, Jason. Editor: *Psychoimmunity and the Healing Process: A Holistic Approach to Immunity and AIDS*. Berkeley: Celestial Arts, 1986.

Siegel, Bernie. *Love, Medicine and Miracles*. New York: Harper and Row Publishers, 1986.

Speight, Phyllis. *Homeopathic Remedies for Women's Ailments*. Essex, England: Health Science Press, 1985.

Standard Homeopathic Co. *Homeopathic Professional Reference Catalog*. Los Angeles, CA: Standard Homeopathic Co., 1975.

Steadman, Alice. *Who's the Matter With Me?* Washington, DC: ESP Inc., 1966.

Stein, Diane. *Casting the Circle: A Women's Book of Ritual*. Freedom, CA: The Crossing Press, 1990.

Stein, Diane. *All Woman Are Healers: A Comprehensive Guide to Natural Healing,* Freedom, CA: The Crossing Press, 1990.

Stein, Diane. *The Women's Book of Healing*. St. Paul, MN: Llewellyn Publications, 1987.

Teeguarden, Iona Marsaa. *Acupressure Way of Health: Jin Shin Do*. New York: Japan Publications, Inc., 1978.

Tenney, Louise, MH. *Health Handbook: A Guide to Family Health*. Provo, UT: Woodland Books, 1987.

Thie, John F., DC. *Touch for Health: A New Approach to Restoring Our Natural Energies*. Marina Del Rey, CA: DeVorss and Co., 1973.

Thomas, Sara. *Massage for Common Ailments*. New York: Simon and Schuster, 1988.

Tisserand, Maggie. *Aromatherapy for Women*. Rochester, VT: Thorson's Publishing Group, 1985.

Trattler, Dr. Ross. *Better Health Through Natural Healing*. New York: McGraw-Hill Book Co., 1985.

Van Straten, Michael, ND, DO. *The Complete Natural Health Consultant*. New York: Prentice Hall Press, 1987.

Wilen, Joan, and Wilen, Lydia. *Chicken Soup and Other Folk Remedies*. New York: Fawcett Columbine Books, 1984.

Index